Computer Applications in Drug Discovery and Development

A. Puratchikody
Anna University, India

S. Lakshmana Prabu
Anna University, India

A. Umamaheswari
Anna University, India

A volume in the Advances in Medical Technologies and Clinical Practice (AMTCP) Book Series

IGI Global
DISSEMINATOR OF KNOWLEDGE

Published in the United States of America by
IGI Global
Medical Information Science Reference (an imprint of IGI Global)
701 E. Chocolate Avenue
Hershey PA, USA 17033
Tel: 717-533-8845
Fax: 717-533-8661
E-mail: cust@igi-global.com
Web site: http://www.igi-global.com

Library of Congress Cataloging-in-Publication Data

Names: Puratchikody, A. (Ayarivan), 1970- editor. | Prabu, S. Lakshmana (Sakthivel Lakshmana), 1974- editor. | Umamaheswari, A. (Appavoo), 1981- editor.
Title: Computer applications in drug discovery and development / A. Puratchikody, S. Lakshmana Prabu, and A. Umamaheswari, editors.
Description: Hershey, PA : Medical Information Science Reference, [2019] | Includes bibliographical references.
Identifiers: LCCN 2018031960| ISBN 9781522573265 (hardcover) | ISBN 9781522573272 (ebook)
Subjects: | MESH: Drug Discovery | Software
Classification: LCC RM301.25 | NLM QV 745 | DDC 615.1/9--dc23 LC record available at https://lccn.loc.gov/2018031960

This book is published in the IGI Global book series Advances in Medical Technologies and Clinical Practice (AMTCP) (ISSN: 2327-9354; eISSN: 2327-9370)

British Cataloguing in Publication Data
A Cataloguing in Publication record for this book is available from the British Library.

For electronic access to this publication, please contact: eresources@igi-global.com.

Advances in Medical Technologies and Clinical Practice (AMTCP) Book Series

Srikanta Patnaik
SOA University, India
Priti Das
S.C.B. Medical College, India

ISSN:2327-9354
EISSN:2327-9370

Mission

Medical technological innovation continues to provide avenues of research for faster and safer diagnosis and treatments for patients. Practitioners must stay up to date with these latest advancements to provide the best care for nursing and clinical practices.

The **Advances in Medical Technologies and Clinical Practice (AMTCP) Book Series** brings together the most recent research on the latest technology used in areas of nursing informatics, clinical technology, biomedicine, diagnostic technologies, and more. Researchers, students, and practitioners in this field will benefit from this fundamental coverage on the use of technology in clinical practices.

Coverage

- Biometrics
- Clinical Data Mining
- Nursing Informatics
- Medical Imaging
- Diagnostic Technologies
- Telemedicine
- E-Health
- Clinical Nutrition
- Neural Engineering
- Patient-Centered Care

IGI Global is currently accepting manuscripts for publication within this series. To submit a proposal for a volume in this series, please contact our Acquisition Editors at Acquisitions@igi-global.com or visit: http://www.igi-global.com/publish/.

The Advances in Medical Technologies and Clinical Practice (AMTCP) Book Series (ISSN 2327-9354) is published by IGI Global, 701 E. Chocolate Avenue, Hershey, PA 17033-1240, USA, www.igi-global.com. This series is composed of titles available for purchase individually; each title is edited to be contextually exclusive from any other title within the series. For pricing and ordering information please visit http://www.igi-global.com/book-series/advances-medical-technologies-clinical-practice/73682. Postmaster: Send all address changes to above address.

Titles in this Series

For a list of additional titles in this series, please visit: www.igi-global.com/book-series

Clinical Costing Techniques and Analysis in Modern Healthcare Systems
Ronald Ma (Austin Health, Australia)
Medical Information Science Reference • ©2019 • 265pp • H/C (ISBN: 9781522550822) • US $235.00 (our price)

Optimized Genetic Programming Applications Emerging Research and Opportunities
Bahrudin Hrnjica (University of Bihac, Bosnia and Herzegovina) and Ali Danandeh Mehr (Antalya Bilim University, Turkey)
Medical Information Science Reference • ©2019 • 310pp • H/C (ISBN: 9781522560050) • US $225.00 (our price)

Design and Development of Affordable Healthcare Technologies
Arindam Bit (National Institute of Technology Raipur, India)
Medical Information Science Reference • ©2018 • 388pp • H/C (ISBN: 9781522549697) • US $245.00 (our price)

Optimizing Health Literacy for Improved Clinical Practices
Vassilios E. Papalois (Imperial College, UK) and Maria Theodosopoulou (Imperial College, UK)
Medical Information Science Reference • ©2018 • 338pp • H/C (ISBN: 9781522540748) • US $235.00 (our price)

Electrocardiogram Signal Classification and Machine Learning Emerging Research and Opportunities
Sara Moein (Mount Sinai School of Medicine, USA)
Medical Information Science Reference • ©2018 • 196pp • H/C (ISBN: 9781522555803) • US $160.00 (our price)

Research Advancements in Pharmaceutical, Nutritional, and Industrial Enzymology
Shashi Lata Bharati (North Eastern Regional Institute of Science and Technology, India) and Pankaj Kumar Chaurasia (LS College Muzaffarpur, India)
Medical Information Science Reference • ©2018 • 549pp • H/C (ISBN: 9781522552376) • US $255.00 (our price)

Microbial Cultures and Enzymes in Dairy Technology
Şebnem Öztürkoğlu Budak (Ankara University, Turkey) and H. Ceren Akal (Ankara University, Turkey)
Medical Information Science Reference • ©2018 • 413pp • H/C (ISBN: 9781522553632) • US $265.00 (our price)

Multifunctional Nanocarriers for Contemporary Healthcare Applications
Md. Abul Barkat (K.R. Mangalam University, India) Harshita A.B. (K.R. Mangalam University, India) Sarwar Beg (Jubilant Generics, India) and Farhan J. Ahmad (Jamia Hamdard, India)
Medical Information Science Reference • ©2018 • 602pp • H/C (ISBN: 9781522547815) • US $265.00 (our price)

IGI Global
DISSEMINATOR OF KNOWLEDGE

701 East Chocolate Avenue, Hershey, PA 17033, USA
Tel: 717-533-8845 x100 • Fax: 717-533-8661
E-Mail: cust@igi-global.com • www.igi-global.com

Table of Contents

Detailed Table of Contents

Modern chemistry foundations were made in between the 18th and 19th centuries and have been extended in 20th century. R&D towards synthetic chemistry was introduced during the 1960s. Development of new molecular drugs from the herbal plants to synthetic chemistry is the fundamental scientific improvement. About 10-14 years are needed to develop a new molecule with an average cost of more than $800 million. Pharmaceutical industries spend the highest percentage of revenues, but the achievement of desired molecular entities into the market is not increasing proportionately. As a result, an approximate of 0.01% of new molecular entities are approved by the FDA. The highest failure rate is due to inadequate efficacy exhibited in Phase II of the drug discovery and development stage. Innovative technologies such as combinatorial chemistry, DNA sequencing, high-throughput screening, bioinformatics, computational drug design, and computer modeling are now utilized in the drug discovery. These technologies can accelerate the success rates in introducing new molecular entities into the market.

Biologically active and approved molecules have attracted great interest from scientists working in the therapeutic area. This has greatly increased the pressure on the pharma and life science industry in fueling new molecules to the market. Chemical structure database, the backbone of cheminformatics and the bioinformatics industry, has warehoused millions of active and non-active molecules/ligands/derivatives of drug compounds. Numerous public and private chemical databases support the drug discovery projects by contributing their data source in terms of 2D, 3D structure, and annotation reports in development of effective therapeutic projects. In this chapter, the authors discuss important chemical structure databases and their diverse dataset utilization in drug discovery projects.

the process of drug discovery (e.g., when the 3D image of the receptor is known, structure-based drug design is recommended). The pharmacophore-based model is advisable when the information about the receptor or any macromolecule is unknown. In this ADME, parameters such as Log P, bioavailability, and QSAR can be used as filters. This chapter shows both models with various representative examples that facilitate the scientist to use computational screening tools in modern drug discovery processes.

Piperine is known for its versatile therapeutic activity. It has been used for various disease conditions (e.g., cold, cough, etc.). Piperine is an alkaloid found in black pepper. It possesses various pharmacological actions like anti-inflammatory, anti-oxidant, anti-cholinergic, and anti-cancerous. The above-mentioned properties will be studied by selecting target proteins COX-2 protein, angiotensin converting enzyme, acetylcholineesterases, and survivin using computational docking study. This chapter explains the inhibition property of piperine against selected target protein from the results of docking studies. Based on the docking scores and protein-ligand interactions, piperine was found to bind well in the active site of the selected target proteins. It ensures the binding efficacy of piperine against selected target proteins. Docking scores and protein-ligand interactions plays an important role in its therapeutic activity.

Target identification has been considered as a chief parameter in drug discovery as it fully characterizes on-target and off-target effects of drug binding. Cell signaling receptors, structural proteins, and post-translational modifications of histones by histone deacetylases are the most widespread targets that are progressively being explored. The FDA approved histone deacetylases inhibitors and the majority of HDACi in and out of clinical trials based on the activities of 11 isoforms of the enzyme in non-selective influence approach. Unfortunately, reported HDACi does not possess a high degree of structural specificity and ultimately lessens the therapeutic index with many dose limiting toxicities. This chapter illustrates how different approaches are incorporated into the novel inhibitors discovery that are truly isoform-selective and which are specifically involved in targeting only a particular isozyme. Further, it highlights the aspects relating to provide a wider therapeutic index with an improved toxicity profile of lead like epigenetic modulators.

Molecular modelling uses theoretical and computational chemistry, which offers insight into the nature of molecular systems. This chapter highlights the theoretical explanation of molecular modelling methods and describes the designing of novel tyrosine COX-2 inhibitors using molecular modelling as an example. As a first step, fragment-based drug design is used to design the novel tyrosine analogues and ligand-based drug design such as QSAR, and pharmacophore was used to identify the descriptors, ensemble of steric and electronic features, which is responsible for the selective COX-2 inhibition. The next step, structure-based drug design, was used to analyses intra- and intermolecular interactions in the drug receptor system to improve the binding affinity and pharmacokinetic properties. Finally, the pharmacokinetic and toxicity properties were predicted quantitatively using rationalization of observed structure-activity relationships and the results are reported.

Chapter 9
Construction and Analysis of Protein-Protein Interaction Network: Role in Identification of Key Signaling Molecules Involved in a Disease Pathway 204
Divya Dasagrandhi, Bharathidasan University, India
Arul Salomee Kamalabai Ravindran, Bharathidasan University, India
Anusuyadevi Muthuswamy, Bharathidasan University, India
Jayachandran K. S., Bharathidasan University, India

Understanding the mechanisms of a disease is highly complicated due to the complex pathways involved in the disease progression. Despite several decades of research, the occurrence and prognosis of the diseases is not completely understood even with high throughput experiments like DNA microarray and next-generation sequencing. This is due to challenges in analysis of huge data sets. Systems biology is one of the major divisions of bioinformatics and has laid cutting edge techniques for the better understanding of these pathways. Construction of protein-protein interaction network (PPIN) guides the modern scientists to identify vital proteins through protein-protein interaction network, which facilitates the identification of new drug target and associated proteins. The chapter is focused on PPI databases, construction of PPINs, and its analysis.

Chapter 10
Quality by Design in Pharmaceutical Formulation 221
Sundaramurthy Vivekanandan, Bluefish Pharmaceuticals Pvt. Ltd, India

Quality by design (QbD) is a systematic, scientific, risk-based approach to product development and manufacturing process to consistently deliver the quality product. In this chapter, application, benefits, opportunities, regulatory requirements involved in quality by design of pharmaceutical products are discussed. In quality by design approach, during development, the developer defines quality target product profile (QTPP) and identifies critical quality attributes (CQA). Critical process parameters (CPP) of unit operations which impacts critical quality attributes need to be identified to understand the impact of critical material attributes (CMA) on quality attributes of the drug product. Quality by design approach is defined in ICH guidelines Q8 – Pharmaceutical Development, Q9 – Quality Risk Management, Q10 – Pharmaceutical Quality System. This chapter describes the implementation of new concepts in quality by design like design of experiments to achieve design space, control strategy to consistently manufacture quality product throughout the product lifecycle.

Next-generation sequencing or massively parallel sequencing describe DNA sequencing, RNA sequencing, or methylation sequencing, which shows its great impact on the life sciences. The recent advances of these parallel sequencing for the generation of huge amounts of data in a very short period of time as well as reducing the computing cost for the same. It plays a major role in the gene expression profiling, chromosome counting, finding out the epigenetic changes, and enabling the future of personalized medicine. Here the authors describe the NGS technologies and its application as well as applying different tools such as TopHat, Bowtie, Cufflinks, Cuffmerge, Cuffdiff for analyzing the high throughput RNA sequencing (RNA-Seq) data.

The ongoing rapid growth of diversity of data and their wide use to solve different complex tasks resulted in a significant number of semantic reference systems enriched with vocabularies, thesauri, terminologies, and ontologies. The extensive use of ontologies stemmed a new approach to build modern intelligent systems in reusing and sharing pieces of declarative knowledge. A lot of effort has been made to produce standard ontologies for medical knowledge representation. This chapter brings an overview of semantic knowledge representation frameworks such as RDF and OWL for developing ontology-based medical systems. The chapter presents the state of the art in ontology resources/systems so that it could be useful for learners and researchers involved in interdisciplinary research areas that include medicine and information technology. Also, a clinical use case is illustrated highlighting the role of ontology in the medical domain.

Preface

Computer Applications in Drug Discovery and Development presents a comprehensive look out to provide a complete source of information on all facets of drug design and discovery for under graduate and post graduate students, Pharma Researchers (Academicians and Industrial persons) in the field of Drug design and development, Medicinal chemistry, Pharmaceutical chemistry, chemical biology, pharmacology, biotechnology, etc.

Due to the rapid and steady growth of available low-cost computer power, the use of computers for discovering and designing new drugs is becoming a central topic in modern molecular biology and medicinal chemistry. Experts in the field of Pharmaceutical Technology considers that synthesizing more number of compounds by conventional methods and finding anyone compound with significant activity is a mere wastage of money, time and chemicals. Alternatively, they provide key techniques of computational approaches to investigate bioactive compounds that reduce the consumption of time and resources.

This book focuses on the current computational methods used in drug design, how a small change in functional group or part of the molecular structure elicit variation in the biological activity and this can be used in a designing a lead molecule. With more restrictions upon animal experimentations, the Pharmaceutical Industries today focuses on new generation of experiments that are considerably more efficient. The integration of computational and experimental strategies has led to the identification and development of novel promising compounds. In the current panorama of drug discovery, where high drug failure rates are a major concern, properly designed virtual screening strategies are time-saving, cost-effective and productive alternatives.

Written by leading experts in the field, chapters guide readers through techniques of the available computational tools. Beginning with an introduction to drug design and discovery, the first four chapters focus on the methods that are commonly used in the early stage of drug discovery, chapters explore detailed methodology and techniques for identification of drug targets, binding sites prediction, high-throughput virtual screening, and prediction of pharmacokinetic properties using computer. In addition to the state-of-the-art theoretical concept, the middle three chapters provide case studies of drug design for a particular disease where in potential drug molecules are optimized with respect to *in vitro* potency and other important parameters reflecting bioavailability and pharmacokinetic or toxicological properties. Protein and peptide drugs are currently the most rapidly expanding class of drugs. An insight into protein- protein interaction network involved in the identification of signaling pathways in a disease pathway by *in silico* techniques is covered in detail in one chapter. Finally, the book concludes with the application of computer based studies an examination of neglected diseases, anticancer agents and anti-inflammatory agents. The editors of this book are sure these chapters will guide the students and researchers with unexplored avenues and future perspectives of the drug design to identify promising compounds that might represent future solutions in critical areas of human health.

ORGANIZATION OF THE BOOK

This book is organized into 12 chapters. A brief description of each of the chapters follows.

Chapter 1 discusses how modern chemistry foundations were made in between 18th and 19th centuries and have been extended in 20th century. R&D towards synthetic chemistry has been introduced during 1960. Development of new molecular drugs from the herbal plants to synthetic chemistry is the fundamental scientific improvement. About 10-14 years are needed to develop a new molecule with an average cost of more than $800 million. Pharmaceutical industries spend highest percentage of revenues, but the achievement of desired molecular entities into the market is not increasing proportionately. As a result, an approximate of 0.01% of new molecular entity is approved by the FDA. The highest failure rate is due to inadequate efficacy exhibited in Phase II of the drug discovery and development stage. Innovative technologies such as combinatorial chemistry, DNA sequencing, high-throughput-screening, bioinformatics, computational drug design and computer modeling are now utilized in the drug discovery. These technologies can accelerate the success rates in introducing new molecular entities into the market.

Chapter 2 reviews how biological active and approved molecules have attracted great interests of scientists working in the therapeutic area. Due to closely end term of patent products have greatly increase the pressure on pharma and life science industry in fueling new molecules to the market, the former analysed data from vast chemical consortium stood as a one of the major stake holder in studying, analysis and repurposing of their therapeutic applications. Chemical structure database, the backbone of cheminformatics and bioinformatics industry has been warehoused with millions of such active and non-active molecules / ligands / derivatives of drug compounds. Numerous public and private chemical databases supports the drug discovery projects by contributing their data source in terms of 2D, 3D structure and annotation reports in development of effective therapeutic projects. In this present chapter we are going to discuss few important chemical structure database and their diverse dataset utilization in drug discovery projects.

Chapter 3 demonstrates how discovering a new drug molecule against disease is the main objective of the drug discovery. Lead Optimization is one of the important step and act as a starting point, over the years it has changed significantly in the drug discovery process. Its main focus is the development of preclinical candidate from "Hit" or "Lead". Lead optimization comprises lead selection and optimization, drug candidate confirmation and preclinical drug characterization. Lead optimization process can improve the effectiveness towards its target potency, selectivity, protein binding, pharmacokinetic parameters and to develop a good preclinical candidate. Lead optimization from high-throughput screening to identification of clinical drug candidate is a seamless process that draws new techniques for accelerated synthesis, purification, screening from iterative compound libraries, validation and to deliver clinical drug candidate with limited human resources. In conclusion, lead optimization phase is done under the suggestion that the optimized lead molecule will have activity against a particular disease.

Chapter 4 establishes how there are many diseases for which suitable drug have not been identified. As the population increases and the environment gets polluted, new infections are reported. Random screening of synthesized compounds for biological activity is time-consuming. QSAR has a prominent role in drug design and optimization. It is derived from the correlation between the physicochemical properties and biological activity. QSAR equations are generated using statistical methods like regression analysis, genetic function approximation. Both, 2D parameters and 3D parameters are involved in generating the equation. Among several QSAR equations generated, the best ones are selected based on statistical parameters. Validation techniques usually verify the predictive power of generated QSAR equations. Once the developed QSAR model is validated to be good, the results of that model may be applied to predict the biological activity of newer analogues. This chapter illustrates the various steps in QSAR and describes the significance of statistical parameters and software used in QSAR.

Chapter 5 presents how virtual screening plays an important role in the modern drug discovery process. The pharma companies invest huge economy in drug discovery and screening. However at final stage of clinical trials, several molecules fail that impacts financial loss at large. To overcome this, the virtual screening tool was developed with super predictive power. The virtual screening tool is not only restricted tool small molecules but also to macromolecules such as protein, enzyme, receptors etc. This gives an insight into structure based and Ligand based Drug Design. VS gives reliable information to direct the process of Drug Discovery e.g. when the 3D image of the receptor is known, structure based Drug Design is recommended. The Pharmacophore based model is advisable when the information about the receptor or any macromolecule is unknown. In this ADME parameters such as Log P, bioavailability and QSAR etc. can be used as filter. This chapter deals both models with various representative examples that facilitate the scientist to use computational screening tool in modern Drug Discovery Process.

Chapter 6 investigates how piperine is known for its versatile therapeutic activity. It has been used for various disease condition cold, cough etc. Piperine is an alkaloid found in black pepper. It possesses various pharmacological actions like anti-inflammatory, anti-oxidant, anti-cholinergic and anti-cancerous. The above mentioned properties will be studied by selecting following target proteins COX-2 protein, angiotensin converting enzyme, acetylcholineesterasesand survivin using computational docking study. This chapter explains the inhibition property of piperine against selected target protein from the results of docking studies. Based on the docking scores and protein-ligand interactions, piperine was found to bind well in the active site of the selected target proteins. It ensures the binding efficacy of piperine against selected target proteins. Docking scores and protein-ligand interactions plays an important role in its therapeutic activity.

Chapter 7 approaches how target identification has been considered as a chief parameter in drug discovery as it fully characterizes on-target and off-target effects of drug binding. Cell signaling receptors, structural proteins and post translational modifications of histones by histone deacetylases are the most widespread targets that are more progressively being explored. The FDA approved histone deacetylases inhibitors and majority of HDACi in and out of clinical trials, based on the activities of eleven isoforms of the enzyme in non-selective influence approach. Unfortunately, reported HDACi does not possess high degree of structural specificity and ultimately lessens the therapeutic index with many dose limiting toxicities. This chapter illustrates how different approaches are incorporated into the novel inhibitors discovery that are truly isoform-selective and which are specifically involved in targeting only a particular isozyme. Further, it highlights the aspects relating to provide a wider therapeutic index with an improved toxicity profile of lead like epigenetic modulators.

Chapter 8 analyses how molecular modelling uses theoretical and computational chemistry which offers insight into the nature of molecular systems. This present chapter highlights the theoretical explanation of molecular modelling methods and describe the designing of novel tyrosine COX-2 inhibitors using molecular modelling as an example. As a first step, fragment based drug design is used to design the novel tyrosine analogues and ligand-based drug design such as QSAR and pharmacophore was used to identify the descriptors, ensemble of steric and electronic features which is responsible for the selective COX-2 inhibition. The next step, structure-based drug design was used to analyse intra- and intermolecular interactions in the drug receptor-system to improve the binding affinity and pharmacokinetic properties.

Finally, the pharmacokinetic and toxicity properties were predicted quantitatively using rationalisation of observed structure-activity relationships and the results are reported.

Chapter 9 reviews how understanding the mechanisms of a disease is highly complicated due to the complex pathways involved in the disease progression. Despite of several decades of research, still the occurrence and prognosis of the diseases is not completely understood even with high throughput experiments like DNA microarray and Next-Generation sequencing. This is due to challenges in analysis of huge data sets. . Systems biology is one of the major divisions of Bioinformatics and has laid cutting edge techniques for the better understanding of these pathways. Construction of protein-protein interaction network (PPIN) guides the modern scientists to identify vital proteins through protein-protein interaction network, which facilitates the identification of new drug target and associated proteins. The current chapter is focused on PPI databases, construction of PPINs and its analysis

Chapter 10 demonstrates how Quality by Design (QbD) is a systematic, scientific, risk-based approach to product development and manufacturing process to consistently deliver the quality product. In this article, application, benefits, opportunities, regulatory requirements involved in Quality by Design of Pharmaceutical product are discussed. In Quality by Design approach during development, the developer defines Quality Target Product Profile (QTPP), identify Critical Quality Attributes (CQA). Critical Process Parameters (CPP) of unit operations which impacts critical quality attributes need to be identified to understand the impact of Critical Material Attributes (CMA) on quality attributes of the drug product. Quality by Design approach is defined in ICH guidelines Q8 - Pharmaceutical Development, Q9 – Quality risk management, Q10 – Pharmaceutical Quality System. This article describes the implementation of new concepts in Quality by Design like Design of experiments to achieve design space, control strategy to consistently manufacture quality product throughout the product lifecycle.

Chapter 11 presents how next generation sequencing or massively parallel sequencing describe DNA sequencing, RNA sequencing or methylation sequencing, which shows its great impact on the Life sciences. The recent advances of these parallel sequencing for the generation of huge amounts of data in a very short period of time as well as reducing the computing cost for the same. It plays a major role in the gene expression profiling, chromosome counting, finding out the epigenetic changes and enabling the future of personalized medicine. Here we describe the NGS technologies and its application as well as applying different tools such as TopHat, Bowtie, Cufflinks, Cuffmerge, Cuffdiff for analyzing the high throughput RNA sequencing (RNA-Seq) data.

Chapter 12 identifies how the ongoing rapid growth of diversity of data and their wide use to solve different complex tasks resulted in a significant number of semantic reference systems enriched with vocabularies, thesauri, terminologies, and ontologies. The extensive use of ontologies stemmed up a new approach to build modern intelligent systems in reusing and sharing pieces of declarative knowledge. A lot of effort has been made to produce standard ontologies for medical knowledge representation. This chapter brings an overview of semantic knowledge representation frameworks such as RDF and OWL for developing ontology based medical systems. The chapter presents the state of the art in ontology resources/systems so that it could be useful for learners and researchers involved in interdisciplinary research areas that include medicine and information technology. Also a clinical use case is illustrated highlighting the role of ontology in medical domain.

Acknowledgment

Whatever endeavor we have put to prepare this work, it would not have been possible without the support of each one of the authors, who sacrificed a lot of their time and contributed much of their expertise to this book and provided the right impetus soulfully to undertake the challenge of this proportional. We wish to express our deep- rooted gratefulness towards each one of the authors for their contribution.

Our special thanks to the valuable contributions of the reviewers regarding the improvement of quality, edifying, enlightening coherence, constructive criticism and discussions especially to Dr. Selvam, Dr. Senthil, Dr. Suresh and Dr. N. Sriram for their review task.

We are elated to place on record with a sense of gratitude to our Editorial Assistant whose crucial help, benevolent attention and precious suggestions, made the book successful.

A sincere expression of the thanks goes to the entire team of IGI Global.

There are many others whose names flashed across our mind when we enlist those who have been with us over the course of the years. It is rather impractical to mention each of them separately, but we are conscious about our obligation and we thank them collectively.

Chapter 1
Drug Discovery:
Current State and Future Prospects

S. Lakshmana Prabu
Anna University, India

ABSTRACT

Modern chemistry foundations were made in between the 18th and 19th centuries and have been extended in 20th century. R&D towards synthetic chemistry was introduced during the 1960s. Development of new molecular drugs from the herbal plants to synthetic chemistry is the fundamental scientific improvement. About 10-14 years are needed to develop a new molecule with an average cost of more than $800 million. Pharmaceutical industries spend the highest percentage of revenues, but the achievement of desired molecular entities into the market is not increasing proportionately. As a result, an approximate of 0.01% of new molecular entities are approved by the FDA. The highest failure rate is due to inadequate efficacy exhibited in Phase II of the drug discovery and development stage. Innovative technologies such as combinatorial chemistry, DNA sequencing, high-throughput screening, bioinformatics, computational drug design, and computer modeling are now utilized in the drug discovery. These technologies can accelerate the success rates in introducing new molecular entities into the market.

INTRODUCTION

Drugs/Active pharmaceutical ingredients are chemicals used to treat disease or helping to restoring the health of diseased individual human being. Active pharmaceutical ingredients are substance or mixture of substances intended to be used in the manufacture of a pharmaceutical dosage form.

Active pharmaceutical ingredients are classified as

- Inorganic substances
- Organic substances (isolated from materials of animal or human origin)
- Organic substances (synthetic or semi-synthetic or isolated from herbal sources or micro-organisms) (Regulatory control of active pharmaceutical ingredients. Version 1, Appendix 14).

The aim of the drug discovery and development process is to identify the compounds with desired pharmacological property to treat the diseases leads to improve the quality of the diseased individual life.

DOI: 10.4018/978-1-5225-7326-5.ch001

Innovation of a new drug begins with a scientific 'idea' from basic research, subsequently discovery and development of a compound followed by approval from regulatory authority. Drug discovery and development are in a parallel situation. Recently drug discovery and development process has considerable changes like discovering the drug from botanicals to synthetic chemistry is a fundamental scientific development. Last few decades majority of new drug molecules are discovered through synthetic chemistry process (Lakshmana Prabu, *et al.*, 2014).

Process involved in the development of new chemical entity is

1. Preclinical
2. Investigational new drug application
3. Phase I
4. Phase II
5. Phase III
6. New drug application
7. New drug approval (Mathieu, 2002)

Objectives of Drug Discovery and Development

- Determination of medical needs by availability of current drugs, disease burden and its epidemiological trends.
- Recent available drug properties such as efficacy, safety and costs.
- Opportunities available through R&D activities.

Stages in Drug Discovery and Development

Drug discovery and development of a new chemical entity for a disease or existing therapeutic area is based on the emergency medical need or market potential of the disease. Drug discovery and development process includes:

1. **Understanding the Disease:** Before discovering a new drug molecule, understand the nature of disease, gene which is responsible for the disease, role in protein, protein encoding and changes in the living tissues.
2. **Target Identification:** Identification of the target gene or protein responsible for disease which can interact with the drug molecule.
3. **Target Validation:** Verifying the interaction between the target gene or protein and the drug molecule (www.slideshare.net/anisha88shah/rd-brochure).

Product Development Team

Product Development Team (PDT) includes the scientist from various disciplines such as

1. **Medicinal Chemist:** Synthesis of new molecule
2. **Animal Toxicology:** To assess the toxicity in the animal models

3. **Pharmacokinetics and Pharmacodynamics:** To assess the absorption, distribution, metabolism, excretion and pharmacological activity.
4. **Clinician:** To assess the toxicity, pharmacokinetic and pharmacodynamic properties in human volunteers.
5. **Regulatory Experts:** To commercializing the new molecule into the market (UNICEF/UNDP/World Bank/WHO Special Programme for Research and Training in Tropical Diseases (TDR), Drug Discovery and Drug Development, 2004).

DRUG DISCOVERY PROCESS

Chemical synthesis is an art to create a new molecule by performing chemical transformations, either by known process or creation of new process. Traditionally medicinal chemist synthesis the compounds in batch wise. In general thousands of compounds will be synthesized and verified through various screening techniques to assess its biological activity or therapeutic response. Recently receptor targeted based research is used to assess its biological activity.

Based on the potential therapeutic response, several key go/no-go 'decision gates', is used in drug discovery and development process. Decision gate is a tool to assess the new molecule properties based on its predetermined specification/criteria to proceeds further or next stage (Lakings, 2009; Lombardino, & Lowe, 2004; Pritchard, *et al.*, 2003).

Steps involved in the drug discovery and developments are

- **Synthesis:** Synthesis of new chemical entity/molecule
- **Non-Clinical Testing:** Identification of the pharmacological properties and toxicological profile of the synthesized compound.
- **Non Clinical Pharmacology Evaluation**: Identification of its mechanism of action, starting dose, efficacy, test species and pharmaceutical combinations
- **Nonclinical Pharmacology Evaluation Through *in vitro* Techniques:** Assess its pharmacological activity through cell line, membrane transport, cellular uptake, drug metabolism (human key liver enzymes - CYP3A4/5, CYP1A2, CYP2C9, CYP2C19 and CYP2D6) and protein binding.
- **Preliminary Animal Pharmacokinetics:** Characterize its absorption and disposition profile through suitable bioanalytical method.
- **Preliminary Drug Metabolism:** Assess its distribution, disposition, metabolism and elimination.
- **Toxicity Studies:** Acute toxicity studies.
- **Nonclinical Pharmacology Evaluation Through in Vivo Studies:** Assess its efficacy, therapeutic index and schedule for dose selection.
- ***In Vitro* and *in Vivo* Correlation:** Compare and correlate *in vitro* and *in vivo* efficacy (Lakshmana Prabu, *et al.*, 2014).

Pharmaceutical Research and Development

Drug discovery and development through innovation is considered as the backbone and indirect strength of any pharmaceutical organization. Research and development of a company has been considered as a part of company's DNA, which has specific strength and weakness. Pharmaceutical Research and development sector is a very complex structural organization involves scientist from variety of disciplines. The R&D activities of the organization have a large impact and the ability to execute the company's targets in time bound manner to maintain their business and technology strategy. The success of the organization is depends on the head of R&D; R&D head should have broad technical skills and managing experience to execute the task within the time frame.

R&D structure of the company is defined as

- Organization structure, i.e., "org. chart."
- Coordination mechanisms, e.g., resource allocation, project planning.
- Culture for innovation, i.e., behavior norms for value creation/capture.
- Strategic mission for R&D activities, i.e., reason for R&D (Thomas, *et al.*, 2006; Agyres, & Silverman, 2004; Allen, & Fusfeld, 1975).

R&D organizational structure is shown in Figure 1. (www.slideshare.net/teresatreasures/drug-development-biotechnology)

Drug innovation through conventional R&D pattern has been started during 1960's. In new drug discovery it is estimated that about one out of 10000 screened compounds is approved by FDA as a new drug molecule that is approximately 0.01%. Drug discovery and development can be initiated not only based on the medical need and commercial market potential of the new drug, but also depends upon the new science in which a new therapeutic opportunities can be created based on the target identification and disease mechanism (Changxiao, *et al.*, 2014).

Figure 1. R&D organizational structure

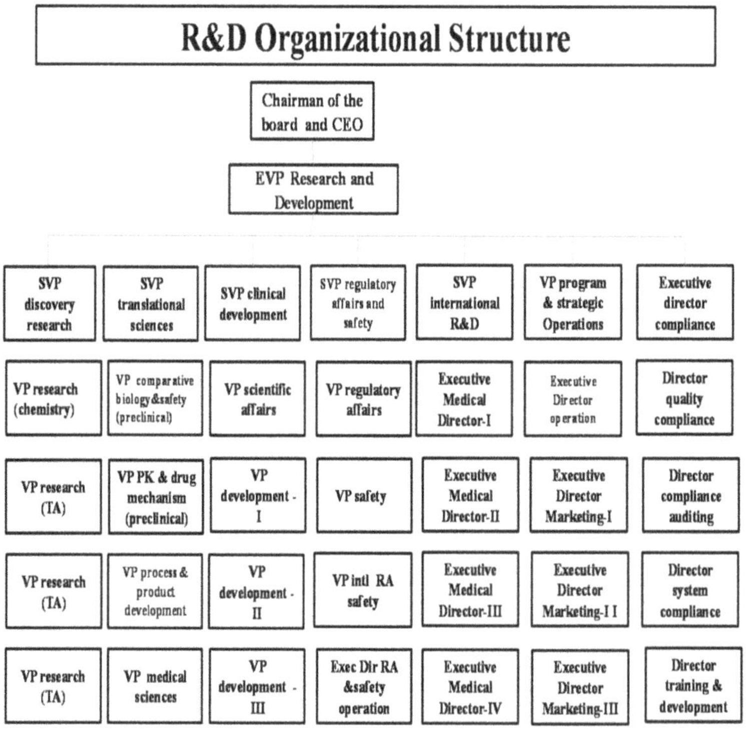

Recently a huge competitive environment in between the pharmaceutical organizations is reflected in developing a new drug molecule. Any pharmaceutical organization will pursue in investing R&D for a new drug is based on the reasonable expectation that the particular new drug molecule will get NDA approval in the market.

For new drug discovery, development, approval and launching the time duration has been increased significantly an average of around 7.9 years in the 1960s, 12.8 years in 1990s and 13.9 years from 2000 onwards. An average of around 12-14 years is required to innovative new drug molecule through drug discovery and development process (Michael, & Jean, 2014; Fabio, *et al.*, 2011). Different time duration for the drug discovery and approval are

- **Drug Discovery Research:** 4.5 years
- **Preclinical Testing:** 1 year
- **Clinical Trial:** Phase I – 1.5 years
- **Phase II:** 2.5 years
- **Phase III:** 2.5 years
- **Submission, FDA Approval and Product Launch:** 1.5 years (DiMasi, 2011).

Different drug discovery and development stages and process are shown in Figure 2 (The Pharmaceutical Innovation Platform, 2004) and Figure 3 (Lakshmana Prabu *et al.*, 2014).

This drug approval process through drug discovery indicates pharmaceutical organizations make huge investments in R&D; these investments exclude the costs of laboratories, buildings, equipment, etc. Many pharmaceutical companies generate and spend maximal revenues in R&D activities, but the

Figure 2. Drug discovery and development stages and process

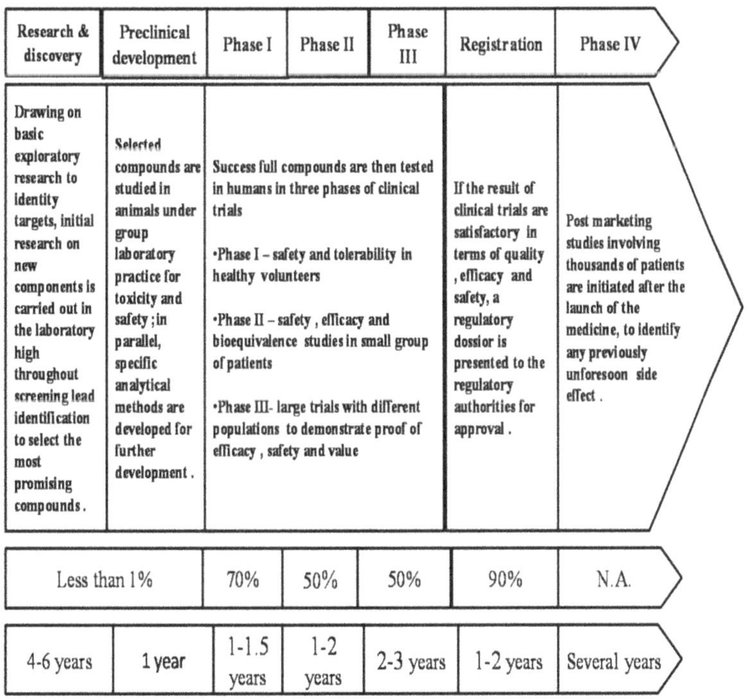

Figure 3. Drug discovery and development stages and process

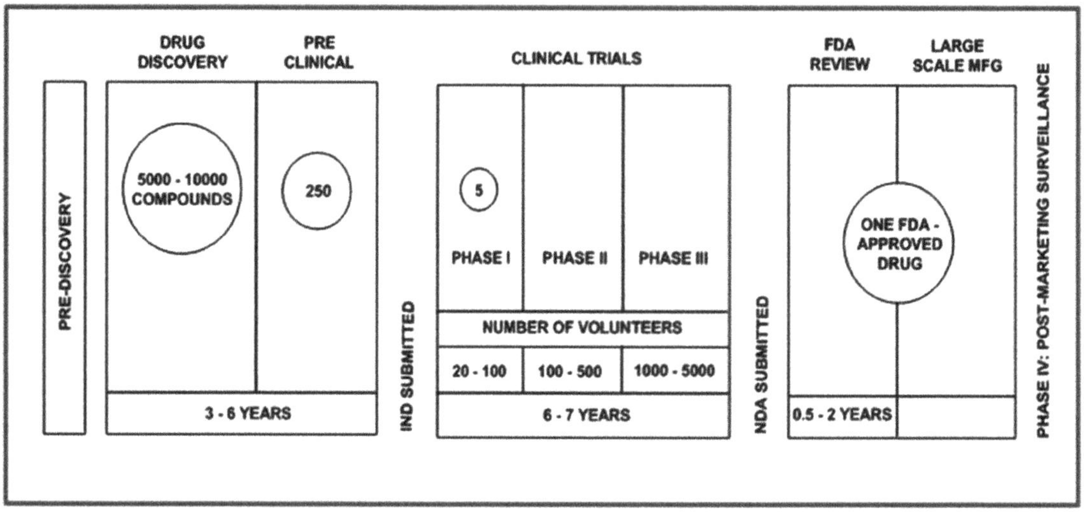

number of new drug molecule achieving the marketing authorization and approval by FDA or regulatory agency did not increase as anticipated level due to higher potential failure of the new drug approval by the regulatory authority. Organizations are trying in different approaches to advance the R&D efficiency for getting drug approval from the regulatory authority (Steven, *et al.*, 2010). Approaches in R&D are varies between organizations and other organizations. Over the past two decades, pharmaceutical industry innovation has directed to a decline position. The investment towards the R&D in 1999 was $55billion whereas in 2009 it is $125 billion; that is 128% increasing in the investment (3 fold) (Changxiao, *et al.*, 2014; The Pharmaceutical Innovation Platform, 2004). The increased investment includes the post market approval expense for assessing the long term safety and efficacy, also tripling the average number patients in the clinical trial phase. Due to stringent drug approval process, the approval of new molecular entity is dropped from 45 New Medical Entity (NME) in 1997 to 25 NME in 2009; that is 44% decline in the NME approval. This decline in the productivity and low approval rate raises the drug development cost. Investment for developing a NME was $250 million before the year 1990 whereas $403 million in 2000 and $873 million in 2010. The above statistics states the cost for the drug approval also increased drastically (Tang, 2013; He, 2013; Liu, 2013; DiMasi, *et al.*, 2003; Munos, 2009; Wiggins, 1987; Ernst, & Young, 2001; Profile Biopharmaceutical Industry, 2016; Tollman, 2001; DiMasi, 1991; Dickson, & Gagnon, 2004; DiMasi, 2003; Morgan, S *et al.*, 2011; Vernon, *et al.*, 2010; Scannell, *et al.*, 2012;, *et al.*, 2011).

The risk and success rate in the different drug discovery stages are 51% in discovery research, 69% in preclinical development, 12.8% in clinical development phases, 91% in submission phase and 4.1% in technical and regulatory approval (Alexander, *et al.*, 2016).

Failure Rates in Drug Discovery and Development

The reports of drug discovery and development of new drug molecule suggest that the 70% of failure in Phase II is due to technical deficiencies which exhibited highest attrition when compared to other phases whereas it is 29% due to non-technical deficiencies (Ish, 2012). During 1991, development of new drug molecule failed due to intolerable pharmacokinetic profile in human being. In order to overcome the pharmacokinetic profile during the developmental stage, pharmaceutical companies adopted different preclinical testing to assess the various pharmacokinetic parameters such as permeability, absorption, distribution, metabolism and excretion for projection of human pharmacokinetic profile.

A survey on analytical study results of drug development database suggested that 71.0% endured new drug molecule in Phase I enters into phase II, and 31.4% endured in phase II will enter into phase III. Overall, 21.5% of a new drug molecule completed phase III will enter into FDA approval. Failure in phase III rose from 30% to 50% in the year 2000. The cost of the R&D investment in Phase III is huge because phase III trial is much larger, more expensive and may not able to get the predicted therapeutic effect from the human beings which raises the cost of the R&D investment. Success rate from Phase III clinical trial to New Drug approval by FDA was 40% during 1999-2003, 34% during 2003-2007, 22% during 2007-2011 and 18% during 2011-2014 (Congressional Budget Office (CBO) study, 2016; Domenico, 2015; DiMasi, 2001; Arrowsmith, & Miller, 2013; DiMasi, 2010; Michael, 2014; Arrowsmith, 2011).

It was shocking that the overall sales of about 12 drugs approved by FDA crossed over more than $11 billion but were withdrawn from the market due to the adverse effects observed in the post marketing. Due to the observation of high failure in clinical trial phases and unexpected adverse effects for the approved drug in the post marketing, FDA have suggested to submit the additional data along with the new drug application from 2001 onwards (Steven, *et al.*, 2010). These declines in the success rate from one stage to another stage in the drug discovery process increases the R&D costs per new drug molecule. Success or failure in the development of NME is based on the selection of target or disease modulation approach. It is the first critical step in the process to decide the success or failure of the project (Vernon, *et al.*, 2010; Scannell, *et al.*, 2012; Pammolli, *et al.*, 2011).

Current Scenario

Currently high cost, risk and low efficiency are the major draw backs in the drug innovation; whereas investment, productivity and challenges are the major difficulties in the pharmaceutical R&D sector. Pharmaceutical sector spends highest amount in research when compare to any other industrial organizational sector. In 2010, pharmaceutical products global revenue was 856 billion dollars that is about 60% of the sales in US and Europe (Thayer, 2011). Pharmaceutical organizations are implementing the rigorous technological assessments to improve the innovation efficiency of the new drugs and to provide their value for the society. In spite of their large investments and assessment, but decline in productivity has been faced by the pharmaceutical industries.

Important Factors in R&D

- How well health care professionals and consumers are informed about the attributes of existing drugs.
- How patents and health insurance coverage affect pharmaceutical companies' revenues and returns on R&D.
- How strong incentives are provided to doctors for choosing among prescription drugs to patients (Congressional Budget Office (CBO) study, 2016).

Investments Towards the Approval of New Drug Molecule

Investments from the different pharmaceutical organization for the approval of new drug molecule is shown in Table 1 (Pammolli, *et al.*, 2011; Evaluate Pharma orphan drug report, 2017; David, *et al.*, 2009; Citeline Pharma R&D annual review, 2014).

Management in Research and Development

Management of the R&D can be classified as

1. Centralized
2. Decentralized.

Pharmaceutical organizations R&D prefer to have centralized approach.
Strength and weakness of the centralized approach are

Strength

- Encourages risk taking and long term thinking.
- Increases likelihood of fundamental technology advances.
- Emphasizes importance of research.
- Helps to fascinate top talent.

Table 1. Pharmaceutical organizations R&D investment towards NME

S. No	Investment amount (USD) for approval of NME during 2006-2014	Pharmaceutical Organization
1	3–4 billion	Boehringer Ingelheim, Bristol-Myers Squibb, Takeda and Glaxo-SmithKline
2	8 billion	Amgen, Novartis, AstraZeneca, Pfizer, Merck & Co., Sanofi and Roche
3	More than 10 billion	Eli Lilly and Abbott/AbbVie
	Future Investments Year 2020	
1	10.5 billion	Novartis
2	9.1 billion	Roche
3	7.5 billion	Pfizer
4	7.1 billion	Merck
5	6.1 billion	Sanofi
6	5.6 billion	AstraZeneca
7	5.4 billion	Glaxo-SmithKline

Weakness

- May cause disconnect between R&D and the company's need.
- Product development cycles can be slow down.
- Accounting for benefits of the R&D program is hard.
- Valley of death can stop technology deployment (Thomas, *et al.*, 2006; Agyres, & Silverman, 2004; Tushman, & O'Reilly, 1996).

New Productivity and Challenges in Drug Discovery and Development

Considering the cost and other related issue, pharmaceutical organizations adopted different strategies and technologies like combinatorial chemistry, DNA sequencing, high-throughput-screening (HTS) or computational drug design in order to improve the R&D productivity, efficiency and success rate in reduced time lime. In the initial stage of drug discovery, organizations utilize bioinformatics tools and computer modeling along with accelerated proof of concept studies to enhance the productivity (Alexander, *et al.*, 2016).

The computer modeling tool High throughput screening provide a meaningful structure activity relationship in lead optimization phase to choose a desirable centric target and to find an effective lead molecule. An effective lead molecule can be identified in short duration by utilizing the technologies in different stages of drug discovery like target identification, target validation, hit generation through X-ray crystallography, structure guided drug discovery, fragment based, virtual screening, high throughput screening to lead optimization by scaffold hopping, allosteric Vs active site modulation, pharmacokinetic parameters such as absorption, distribution, metabolism and excretion, selectivity and toxicological profile (Andersson, *et al.*, 2009; Meanwell, 2012; Gleeson, 2008; DiMasi, 2002; Andersen, 2011).

COMPUTER AIDED DRUG DESIGN AND DEVELOPMENT/ IN SILICO DRUG DESIGN

The term *in silico* was created in 1989 as an analogy to the Latin phrases *in vivo*, *in vitro*, and *in situ* (Le, *et al.*, 2015). Nowadays computational methods have been considered to have a significant role in drug discovery and development through marketing of new drug molecules. The main goal of the computational method is to get best new drug molecules which are having desirable properties such as active, drug-like and lead-like; eliminate compounds which are having undesirable properties such as inactive, reactive, toxic and poor ADMET/PK, significantly reduce the time, resources in synthesis of drug molecules and its biological testing. With the available software and hardware, advances in computing technologies empowered the computational methods are reliable one. In simple way the current trend in the drug discovery is shifted from "drug discovery" to "drug design". These computational models can help to predict, suggest hypotheses and provide information virtually in every phase of drug discovery and development to choose a suitable drug molecule with its desired therapeutics. Different terms has been applied to this computer aided drug design and development includes computer-aided drug design (CADD), computational drug design, computer-aided molecular design (CAMD), computer-aided molecular modeling (CAMM), rational drug design, *in silico* drug design and computer-aided rational drug design. In these techniques, computational power is applied in the combination of chemical and biological system in order to streamline the design, drug discovery, development and optimization from the existing knowledge (Kumar, *et al.*, 2006; Ekins, & Wang, 2006; Roche, & Guba, 2005; Lakshmana Prabu *et al.*, 2016; Kapetanovic, 2008; Jorgensen, 2004; Kubinyi, 2006).

In computational methods basic knowledge of the biochemical role in the particular disease, protein which causes the diseases, pathway, compounds which can able to act and modify the role of the disease causing protein are need to be identified. Computer aided biological system includes identification of hit, hit-to-lead selection, optimization of the absorption, distribution, metabolism, excretion, toxicity profile and avoid safety issues. Biological system includes functional proteins, monocellular organisms, multicellular organisms, cells isolated from tissues and organs. Chemical system includes ligand-based drug design, structure-based drug design, quantitative structure-activity and quantitative structure-property relationships to improve their physicochemical, pharmaceutical and pharmacokinetic properties. Bioinformatics and cheminformatic are the two major branches of CADD in modern drug discovery. Application of both cheminformatics and bioinformatics we can able to study the interactions of the chemical structures of the drug in the molecular level within a cell and DNA in the nucleus (Roche, & Guba, 2005; Kapetanovic, 2008; Jorgensen, 2004; Kubinyi, 2006).

Bioinformatics is a scientific field that holds large computer networks hanger (called *GRID)* and dedicated energy facilities with power back-up (called *APS*), more than a performant software with ultra-fast rendering capacity and several webbased applications for the final end-user (Ouzounis, 2012). It holds lot of potential in identification of target (generally proteins/enzymes), validation of target, protein understanding, evolution and phylogeny and modeling of protein (Lengauer, 2004).

Cheminformatic is a scientific field having lot of potential in storage management and maintaining the chemical compounds and related property information. It is utilized in the novel bioactive compounds identification, lead optimization, ADME (Absorption, Distribution, Metabolism and Elimination) prediction and related issues. This cheminformatics can display any drug molecular structure from the computer data base and allowing slight molecular changes to predict the influence in absorption, metabolism, half-life, therapeutic effect or side effects (Kapetanovic, 2008; Hohman, *et al.*, 2009). Also provides the information that drug molecule which does not have any significant therapeutic effect for a particular disease.

Multiple stages are involved in the *in silico* drug design. They are

1. Protein structure determination.
2. Determination of structure of the target in complex with a promising lead.
3. Synthesis of the optimized lead, determination of structure of the new target: lead complex.
4. Optimization of the lead compound (Deepali, *et al.*, 2016; Sumudu, & Steffen, 2016).

Structure/Receptor Based Drug Design

In this drug design, drug targets molecules has a key role for a specific disease through cell signaling or metabolic pathway. Drug target molecules are often protein and enzymes play a significant role in disease development through either protein-nucleic acid or protein-protein interaction leads to interruption or alteration in the metabolic pathway process. Designing the drug molecules to interact with the drug targets, inhibit or modify or restore the target protein structure or enzymes.

Protein Structure Determination

Protein target 3D structure is derived from X-ray crystallography and NMR spectroscopy. Recently, cryo-electron microscopy (cryoEM) is used to increase the near atomic resolution structure numbers. X-ray crystallography technique is applicable only if the target protein can be crystallized, whereas NMR technique is appropriate only to smaller proteins (Sumudu, & Steffen, 2016).

Homology Modeling

This technique is frequently applied in Structure/Receptor based drug design to predict the structure of target that are important in diseases. If the crystallographic coordinates or 2D NMR models are not available, then Homology modeling is a technique used to predict the 3D coordinates structure. In homology modeling, three-dimensional protein structure is made up from fragments of crystallographic models (Le, *et al.*, 2015; Kapetanovic, 2008; Ekins, *et al.*, 2007).

The first task is to identification of a homologous structure to the sequence of interest. To find the homologous structure, known three dimensional protein structure sequence is compared from the protein database. While choosing the homologous structure amino acid sequences to the target sequence of interest need to be considered. Binding and function sites will assist for selecting the homologous structure. If not the homologous structure is built by, α-helix shape is taken from one crystal structure, β-sheet shape is taken from another structure and loops can be taken from other structures. These, selected α-helix, β-sheet and loop pieces are put together to give a complete protein structure and then optimized. Optimization is done by assessing the protein structure through general stereochemistry which includes satisfaction of angle restraints and bond lengths of generated models. Once it is optimized and verified for its acceptability in terms of its stereochemistry, then it will be evaluated for its 3D profile. For built up at least 40% of identity to a protein sequence of a known three dimensional structure is required, if the similarity less than 30% may not give reliable structure prediction. Homology models may be very precise or very marginal, which depends on the degree of identity of the chosen protein sequence. Software such as 3D-JIGSAW, MODELLER, HHpred, RaptorX, Swiss model and Phyre2 are used in this modeling (Le, *et al.*, 2015; Sumudu, & Steffen, 2016; Xiang, 2006; Bourne, & Weissig, 2005; Schwede, *et al.*, 2003; Eswar, *et al.*, 2006; Soding, *et al.*, 2005).

Protein Folding

This method is used when the target protein don't have any sequence similarities, target proteins are identified based on its similar fold recognition or threading methods. In this method, known protein sequence is replaced by the interested target protein sequence for which the structure is unknown. This new threaded structure is evaluated by various scoring methods. Process is continued until best fit structure for the query sequence is obtained and optimized. Sometime this protein folding technique gives a precise model and occasionally it gives relatively a poor model. Software such as GenTHREADER, MUSTER, I-TASSER and DescFold are used in this technique. The disadvantage of this protein folding method is whether the given model is accurate or not (Le, *et al.*, 2015; Sumudu, & Steffen, 2016; Young, 2009; Ingles-Prieto, *et al.*, 2013; McGuffin, 2008; Jones, 1992; Jones, 1999).

Ab Initio (de novo) Modeling

This technique is used when there is no adequate homologous structures are available for comparison. This modeling is depends on the sequence not by the template structure. In this method protein like structure having centroid atoms to represent the side chain will be generated. Generated structure is relaxed by refining the centroid based structure through all-atom refinement function. Software such as QUARK, Rosetta/Robetta, I-TASSER, CABS-FOLD and EVfold are used in this modeling (Le, *et al.*, 2015; Sumudu, & Steffen, 2016; Loew, *et al.*, 1993; Mason, *et al.*, 2001; Englebienne, & Moitessier, 2009; Gohlke, *et al.*, 2009; Leonardo, *et al.*, 2015; da Silva *et al.*, 1999).

Ligand-Based Drug Design (LBDD)

Ligand based drug design is an alternative approach to the structure based drug design. When the structure of target is unknown or unable to predict through homology modeling, protein folding and Ab initio modeling, ligand based drug design is an alternative technique. This method depends on the previous study results and knowledge of a small molecule that interacts and binds to the interested target or very similar targets which has at least marginal activity. Further slight modification is to be done on the molecular structure to improve its activity (Sumudu, & Steffen, 2016; Loew, *et al.*, 1993; Mason, *et al.*, 2001).

Virtual Screening

Identification of novel chemotype from the large chemical compound databases/chemical libraries based on the process of scoring, ranking and affinity for a certain target is referred as Virtual screening. Target based virtual screening is depends on the availability of the information of target structure (determined either experimentally or modeling techniques). Number of compounds to be verified experimentally can be reduced based on the virtual screening, which helps to identify leads and its optimization (Ish, 2012; Le, *et al.*, 2015; Kapetanovic, 2008; Koh, 2003; Koppen, 2009; Subramaniam, *et al.*, 2008; Rester, 2008; Oprea, & Matter, 2004; Green, 2003; Stahura, & Bajorath, 2004; Bajorath, 2002; Klebe, 2006; Jain, 2004). Virtual screening is performed in two categories.

Structure Based Virtual Screening (SBVS)

In SBVS, the selected chemical compound is docked into the selected target protein binding site. SBVS provides a ranking for the docked molecules. Based on the ranking, promising chemical compound will be selected and tested experimentally for its biological activity on the target. Chemical database used in structure based virtual screening are Zinc, PubChem, ChemSpider, ChEMBL, NuBBE DB, ChemBank, eMolecules, DrugBank and Binding DB (Leonardo, *et al.*, 2015; Lionta, *et al.*, 2014; Gangwal, *et al.*, 2015).

Steps involved in the SBVS are

1. Molecular target preparation
2. Compound database selection
3. Molecular docking
4. Post-docking analysis (Scior, *et al.*, 2012).

Ligand Based Virtual Screening (LBVS)

Ligand based virtual screening is performed when receptor structural information is unknown or unable to predict, one or more bioactive compounds are available. Three approaches are used in the virtual screening technique. They are

1. Similarity search
2. Pharmacophore-based virtual screening
3. Quantitative Structure–Activity Relationship

Similarity Search

The similarity search or fingerprint based approach is performed when a single bioactive compound is available. The main principle of this technique is to screen databases based on its physical and chemical similarity with the backbone of the lead molecule for the target. The lead molecule is selected based on similarity score which includes 2D score and a 3D structure similarity. Chemical databases used in similarity search or fingerprint based approach are Molinspiration, OSIRIS Property Explorer, Molsoft and MoKa (Le, *et al.*, 2015; Kapetanovic, 2008; Sumudu, & Steffen, 2016; Leonardo, *et al.*, 2015; Vogt, & Bajorath, 2011; Bologa, *et al.*, 2006; Lindert, *et al.*, 2013; Zhu, *et al.*, 2013).

Pharmacophore-Based Virtual Screening

Pharmacophore-based virtual screening is another approach in LBVS, this approach is performed when one or several bioactive compounds are available. Screening is performed based on the structural features collected from known ligands to generate pharmacophore models that bind to a target. Pharmacophoric features include H-bond acceptors, H-bond donors, aromatic, hydrophobic, positive and negative ionizable groups (Kapetanovic, 2008).

IUPAC defines pharmacophore as: "the ensemble of steric and electronic features that is necessary to ensure the optimal supramolecular interactions with a specific biological target structure and to trigger (or to block) its biological response". In another way "Pharmacophore" is the three-dimensional geometry of interaction features that a molecule must have in order to bind in a protein's active site (Sumudu, & Steffen, 2016).

The principle behind of the Pharmacophore-based virtual screening is a set of chemical features and the 3-Dimensional space arrangement is responsible for the bioactivity of the compound. The aim of the pharmacophore mapping is the transform from 2D structure-activity information into the 3D requirements for binding to the target biomolecule. This pharmacophore mapping allows searching molecules from 3D database that match these 3D properties, identify the bioactive confirmation of the active molecule with how it is superimposed. This mapping also identifies the types of points match with what type of conformation of the compounds. A pharmacophore model is made based on its chemical features (H-bond acceptors, H-bond donors, aromatic, hydrophobic, positive and negative ionizable groups) (Lin, 2005; Langer, & Krovat, 2003; Patel, *et al.*, 2002).

Generating a 3D Pharmacophore model comprises the following steps

1. The active compounds known to be binding to the desired target.

2. For a 2D pharmacophore model, essential atom types and their connectivity are defined whereas for a 3D pharmacophore model, the conformations are defined using IUPAC nomenclature.
3. Alignment of ligand or superimposition is used to identify common feature property required in binders.
4. Generating the Pharmacophore model.
5. Ranking of the pharmacophore models and selecting the best models.
6. Validation of pharmacophore models (Sumudu, & Steffen, 2016).

Programme used for pharmacophore generation in commercial are Hiphop, HypoGen, HypoRefine, GASP, DiscoTech, GALAHAD, LigandScout, MOE, PHASE and XED; whereas programme used for pharmacophore generation in Academic are PharmaGist, ALADDIN, RAPID, DANTE, APOLLO, CLEW, MPHIL, GAMMA, SCAMPI, Apex-3D and LigBuilder (Leonardo, *et al.*, 2015).

Quantitative Structure–Activity Relationship

Quantitative Structure–Activity Relationship is another approach in LBDD. This QSAR is based on the computational statistics method that correlates relationship between molecular descriptors (physico-chemical properties includes molecular weight, number of rotatable bonds, LogP etc.) of the molecules of ligand and binding to a target corresponds to its biological activity (Verma, *et al.*, 2010). The QSAR basis is that similar structural molecules tend to have similar biological activity. The assumption of QSAR is that the activity, property and toxic effect are related to ligand structural features. This technique is used to forecast the activity of any new molecules without performing the *in vitro* or *in vivo* experiments, which saves the times and resources. For quantification of the biological activity, half maximal inhibitory concentration (IC_{50}) and inhibition constant (*K*i) values are commonly used. QSAR is used to determine the positive or negative effect of a particular feature of a drug molecule with respect to its biological activity; ranges from 1D QSAR to 6D QSAR are available. In 1D-QSAR affinity correlates with pKa, molecular volume etc; 2D-QSAR affinity correlates with physicochemical properties such as electronic hydrophobic and steric features of compounds; 3D-QSAR affinity correlates with its physical, geometric features of active drug molecules and quantum chemical features; 4D-QSAR Ligands are represented as orientations, ensemble of conformers, protonation states, tautomers and stereoisomers; 5D-QSAR is similar to 4D, with additional consideration of different induced-fit models and 6D-QSAR is similar to 5D, with additional consideration of different solvation scenarios (Deepali, 2016; Verma, *et al.*, 2010; Verma, & Hansch, 2009; Gupta, S. P. & Kumaran, 2005; Kontogiorgis, & Hadjipavlou-Litina, 2003; Satya, 2003; Mendenhall, & Meiler, 2016; Bleckmann, & Meiler, 2003; Adl, *et al.*, 2016).

Basic steps in QSAR method are

1. Through a database search or literature search or HTS experiments activities are identified between the drug molecules that attach to the desired drug target.
2. Determination of the biological activity based on structural (e.g. bond, atom, functional group counts, surface area etc.) or physicochemical features of the molecule.
3. Built up of a QSAR between the identified features of the drug molecule and biological activity.
4. Validation of the QSAR for its biological activity.
5. Optimize the QSAR model to maximize the biological activity based on the known active compounds.

6. Test experimentally the optimized drug molecule for its biological activity (Sumudu, & Steffen, 2016).

Selection of the molecular physicochemical properties is having an important role in the QSAR model to get the desired predicted biological activity. Linear QSAR is used to pick molecular descriptors that are important in predicting the biological activity. Molecular descriptors that have a good correlation with the target–ligand biological activity can be predicted by Multivariable linear regression (MLR). Relationship between the molecular descriptors and biological activity are always not in linear.

The difference between the pharmacophore model and QSAR model is in pharmacophore model necessary or essential features of an active ligand is used for determining the activity; whereas in QSAR model not only the essential features but also the other features that affect the activity are taken into the consideration. But volume of the binding site is considered in both models (Dudek, *et al.*, 2006; Kurup, 2003; Sippl, 2002).

Drugs such as Norfloxacin (used to treat urinary tract infections), Zolmitriptan (used to treat migraine) and Losartan (used to treat hypertension) are discovered through ligand based drug design through QSAR model and approved by the FDA (Koga, *et al.*, 1980; Duncia, *et al.*, 1990; Buckingham, *et al.*, 1995).

Molecular Docking

Molecular docking is an automated computer algorithm, frequently used in drug design. Docking predicts how a ligand will bind with the appropriate binding site of the target (active site of protein) through orientation, conformational geometry, binding energetics and provide ranking based on the binding affinity of ligand-receptor complexes. Conformation of docking and scoring include the electrostatic interactions, Van der Waals interactions, solvation effects and entropic effects (Le, *et al.*, 2015; Kapetanovic, 2008; Meng, *et al.*, 2011; Yuriev, *et al.*, 2011).

Docking algorithm is divided into 3 types based on the flexibility of protein and ligand. They are

1. Rigid docking: protein and ligand are consider to be rigid
2. Semi-flexible docking: protein is fixed and ligand is flexible
3. Flexible docking: both protein and ligand are flexible (Moitessier, *et al.*, 2008)

Binding confirmation between the ligand and with the active site of protein is identified in two steps.

1. Accurate pose prediction or binding conformation of the ligand inside the binding site of the target protein.
2. Accurate binding free energy prediction (Le, *et al.*, 2015).

Ligand conformation in molecular docking is verified by specific scoring function through several cyclical processes. They are

1. Conformational Search
2. Evaluation of Binding Energetics
3. Covalent Bonds in Molecular Docking

4. Molecular Dynamics
5. Structural Water
6. Protein-Protein Interaction Inhibitors and Molecular Docking

Conformational Search

Ligands structural parameters like torsional, translational and rotational degree of freedom are incrementally modified in the conformational search. Conformational search is performed by applying systematic and stochastic search. Both search methods are used in molecular docking programme (Leach, *et al.*, 2006; Agrafiotis, *et al.*, 2007).

Systematic Search

This search method gradually changes the ligands conformation by slight structural variations. In systematic search, all the probable combinations of the structural parameters through combinatorial explosion are explored. Algorithm used in the systematic search are eHiTS, FRED, Surflex-Dock, DOCK, GLIDE, EUDOC, FlexX, Hammerhead, Flog, SLIDE and ADAM (Leonardo, *et al.*, 2015; Sousa, *et al.*, 2006; Zsoldos, *et al.*, 2007).

Stochastic Search

This search method randomly modifies the ligands structural parameters and performs the conformational search. Genetic algorithms include AutoDock and Gold programs are applied in stochastic search. Encode the structural parameters of the initial structure of the chromosome is called as vector is the first step in the algorithm. Initial population of chromosomes covering a wide area of the energy landscape is generated by random search algorithm. Suitably adapted chromosomes are selected as template based on the evaluation in the initial population to the next population which provides transmitting favorable structural characteristics and conformational space will be explored. Algorithm used in the stochastic search are AutoDock, Gold, PRO_LEADS, EADock, ICM, LigandFit, Molegro Virtual Docker, CDocker, GlamDock, PLANTS, MolDock and MOE_Dock (Leonardo, *et al.*, 2015; Gorelik, & Goldblum, 2008; McGann, 2012).

Evaluation of Binding Energetics

Scoring functions are used in molecular docking programme to calculate the binding energetics between ligand and receptor complex. The energy variation is given by binding constant (*K*d) and the Gibbs free energy (ΔGL), due to the formation of the ligand-receptor structure. The binding energy of ligand – receptor complex is evaluated based on its physicochemical phenomena involved in intermolecular interactions, ligand-receptor binding, desolvation and entropic effects (Foloppe, & Hubbard, 2006; Jain, 2006).

Energy scoring functions are characterized into three types. They are

1. Force-field based scoring function.
2. Empirical scoring function
3. Knowledge based scoring function (Huang, *et al.*, 2010)

Force-Field Based Scoring Function

Estimates the binding energy by adding the contributions of bonded and (bond stretching, angle bending, and dihedral variation) and non-bonded terms (electrostatic and van der Waals interactions) in a general master function. Inaccuracy in estimating the entropic contributions is the limitation of this method. Algorithm used in the Force-field based scoring function are DOCK, AutoDock, GoldScore, ICM, LigandFit, Molegro Virtual Docker, SYBYL_G-Score, SYBYL_D-Score and MedusaScore (Leonardo, *et al.*, 2015). Formula for the Force-field based scoring function is

$$E_{total} = E_{bonded} + E_{nonbonded}$$

$$E_{bonded} = E_{bond} + E_{angle} + E_{dihedral}$$

$$E_{nonbonded} = E_{electrostatic} + E_{Van\ der\ Wals}$$

E_{bond} represent potential energy of covalent bonds.

E_{angle} represent potential energy between angled bonds.

$E_{dihedral}$ represent potential energy of tortion of bonded atoms.

$E_{electrostatic}$ represent potential energy of electrostatic forces.

$E_{Van\ der\ Waals}$ represent potential energy of Van der Waals forces (Le, *et al.*, 2015).

Empirical Scoring Function

Empirical scoring function is based on the formation of ligand-receptor complex. Formation of this complex includes hydrogen-bonding, ionic and apolar interactions, as well as desolvation and entropic effects. Depends on the data accuracy used in the development of the model is the drawback of this scoring functions. Algorithm used in the empirical scoring function are AutoDock, GlideScore, Chem-Score, X_Score, F_Score, Fresno, SCORE, LUDI, SFCscore, HYDE, LigScore and PLP (Le, *et al.*, 2015; Leonardo, *et al.*, 2015; Murray, *et al.*, 1998; Eldridge, *et al.*, 1997; Bohm, 1994). Formula for the Empirical scoring function is

$$\Delta G_{bind} = \Delta G_{desolvation} + \Delta G_{motion} + \Delta G_{configuration} + \Delta G_{interaction}$$

desolvation – enthalpic penalty for removing the ligand from solvent.

motion – entropic penalty for reducing the degrees of freedom when a ligand binds to its receptor.

configuration – conformational strain energy required to put the ligand in its “active” conformation.

interaction – enthalpic gain for “resolvating” the ligand with its receptor.

Knowledge Based Scoring Function

Based on the pairwise energy, potential extracted from the known ligand-receptor complex. Various types of interactions observed in the dataset are classified and weighted according to their frequency of occurrence. The final score is the sum of all individual interactions. Algorithm used in the knowledge based scoring function are SMoG, DrugScore, PMF_Score, MotifScore, RF_Score, PESD_SVM and PoseScore (Leonardo, *et al.*, 2015; Huang, & Zou, 2006; Gohlke, *et al.*, 2000).

Covalent Bonds in Molecular Docking

Drug molecules which have covalent bonds are favorable one for the therapeutic treatment of the diseases such as cancer, diabetes, infectious, cardio-vascular, gastro-intestinal and neurologic disorder. Protein targets are irreversibly inactivated by the covalent bonds leads to re-synthesis of the target protein and regaining its biological function. These covalent molecules with high affinity it bind with the target protein, leads to produce long lasting pharmacological action and reduced frequency of drug administration. Covalent interaction and non-covalent interaction of drugs with the target protein differ with respect to its binding thermodynamics (Kumalo, *et al.*, 2015; Ouyang, *et al.*, 2013). Program used in the covalent bonds in molecular docking are DOCK, AutoDock and Gold (Leonardo, *et al.*, 2015; Ewing, *et al.*, 2001; Morris, *et al.*, 1996).

Molecular Dynamics

In molecular docking, flexibility of the target binding site is essential one. During the molecular recognition process, target site (enzymes and receptors) can undergo some conformational changes leads to have secondary and tertiary structure. In molecular recognition process, the ligand fit to the target site with little mobility. Molecular dynamics is a technique specifically used when the conformational changes in the target site. A set of convenient structure for docking is generated by the molecular dynamics when the molecular targets are not having suitable crystallographic structures (i.e. structures with inaccessible or poorly defined binding sites). Ligand-receptor complex stability proposed by molecular docking can be assessed by this molecular dynamics.

Newton's equation of motion is applied in molecular dynamics to specify the position and speed of each atom in the study system which helps to examine the trajectory and temporal evolution of ligand-receptor complex (Salsbury, 2010; Durrant, & McCammon, 2011; Harvey, & de Fabritiis, 2012; Nichols, *et al.*, 2011). Simulations such as AMBER, CHARMM and GROMOS are widely used in molecular dynamics (Leonardo, *et al.*, 2015; Cornell, *et al.*, 1995; Christen, *et al.*, 2005).

Structural Water

Crystallographic water is strongly bound to the receptor and it is major challenging one in the molecular docking. At least one water molecule is involved in the ligand-receptor complex. In general structural water facilitate between ligand and the binding site of protein through multiple hydrogen bonding. By designing the ligand or part of the target structure, this structural water can be displaced. This displacement is the entropically favorable, cause enthalpy loss. This enthalpy loss can be compensated by designing specific moiety to mimic the interaction of the displaced water and creation of hydrogen bond with the protein. Otherwise, hydrogen bond between the ligand and the target binding site can be created by inclusion of structural water in the molecular docking (Leonardo, *et al.*, 2015; Michel, *et al.*, 2009; Amadasi, *et al.*, 2008; Amadasi, *et al.*, 2006; Kellogg, & Chen, 2004).

Protein-Protein Interaction Inhibitors and Molecular Docking

Interaction between the dissimilar classes of protein can control the cellular and biochemical process. Small-molecule compounds that directly contest with one of the protein partners are called as protein-protein interaction (PPI) inhibitors. Disease like cancer is attributed due to defective protein-protein interactions, and it has an attractive target in drug discovery. Identification and characterization of binding sites, assessment of their potential interaction with small molecule compounds are the major challenges in the molecular docking (Leonardo, *et al.*, 2015; Arkin, & Wells, 2004; Wells, & McClendon, 2007).

Computational methodologies, Q-SiteFinder and ANCHOR are used in assessing the PPI inhibitors (Laurie, & Jackson, 2005; Meireles, *et al.*, 2010). Q-SiteFinder algorithm is an energy-based method to predict the protein binding sites, based on the interaction energy of each interface pocket in molecular modeling. ANCHOR algorithm search for amino acid side chains deeply suppressed at protein-protein interfaces to locate potential binding pockets carrying druggable properties (Meireles, *et al.*, 2010).

Molecular Lipophilicity

Molecular lipophilicity is quantified as log P, is the molecular characteristics of the chemical compound. Molecular lipophilicity is a key physicochemical parameter of a drug molecule which has an important role in permeability, bioavailability and toxicity. Also determine the ability of the drug molecule to interact with the biological target site. The log P is used to quantify the lipophilicity, also it determines the pharmacokinetic properties and bioavailability of the drug molecule. Drug molecule before reaching the systemic circulation, it should cross the biological barriers through active diffusion or passive diffusion or endocytosis (Kujawski, *et al.*, 2012).

Partition coefficient *n*-octanol/water system has been used for many years to measure the lipophilicity/hydrophobicity. Molecular lipophilicity helps to determine the distribution within the organ. Drug molecule ability to aggregation with water is described as Hydrophobicity whereas ability to aggregation with between drug molecule and solvent is described as lipophilicity. In general the hydrophobic drugs are distributed to hydrophobic compartments (lipid bilayers of cells), while hydrophilic drugs are distributed to hydrophilic compartments (blood serum) (Kujawski, *et al.*, 2012).

Drug like molecule standard properties are identified by Lipinski in the "rule of five". Actually four rules are governed in the Lipinski rule with cut-off numbers that are 5 or multiples of 5. Lipinski rule is

1. Hydrogen bond donors (sum of hydroxyl and amine groups) less than 5.
2. Hydrogen bond acceptors (sum of nitrogen and oxygen atoms) less than 10.
3. A molecular weight under 500 daltons.
4. A log P coefficient of less than 5 (Lipinski, *et al.*, 2001).

Interaction between the drug molecule and biological target can be predicted through log p.

At least three reasonable answers could be possible

1. log *P* is essentially an experimental reproducible measurement.
2. Partition experiments are cheap and relatively no time-consuming.
3. log *P* is directly related to the free energy of binding and solvation/desolvation effects.

Different computational procedures have been developed for calculation of log *P*.
Two methods are used for the calculation of log *P*.
They are

1. The *substructure-based* methods – In this method disconnecting the molecules into atoms (*atom contribution methods*) and utilize multiple regression equations. Algorithm AlogP98 is based on this substructure.
2. Groups (*fragmental methods*); by adding the single-atom or fragmental contributions (supplemented by applying correction rules in the latter case) utilizing additive contributions of functional groups and fragments, then log *P* can be calculated. Algorithms ClogP, log- Kow ACD/logP DB and KlogP are based on this fragmental method.
3. The *whole molecule approaches* – In this method the entire molecule using *molecular lipophilicity potentials (MLP),* VlogP, *topological indices* or *molecular properties* are used to quantify log *P* (Mannhold, & van de Waterbeemd, 2001)

These methods are not suitable for molecule having complex structures due to complexity of quantum mechanical methods.

Softwares for calculation of log *P*

1. CLOGP program breaks the molecules into fragments and calculate these constant fragment values and structure-dependent correction values taken from Hansch and Leo's database, to predict log *P* of several organic molecules.
2. HINT (**H**ydropathic **INT**eractions) program directly calculate the hydrophobic atomic constants for small molecules or acquire them from a residue-based dictionary.
3. KOWWIN program uses the *atom/fragment contribution method* (AFC)
4. XLOGP algorithm is essentially an atom-additive model which is supplemented by a small number of the correction factors.
5. XLOGP2 program uses a total of 90 types of atom to classify atoms in neutral organic compounds. Atoms are classified according to element, hybridization state, solvent accessibility, nature of the neighboring atoms and adjacency to π-systems.
6. The XLOGP3 program adopts 87 atom/group types from optimized classification scheme and internal H-bonds and amino acids as the other two correction factors.
7. ACD/logP packages is *constructionistic* approaches – From measured log *P* data of simple molecules the basic fragment values are derived, then the remaining fragment set is constructed.

Other programmes in the prediction of log P are MiLog P, IA_logP, ALOGPS, AB/LogP and ACD Lab/ChemSketch (Kujawski, *et al.*, 2012).

Recently the computational methods VCCLAB platform and ALOGPS2.1 package are used.

1. The VCCLAB programme include three main parts

a. Applet Clients - A front-end part of the site allows the users to provide data, specify parameters, execute tasks and collect calculated results
b. Super Server - Execute the tasks submitted by the clients.
c. Calculation Servers - Link between the Applet Clients and Calculation Servers (Tetko, *et al.*, 2005).

2. ALOGPS 2.1 package is built on the *Associative Neural Network* (ASNN) pattern; it is a combination of *k*-nearest neighbor and artificial neural network methods (Tetko, Associative Neural Network, CogPrints archive code: cog00001441).

Pharmacokinetic Properties (ADME)

Pharmacokinetic properties such as absorption, distribution, metabolism and excretions are need to be measured in the new drug development stage itself to avoid the failure in the drug design stage which leads to save time and money. Last two decades automated and microprocess controlled robotic techniques combined with mathematic methods (High Throughput Screening) is used to assess the pharmacokinetic properties of the new drug molecules (Alexander, *et al.*, 2016; Domenico, 2015; Le, *et al.*, 2015; Ranganatha, & Kuppast, 2012). These techniques are developed based on the information of physicochemical properties, tridimensional structural information, biology, engineering and informatics of a few illustrative substances assuming that the alike chemical structures often have comparable properties.

The principle behind the HTS is based on the interaction between the ligand and biological compound which is measured as luminescence based binding assay. Different luminescence based binding assay techniques are

1. Fluorescence Anisotropy (FA)
2. Fluorescence Correlation Spectroscopy (FCS)
3. Fluorescence Intensity (FI)
4. Fluorescence Lifetime Imaging Microscopy (FLIM)
5. Fluorescence Resonance Energy Transfer (FRET)
6. Total Internal Reflection Fluorescence (TIRF)
7. Time Resolved Resonance Anisotropy (TRRA).

Other nano-bead based techniques are

1. Scintillation Proximity Assay (SPA)
2. Amplified Luminescence Proximity Homogeneous Assay (ALPHA) (Ranganatha, & Kuppast, 2012).

Bioavailability is defined as the amount of drug which reaches the systemic circulation. Different factors such as absorption, liver first pass metabolism, volume of distribution, rate of clearance, drugs half-life and dosage form affects the bioavailability. Other biopharmaceutical factors like poor aqueous solubility and slow dissolution rate also affect the bioavailability (Nuez, & Rodriguez, 2008).

In drug design and discovery *in silico* ADME models commonly utilize quantitative structure-activity relationship (QSAR) and quantitative structure-property relationship (QSPR) approaches includes several quantitative descriptors based on 2-dimensional or 3-dimensional molecular structures, fragment, topological and global physicochemical properties (Buchwald, & Bodor, 2002).

The mathematical method includes linear methods (multiple linear regression and partial least squares), non-linear methods (feedforward artificial neural network), neural networks, self-organizing maps, recursive partitioning and support vector machines. The similarity/dissimilarity of the drug molecule can be assessed by *k*-nearest neighbor method and stochastic artificial neural network (Nuez, & Rodriguez, 2008).

Physicochemical Properties includes

1. pKa
2. LogP and LogD
3. Polar surface area
4. Lipophilicity
5. Solubility
6. Permeability

pKa

It is the negative logarithm of the acid ionization constant (pKa) and defined as the ability of an ionizable group of an organic compound to donate a proton in an aqueous medium. Solubility, lipophilicity, permeability and absorption of a compound can affect the pKa. Natures of chemical structure and acid strengthening or base weakening factors of the substitutes are considered for the development of algorithms in the calculation of pKa (Nuez, & Rodriguez, 2008; Wang, *et al.*, 2015).

logP and logD

logP is the logarithm of the partition coefficient in an octanol/water system and logD is the pH dependent distribution coefficient. Distribution coefficient (logD) is related to partition coefficient (logP) and ionization constant (pKa). Different algorithms are developed to calculate logP are ClogP, log- Kow, ACD/logP DB, KlogP AlogP98, MlogP and VlogP (Kujawski, *et al.*, 2012; Nuez, & Rodriguez, 2008; Wang, *et al.*, 2015).

Polar Surface Area

Polar surface area is based on the van der Waals surface area which includes nitrogen, oxygen and attached hydrogen atoms. These PSA reflect the ability of the solute to leave the hydrogen binding environment. Calculation of PSA is based on the all three dimensional conformations of the compounds and calculated the PSA as the Boltzmann weighted average (Nuez, & Rodriguez, 2008).

If the polar surface area value greater than 140 Å2 shows poor intestinal absorption whereas the value between 60 and 90 Å2 shows blood-brain partition (Palm, *et al.*, 1997; Kelder, *et al.*, 1999; Folkers, *et al.*, 1998).

Lipophilicity

The drug molecule prefers to have lipidic to an aqueous one. Lipophilicity of a drug is a key parameter for drug permeability (drug absorption and distribution) and elimination (Kujawski, *et al.*, 2012; Nuez, & Rodriguez, 2008).

Solubility

Solubility in the aqueous medium is a most important factor which affects the bioavailability of the drug. *In silico* solubility models are based on the QSPR equation. QSPR equation incorporates molecular lipophilicity (logP) and melting point temperature of the new molecule (Nuez, & Rodriguez, 2008; Jain, & Yalkowsky, 2001).

Permeability

Permeability is the key parameter for any drug molecule absorption (oral, transdermal, ocular, pulmonary); distribution (across the blood-brain barrier or blood retina barrier) and elimination. Human intestinal absorption is an important parameter for oral dosage form whereas drug permeation through blood brain barrier is important for drugs which act via the central nervous systems. Factors such as lipophilicity, hydrogen bonding capacity, size and charge are having role in permeation of drugs through biological membrane (Nuez, & Rodriguez, 2008; Camenisch, *et al.*, 1996).

Prediction of ADME and Related Properties

ADME Prediction Models

Interaction between human body and drug is a bidirectional process. Administration of drug into the human body and the desired activity produced by drugs take place by the inhibition of receptors, activation, blocking of signal pathway via absorption, distribution and metabolism and finally disposes the drug by excretion. These processes between the drug and human body are simultaneous and interactional leads to produce desired therapeutic effect or side effects.

Absorption

Numerous factors influence the drugs absorption in the gastrointestinal tract. They are

1. **Physicochemical:** pKa, lipophilicity, solubility, diffusivity, stability and salt form.
2. **Physiological:** Gastrointestinal pH, gastric passage, transit time of small and large intestine, active transport, efflux and gut wall metabolism.
3. **Formulation Factors:** Drug particle size, crystal form, and dosage form such as tablet, capsule, solution, emulsion, suspension, gel and modified release (Nuez & Rodriguez, 2008; Yamashita, & Hashida, 2004).

Among the above said factors, physicochemical factors are having the major role in the prediction of absorption; formulation factors are characterized and optimized experimentally whereas physiological factors cannot be controlled.

Majority of the drugs are administered through oral route, solubility and human intestinal absorption are the most important parameters affects the drug absorption. Drugs are absorbed in the intestine by passive diffusion. Polar surface area is used as a descriptor for the prediction of intestinal absorption. Caco-2 permeability in combination with kinetic solubility data can be used to calculate the Human intestinal absorption (HIA) (Thomas, *et al.*, 2008). Other molecule descriptors used in the prediction of absorption are

1. Sum of the net atomic charges of oxygen atoms.
2. Sum of the net atomic charges of nitrogen atoms with net negative atomic charges.
3. Sum of the net atomic charges of hydrogen atoms attached to oxygen or nitrogen atoms.
4. Number of carboxyls.
5. Topological polar surface area (TPSA).
6. Predicted apparent octanol-water distribution coefficient at pH 6.5 (logD6.5) (Nuez, & Rodriguez, 2008).

Different pharmacokinetic model for drug absorption includes

1. Metabolism by CYP3A4 inside the epithelial cell.
2. Pgp- mediated model efflux into the lumen.
3. Intracellular diffusion from luminal side to basal side and subsequent permeation through the basal membrane (Nuez, & Rodriguez, 2008).

Models used in the calculation of intestinal absorption are CoMFA, P-gp pharmacophore model and QSAR P-gp model. Algorithm used in the calculation of intestinal absorption are GlastroPlus and iDEA (Nuez, & Rodriguez, 2008; Swaan, *et al.*, 1997; Ekins, *et al.*, 2002). Algorithm GastroPlus simulates gastrointestinal absorption and pharmacokinetics for drugs administered orally or intravenous in humans and animals whereas iDEA simulates human physiology and accounts for regional variations in solubility, surface area, intestinal permeability and fluid movement (Nuez, & Rodriguez, 2008).

Distribution

Once the drug is absorbed by the human body, it should be distributed and reach the target site. Molecular structure and physicochemical parameters are the two parameters affect the drug distribution. During the distribution, the absorbed drug molecules are interacting with the plasma proteins like albumin, alpha1-acid glycoprotein, lipoproteins, erythrocytes, alpha, beta and gamma-globulins; these plasma proteins influence the drug distribution. Albumin influence acidic drugs, alpha1-acid glycoprotein influence basic drugs and lipoproteins influences neutral and basic drugs (Nuez, & Rodriguez, 2008; Kratochwil, *et al.*, 2002).

Blood-Brain Barrier Penetration

Brain consists of tight junctions between microvascular endothelial cell layers; it plays a vital role in separating the brain from the blood (Begley, 1996). Drugs used for targeting the central nervous system, need to have high penetration, whereas non-CNS drugs should be minimized to avoid any CNS side effects. Drug penetrates the Blood brain barrier through either passive diffusion or specific transport mechanism (P-glycoprotein or receptor-mediated transport, peptide transporters, carrier-mediated transport, receptor-mediated transcytosis and other transport systems such as GLUT-1, system L1 and system ASC) (Clark, 2003). Passive membrane transport is predicted based on the molecular descriptors like lipophilicity, hydrophilic and hydrophobic surface areas, structural parameters and net charge at physiological pH.

Methods to determine BBB

Blood brain barrier penetration is evaluated based on the determination of logBB (logarithm value of brain to plasma concentration ratio).

1. **QSAR Statistical Method:** Based on physicochemical properties like logP, pKa and fraction of unbound on the plasma are used to predict logBB (Lanevskij, *et al.*, 2011).
2. Set of 5 COSMO-RS sigma-moments (from quantum chemical calculations) are used as descriptors to predict logBB (Wichmann, *et al.*, 2007).
3. ANN model based on molecular structural parameters and P-glycoprotein (P-gp) substrate probability of compounds (Garg, & Verma, 2006).

Plasma Protein Binding (PPB)

Binding of the drug with the plasma protein leads to have less bioavailability and may produce drug-drug interactions (Trainor, 2007). *In silico* models are developed to determine the PPB based on

1. **Binding Rate and Affinity:** Evaluate how tightly drug binds to human serum albumin.
2. **Binding Sites and Poses:** Provide useful information about structure modification requirement.

SVM aided docking model is used to predict PPB and provide information to predict

1. Binding of albumin with query ligand.
2. Probable ligand binding site.
3. Albumin X-ray structure in complex with ligand
4. Calculation of putative complex (Wang, *et al.*, 2015; Zsila, *et al.*, 2011).

Metabolism

Prediction of metabolism is a priority research and the metabolic fate of a compound is depends on both the chemical properties (molecular structure and physicochemical properties) and biological system (enzyme and its environment). This metabolic problem creates the issues like enhanced clearance leads to poor bioavailability; accumulation of drug leads to produce toxic effects and drug-drug interaction, inhibition enzyme activity, induction and mechanism based inactivation. In general drugs are metabolized in two phases.

Phase I: Key enzymes involved in the metabolism of Phase I are cytochrome P450 (CYP) family. Cytochrome P450 family includes CYP1A2, CYP2A6, CYP2C9, CYP2C19, CYP2D6, CYP2E1 and CYP3A4, of which CYP3A4, CYP2C9, CYP2C19 and CYP2D6; about 80% of drugs are metabolized by these CYP families (Williams, *et al.*, 2004).

Phase II: Key enzymes involved in the metabolism of Phase II are phenol sulfotranferase (PST), UDP-dependent glucuronosyl transferase (UGT), estrogen sulfotransferase (EST) and glutathione-S-transferase (GST) (Nuez, A. & Rodriguez, 2008).

Various models are used to calculate the metabolism related issues based on

1. Interaction models of enzymes with xenobiotic (predict the xenobiotic is a substrate or inhibitor of CYP450).
2. Quantitative prediction of metabolic stability of xenobiotic based on clearance model.
3. Site of metabolism.
4. Metabolite prediction (Nuez, & Rodriguez, 2008).

In silico metabolism prediction models are

1. Gaussian kernel weighted k-nearest neighbor models based on CYP2D6 and CYP3A4 inhibition.
2. CoMFA models based on CYP1A2, CYP2A5, CYP2A6, CYP2C9, CYP2D6 and rat MAO A and b ((Nuez, & Rodriguez, 2008).
3. Pharmacophore models based on UGT1A1 and UGT1A4 (Sorich, *et al.*, 2002; Smith, *et al.*, 2002).
4. COMPACT (Computer-Optimized Molecular Parametric Analysis of Chemical Toxicity) model utilizes sterical and electronic parameters to assess the capability of formation of enzyme substrate complexes with xenobiotics and metabolic activation by the CYP1A and CYP2E subfamilies of cytochromes P450 (Lewis, *et al.*, 1998; Lewis, 2001).

Site of Metabolism (SOM) Prediction

Site of metabolism is the soft sites and most probable metabolized sites of the drug molecules. Prediction and modification of these sites can improve drug molecules metabolic stability. Around 80% of the drugs are metabolized by CYP families, therefore predicting the CYPSOMs can improve the metabolic stability of the molecules.

SOM calculation models are categorized based on

1. Reactivity based
2. Structure based
3. Statistical learning models (Wang, *et al.*, 2015).

Different models in SOM prediction are

1. **Semi-Empirical QM Calculations:** Based on the site with a hydrogen abstraction energy and solvent accessible surface area (Singh, *et al.*, 2003).

2. **SMARTCyp:** Based the 2D structure of a molecule (Rydberg, *et al.*, 2010).
3. **MLlite:** Based on docking methods and quantum chemistry calculations (Oh, *et al.*, 2008).

Metabolite Prediction

Metabolite prediction is to recognize the primary metabolites for xenobiotics and to identify the metabolite related toxicity. Metabolite prediction methods are developed based on expert systems and statistical-based methods.

Different algorithms for metabolite prediction are

1. MetaPrint2D
2. SmartCYP
3. MetaDrug
4. MetaSite
5. SOME (Wang, *et al.*, 2015; Adams, 2010; Voronkov, *et al.*, 2013).

Excretion

After metabolism of the drug, it is excreted from the body by excretion process. Renal and bile excretion are the two major routes of drug elimination. Large molecules conjugate with glucuronic acid and excreted through bile. Drug molecules metabolized by liver, is eliminated through kidney. Active transport system such as organic anion transporting polypeptides, peptide

transporters, organic anion transporters and organic cation transporters helps to transport their metabolites across the basolateral surface of renal and assist the drug elimination. Other transporters such as P-gp, BCRP and MDR, facilitate the drug elimination (Nuez, A. & Rodriguez, 2008; Lee, & Kim, 2004).

Very few *in silico* modeling work has been carried out for prediction of excretion. *In silico* model like P-gp substrates and inhibitor are used to predict the excretion (Launay-Vacher, *et al.*, 2006). Tissue distribution based on blood flow, protein binding, lipophilicity and pKa can assist to predict the passive excretion. However, significance of the renal excretion route can be determined only by initial animal pharmacokinetic study results (Boobis, *et al.*, 2002).

Toxicity

Desirable drug should have a good therapeutic effect and not to produce any toxicity. Toxicity is defined as damage on organism or substructure of organisms includes cells and organs, it can be determined only in the clinical trial stage. Assessing the toxicity in the last stage leads to failure in the drug development process. Predicting the toxicity in the earlier stage can enhance the drug development process (Wang, *et al.*, 2015). Presence of some substructures includes arylpropionic and arylacetic acids, aryl hydroxamic acids, anilines, oximes, anilides, hydrazides, hydrazines, hydantoins, nitroaromatics, quinones, quinone methides, hetero aromatics, halogenated hydrocarbon and some halogenated aromatics in the molecular structure can form metabolites which are involved to produce the toxicity (Nassar, *et al.*, 2004).

Determination of undesirable side effects for the compounds is an objective in the pharmaceutical organization.

The following five steps are considered while developing the prediction models. They are

1. Collection of biological data based on the relationship between chemicals and toxicity endpoints.
2. Molecular descriptors calculation for the chemicals.
3. Developing a prediction model.
4. Performance evaluation of the developed model
5. Interpreting the observed results with the model (Devillers, 2013; Raies & Bajic, 2016; Hannu, 2011; Valerio, 2009; Zhu, 2013; Benigni, *et al.*, 2013; Venkatapathy & Wang, 2013; Roncaglioni, *et al.*, 2013).

Numerous toxicity prediction softwares are developed to assess the toxicity of the drug molecule in the drug discovery during the early stage. The softwares are

1. Deductive Estimation of Risk from Existing Knowledge for Windows (DEREK) provides a qualitative assessment of toxicity potential using structure-based alerts that define toxophores (Sanderson & Earnshaw, 1991).
2. ToxAlerts, a web server of structural alerts for toxic chemicals with potential adverse effects (Sushko, *et al.*, 2012).
3. TOPKAT (Toxicity Prediction by Komputer Assisted Technology) system based on the cross validated QSTR models, predicts toxicity includes rodent carcinogenicity, Ames mutagenicity, rat baoral LD50, rat chronic lowest-observable adverse effect level, developmental toxicity potential and skin sensitization (Prival, 2001; Enslein, *et al.*, 1994; http://accelrys.com/products/discovery-studio/admet.html).
4. The MultiCASE (multiple computer automated structure evaluation) approach evaluates a data set by trying to identify the structural features associated with observed (biophores) (Klopman, 1992; Klopman, *et al.*, 2003).
5. HazardExpert is a toxicity prediction system based on the structure of the compounds and predicts different effects such as: carcinogenic, mutagenic, teratogenic, and neurotoxic (Lewis, *et al.*, 1998; Prieto, *et al.*, 2013).

OTHER TOXICITY STUDIES

Acute Toxicity

Acute toxicity is defined as the toxicity due to exposure of drug for a short period of time; it is an important indicator to assess the drug safety. Determination of LD_{50} is the common criteria to measure the acute toxicity.

Methods to predict the acute toxicity are

1. Global QSAR model based on MLR method and non-congeneric datasets.
2. Classification models were constructed based on five different types of machine-learning methods (SVMOAO, C4·5, RF, kNN and NB) and MACCS and FP4 fingerprints (Wang, *et al.*, 2015; Benfenati, *et al.*, 2009).

Genotoxicity

Genotoxicity is an important toxicity study in the pre-clinical toxicity tests of drug design. Different carcinogenicity datasets are available to predict the toxicity are Chemical Carcinogenesis Research Information System (CCRIS), EPA Gene-tox, the National Toxicology Program (NTP), IARC, Tokyo-Eiken, Mutants, the Carcinogenic Potency project (CPDB) and ISSCAN (Nuez, A. & Rodriguez, 2008; Wang, *et al.*, 2015).

Different models are developed to predict the genotoxicity based on the ligand-based machine learning QSAR/QSPR. Different models are Leadscope FDA Model Applier, Derek from Lhasa, toxicity prediction by computer-assisted technology (TOPKAT), MultiCASE, SciQSAR, OncoLogic and lazy structure-activity relationships (LAZAR) (Nuez, A. & Rodriguez, 2008; Wang, *et al.*, 2015; Arono, 2005).

hERG Toxicity

Sudden death induced by a blockage of human Ether-a-go-go Related Gene (hERG), potassium channel blockage is widely considered as the major cause due to cardiac toxicity. Different range of chemical structure in the drug molecule can cause Cardiac toxicity through hERG. Data bases WOMBAT-PK and PubChem BioAssay are having huge amount of hERG toxicity data for prediction of toxicity (Wang, *et al.*, 2015).

Major complications in the development of hERG blocker models are

1. An unclear mechanism for the hERG blocker.
2. Lack of reliable and extensive experimental data.

Different models used to calculate the genotoxicity are

1. NB classification
2. Recursive partitioning techniques
3. Laplacsian-corrected Bayesian classification (Wang, *et al.*, 2015; Arono, 2005; Seierstad, & Agrafiotis, 2006; Sun, 2006; Wang, *et al.*, 2012; Wang, *et al.*, 2013; Liu, *et al.*, 2014).

OVERVIEW OF DRUG DISCOVERY AND DEVELOPMENT

The drug discovery process has undergone enormous changes during the few years. After synthesizing the new molecules and purification it is evaluated for its physicochemical properties. Then it will be evaluated for its therapeutic activity by *in vitro* and *in vivo* models.

Four stages are involved in the drug discovery and development.

In the first stage, optimized lead compound is explored in animal model to assess acute toxicity, preliminary pharmacokinetics and its therapeutic effect.

In the second stage, subchronic toxicity is assed to ensure the drug safety and pharmacokinetic properties. Based on the pharmacokinetic properties, dosage form and its frequency are optimized.

In the third stage, optimized lead compound is assessed for its therapeutic effect in the patients.

In the final stage, the developed new chemical entity is asses for its definite safety and efficacy in human beings through clinical studies; different toxicity such as carcinogenicity, mutagenicity and reproductive toxicology study etc are performed. *In Silico* intervention process for drug discovery and development is shown in Figure 4. (http://www.allesh.com/solutions.html)

CONCLUSION

Defined organizational structure of R&D activities has large impact in achieving the organizational goal. Currently, high cost for the drug approval, risk, as well as low efficiency and productivity are the main drawbacks in drug innovation. Approval of NME has become more expensive because the investigating diseases are more complex and numbers of biological target are also differing. Investing towards the R&D activity is increasing every year whereas the approval of NME is not a proportionate one. Delivery of the NME with desired property is a critical parameter for the success of any organization. Pharmaceutical industrial R&D sectors adopt various strategies to improve R&D efficiency and productivity. Now computer modeling along with different algorithms are used as concept studies in drug design and development, to enhance the input and output as commercial product into the market. Ultimately to improve the R&D productivity, pharmaceutical industries make the joint ventures and collaborations with academic, universities/ research institutes, contract development and manufacturing organizations (CDMO) and other partners. In near future pharmaceutical R&D can overcome the barriers like difficult task, high cost for the drug approval and risk in the pharmaceutical R&D in discover new drug molecules to the patients around the world. There is no doubt that the industry will boom and establish new landmarks in near future.

Figure 4. In Silico intervention process for drug discovery and development

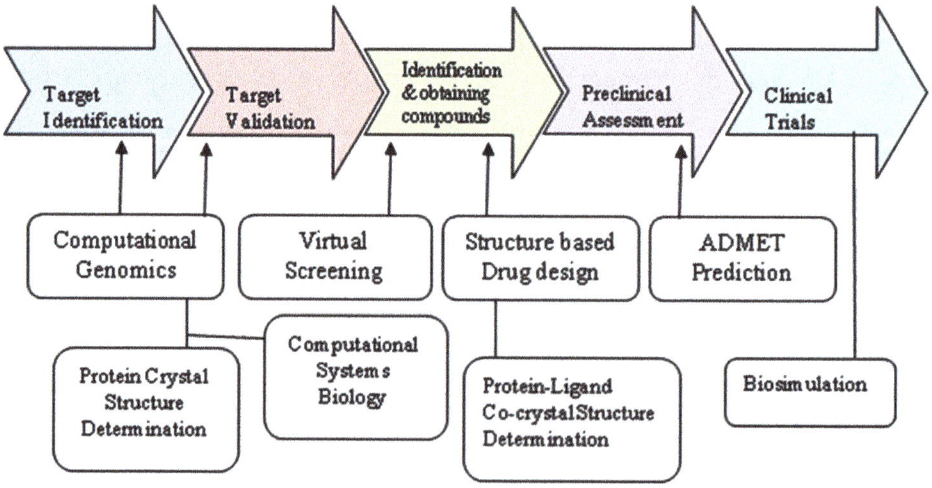

REFERENCES

Accelrys. TOPKAT (TOxicity Prediction by Komputer Assisted Technology). (2015). Available at: http://accelrys.com/products/discovery-studio/admet.html

Adams, S. E. (2010). *Molecular Similarity and Xenobiotic Metabolism* (Ph.D. thesis). University of Cambridge.

Adl, A., Zein, M., & Hassanien, A. E. (2016). PQSAR. Expert System with application. *International Journal (Toronto, Ont.)*, *54*, 219–227.

Agrafiotis, D. K., Gibbs, A. C., Zhu, F., Izrailev, S., & Martin, E. (2007). Conformational sampling of bioactive molecules: A comparative study. *Journal of Chemical Information and Modeling*, *47*(3), 1067–1086. doi:10.1021/ci6005454 PMID:17411028

Agyres, N., & Silverman, B. (2004). R&D, Organizational Structure, and the Development of Corporate Technological Knowledge. *Strategic Management Journal*, *25*(8–9), 929–958. doi:10.1002mj.387

Agyres, N., & Silverman, B. (2004). R&D, Organizational Structure, and the Development of Corporate Technological Knowledge. *Strategic Management Journal*, *25*(8–9), 929–958. doi:10.1002mj.387

Alexander, S., Oliver, G., & Markus, H. (2016). Changing R&D models in research-based pharmaceutical companies. *Journal of Translational Medicine*, *14*(1), 105. doi:10.118612967-016-0838-4 PMID:27118048

Allen, T. J., & Fusfeld, A. (1975). Research laboratory architecture and the structuring of communications. *R & D Management*, *5*(2), 153–163. doi:10.1111/j.1467-9310.1975.tb01230.x

Amadasi, A., Spyrakis, F., Cozzini, P., Abraham, D. J., Kellogg, G. E., & Mozzarelli, A. (2006). Mapping the energetics of water-protein and water-ligand interactions with the "natural" HINT forcefield: Predictive tools for characterizing the roles of water in biomolecules. *Journal of Molecular Biology*, *358*(1), 289–309. doi:10.1016/j.jmb.2006.01.053 PMID:16497327

Amadasi, A., Surface, J. A., Spyrakis, F., Cozzini, P., Mozzarelli, A., & Kellogg, G. E. (2008). Robust classification of "relevant" water molecules in putative protein binding sites. *Journal of Medicinal Chemistry*, *51*(4), 1063–1067. doi:10.1021/jm701023h PMID:18232647

Andersen, M. R., Almen, M. S., & Schioth, H. B. (2011). Trends in the exploitation of novel drug targets. *Nature Reviews. Drug Discovery*, *10*(8), 579–590. doi:10.1038/nrd3478 PMID:21804595

Andersson, S., Armstrong, A., Bjore, A., Bowker, S., Chapman, S., Davies, R., ... Whittamore, P. (2009). Making medicinal chemistry more effective – application of lean sigma to improve processes, speed and quality. *Drug Discovery Today*, *14*(11-12), 598–604. doi:10.1016/j.drudis.2009.03.005 PMID:19508922

Arkin, M. R., & Wells, J. A. (2004). Small-molecule inhibitors of protein-protein interactions: Progressing towards the dream. *Nature Reviews. Drug Discovery*, *3*(4), 301–317. doi:10.1038/nrd1343 PMID:15060526

Arono, V. A. M. (2005). Predictive *in silico* modeling for hERG channel blockers. *Drug Discovery Today*, *10*(2), 149–155. doi:10.1016/S1359-6446(04)03278-7 PMID:15718164

Arrowsmith, J. (2011). Phase II failures: 2008–2010. *Nature Reviews. Drug Discovery*, *10*(5), 328–329. doi:10.1038/nrd3439 PMID:21532551

Arrowsmith, J., & Miller, P. (2013). Trial Watch: Phase II and Phase III attrition rates 2011–2012. *Nature Reviews. Drug Discovery*, *12*(8), 569. doi:10.1038/nrd4090 PMID:23903212

Bajorath, J. (2002). Integration of virtual and high-throughput screening. *Nature Reviews. Drug Discovery*, *1*(11), 882–894. doi:10.1038/nrd941 PMID:12415248

Begley, D. J. (1996). The blood-brain barrier: Principles for targeting peptide and drugs to the central nervous system. *The Journal of Pharmacy and Pharmacology*, *48*(2), 136–140. doi:10.1111/j.2042-7158.1996.tb07112.x PMID:8935161

Benfenati, E., Benigni, R., Demarini, D. M., Helma, C., Kirkland, D., Martin, T., ... Yang, C. (2009). Predictive models for carcinogenicity and mutagenicity: Frameworks, state-of-the-art, and perspectives. *Journal of Environmental Science and Health. Part C, Environmental Carcinogenesis & Ecotoxicology Reviews*, *27*(2), 57–90. doi:10.1080/10590500902885593 PMID:19412856

Benigni, R., Battistelli, C. L., Bossa, C., Colafranceschi, M., & Tcheremenskaia, O. (2013). Mutagenicity, carcinogenicity, and other end points. In B. Reisfeld & A. N. Mayeno (Eds.), *Computational Toxicology* (Vol. 930, pp. 67–98). New York: Humana Press. doi:10.1007/978-1-62703-059-5_4

Bleckmann, A., & Meiler, J. (2003). Quantitative structure activity relations studied by support vector machines and artificial neural networks. *QSAR & Combinatorial Science*, *22*(7), 722–728. doi:10.1002/qsar.200330837

Bohm, H. (1994). The development of a simple empirical scoring function to estimate the binding constant for a protein-ligand complex of known three-dimensional structure. *Journal of Computer-Aided Molecular Design*, *8*, 243–256. doi:10.1007/BF00126743 PMID:7964925

Bologa, C. G., Revankar, C. M., Young, S. M., Edwards, B. S., Arterburn, J. B., Kiselyov, A. S., ... Prossnitz, E. R. (2006). Virtual and biomolecular screening converge on a selective agonist for GPR30. *Nature Chemical Biology*, *2*(4), 207–212. doi:10.1038/nchembio775 PMID:16520733

Boobis, A., Gundert-Remy, U., Kremers, P., Macheras, P., & Pelkonen, O. (2002). *In silico* prediction of ADME and pharmacokinetics. Report of an expert meeting organised by COST B15. *European Journal of Pharmaceutical Sciences*, *17*(4-5), 183–193. doi:10.1016/S0928-0987(02)00185-9 PMID:12453607

Bourne, P. E., & Weissig, H. (2005). *Structural Bioinformatics*. Hoboken, NJ: John Wiley & Sons, Inc.

Buchwald, P., & Bodor, N. (2002). Computer aided drug design: The role of quantitative structure-property, structure-activity and structure-metabolism relationships (QSPR, QSAR, QSMR). *Drugs of the Future*, *15*(6), 577–588. doi:10.1358/dof.2002.027.06.856934

Buckingham, J., Glen, R. C., Hill, A. P., Hyde, R. M., Martin, G. R., Robertson, A. D., ... Woollard, P. M. (1995). Computer-Aided Design and Synthesis of 5-Substituted Tryptamines and Their Pharmacology at the 5-HT1D Receptor: Discovery of Compounds with Potential Anti-Migraine Properties. *Journal of Medicinal Chemistry*, *38*(18), 3566–3580. doi:10.1021/jm00018a016 PMID:7658443

Camenisch, G., Folkers, G., & van de Waterbeemd, H. (1996). Review of theoretical passive drug absorption models: Historical background, recent developments and limitations. *Pharmaceutica Acta Helvetiae*, *71*(5), 309–327. doi:10.1016/S0031-6865(96)00031-3 PMID:8973162

Changxiao, L., Panayiotis, P. C., & Yazhuo, L. (2014). Research and development in drug innovation: Reflections from the 2013 bioeconomy conference in China, lessons learned and future perspectives. *Acta Pharmaceutica Sinica. B*, *4*(2), 112–119. doi:10.1016/j.apsb.2014.01.002 PMID:26579372

Christen, M., Hunenberger, P. H., Bakowies, D., Baron, R., Burgi, R., Geerke, D. P., ... van Gunsteren, W. F. (2005). The GROMOS software for biomolecular simulation: GROMOS05. *Journal of Computational Chemistry*, *26*(16), 1719–1751. doi:10.1002/jcc.20303 PMID:16211540

Citeline Pharma R&D annual review. (2014). Retrieved from http://maxicool5.free.fr/Bourse/Valo%20 Pharma/Annual-Review-2014b.pdf

Clark, D. E. (2003). *In silico* prediction of blood-brain barrier permeation. *Drug Discovery Today*, *8*(20), 927–933. doi:10.1016/S1359-6446(03)02827-7 PMID:14554156

Congressional Budget Office (CBO) study. (2016). *Research and Development in the Pharmaceutical Industry*. Retrieved from https://www.cbo.gov/sites/default/files/109th-congress-2005-2006/reports/10-02-drugr-d.pdf

Cornell, W. D., Cieplak, P., Bayly, C. I., Gould, I. R., Merz, K. M., Ferguson, D. M., ... Kollman, P. A. (1995). A second generation force field for the simulation of proteins, nucleic acids, and organic molecules. *Journal of the American Chemical Society*, *117*(19), 5179–5197. doi:10.1021/ja00124a002

da Silva, C., da Silva, E. C., & Nascimento, M. A. C. (1999). Ab Initio Calculations of Absolute pKa Values in Aqueous Solution I. Carboxylic Acids. *The Journal of Physical Chemistry A*, *103*(50), 11194–11199. doi:10.1021/jp9836473

David, E., Tramontin, T., & Zemmel, R. (2009). Pharmaceutical R&D: The road to positive returns. *Nature Reviews. Drug Discovery*, *8*(8), 609–610. doi:10.1038/nrd2948 PMID:19644471

Deepali, G., Gauri, S., & Ashish, M. (2016). Re-thinking drug discovery: *In silico* method. *Journal of Chemical and Pharmaceutical Research*, *8*(8), 1092–1099.

Devillers, J. (2013). Methods for building QSARs. In B. Reisfeld & A. N. Mayeno (Eds.), *Computational Toxicology* (pp. 3–27). New York: Humana Press.

Dickson, M., & Gagnon, J. P. (2004). Key factors in the rising cost of new drug discovery and development. *Nature Reviews. Drug Discovery*, *3*(5), 417–429. doi:10.1038/nrd1382 PMID:15136789

DiMasi, J., Hansen, R., & Grabowski, H. (2003). The price of innovation: New estimates of drug development costs. *Journal of Health Economics*, *22*(2), 151–185. doi:10.1016/S0167-6296(02)00126-1 PMID:12606142

DiMasi, J. A. (2001). Risks in new drug development: Approval success rates for investigational drugs. *Clinical Pharmacology and Therapeutics*, *69*(5), 297–307. doi:10.1067/mcp.2001.115446 PMID:11371997

DiMasi, J. A. (2001). Risks in new drug development: Approval success rates for investigational drugs. *Clinical Pharmacology and Therapeutics*, *69*(5), 297–307. doi:10.1067/mcp.2001.115446 PMID:11371997

DiMasi, J. A. (2002). The value of improving the productivity of the drug development process. *PharmacoEconomics, 20*(S3), 1–10.

DiMasi, J. A., Feldman, L., Seckler, A., & Wilson, A. (2010). Trends in risks associated with new drug development: Success rates for investigational drugs. *Clinical Pharmacology and Therapeutics*, *87*(3), 272–277. doi:10.1038/clpt.2009.295 PMID:20130567

DiMasi, J. A., Hansen, R. W., & Grabowski, H. G. (2003). The price of innovation: New estimates of drug development costs. *Journal of Health Economics*, *23*(2), 151–185. doi:10.1016/S0167-6296(02)00126-1 PMID:12606142

DiMasi, J. A., Hansen, R. W., Grabowski, H. G., & Lasagna, L. (1991). Cost of innovation in the pharmaceutical industry. *Journal of Health Economics*, *10*(2), 107–142. doi:10.1016/0167-6296(91)90001-4 PMID:10113009

Domenico, F. (2015). Hypothesis for changing models: Current pharmaceutical paradigms, trends and approaches in drug discovery. *PeerJ PrePrints, 813*(1).

Drug Discovery and Development. (n.d.). Retrieved from http://www.slideshare.net/anisha88shah/rd-brochure

Dudek, A. Z., Arodz, T., & Galvez, J. (2006). Computational methods in developing quantitative structure–activity relationships (QSAR): A review. *Combinatorial Chemistry & High Throughput Screening*, *9*(3), 213–228. doi:10.2174/138620706776055539 PMID:16533155

Duncia, J. V., Chiu, A. T., Carini, D. J., Gregory, G. B., Johnson, A. L., Price, W. A., ... Timmermans, P. B. M. W. M. (1990). The discovery of potent nonpeptide angiotensin II receptor antagonists: A new class of potent antihypertensives. *Journal of Medicinal Chemistry*, *33*(5), 1312–1329. doi:10.1021/jm00167a007 PMID:2329553

Durrant, J. D., & McCammon, J. A. (2011). Molecular dynamics simulations and drug discovery. *BMC Biology*, *9*(1), 71. doi:10.1186/1741-7007-9-71 PMID:22035460

Ekins, S., Kim, R. B., Leake, B. F., Dantzig, A. H., Schuetz, E. G., Lan, L. B., & ... . (2002). Three-dimensional quantitative structure-activity relationships of inhibitors of P-glycoprotein. *Molecular Pharmacology*, *61*(5), 964–973. doi:10.1124/mol.61.5.964 PMID:11961113

Ekins, S., Mestres, J., & Testa, B. (2007). *In silico* pharmacology for drug discovery: Methods for virtual ligand screening and profiling. *British Journal of Pharmacology*, *152*(1), 9–20. doi:10.1038j.bjp.0707305 PMID:17549047

Ekins, S., & Wang, B. (2006). *Computer Applications in Pharmaceutical Research and Development*. Wiley-Interscience. doi:10.1002/0470037237

Eldridge, M. D., Murray, C. W., Auton, T. R., Paolini, G. V., & Mee, R. P. (1997). Empirical scoring functions: I. The development of a fast empirical scoring function to estimate the binding affinity of ligands in receptor complexes. *Journal of Computer-Aided Molecular Design*, *11*(5), 425–445. doi:10.1023/A:1007996124545 PMID:9385547

Englebienne, P., & Moitessier, N. (2009). Docking ligands into flexible and solvated macromolecules. 5. Force-field-based prediction of binding affinities of ligands to proteins. *Journal of Chemical Information and Modeling*, *49*(11), 2564–2571. doi:10.1021/ci900251k PMID:19928836

Enslein, K., Gombar, V. K., & Blake, B. W. (1994). Internation commission for protection against environmental mutagens and carcinogens. Use of SAR in computer-assisted prediction of carcinogenicity and mutagenicity of chemicals by the TOPKAT program. *Mutation Research*, *305*, 47–61. doi:10.1016/0027-5107(94)90125-2 PMID:7508547

Ernst, & Young, L.L.P. (2001). *Pharmaceutical Industry R&D Costs: Key Findings about the Public Citizen Report*. Retrieved from http://www.cptech.org/ip/health/econ/phrmaresponse.pdf

Eswar, N., Webb, B., Marti-Renom, M. A., Madhusudhan, M. S., Eramian, D., Shen, M. Y., & .... (2006). Comparative Protein Structure Modeling Using Modeller. *Current Protocols in Bioinformatics*, *5*(5-6). doi:10.1002/0471250953.bi0506s15 PMID:18428767

Evaluate Pharma orphan drug report. (2017). Retrieved from http://info.evaluategroup.com/rs/607-YGS-364/images/wp15.pdf

Ewing, T. J., Makino, S., Skillman, A. G., & Kuntz, I. D. (2001). DOCK 4.0: Search strategies for automated molecular docking of flexible molecule databases. *Journal of Computer-Aided Molecular Design*, *15*(5), 411–428. doi:10.1023/A:1011115820450 PMID:11394736

Fabio, P., Laura, M., & Massimo, R. (2011). The productivity crisis in pharmaceutical R&D. *Nature Reviews. Drug Discovery*, *10*(6), 428–438. doi:10.1038/nrd3405 PMID:21629293

Folkers, G., Chretien, J. R., & Raevsky, O. A. (1998). Estimation of blood-brain barrier crossing of drugs using molecular size and shape, and H-bonding descriptors. *Journal of Drug Targeting*, *6*(2), 151–165. doi:10.3109/10611869808997889 PMID:9886238

Foloppe, N., & Hubbard, R. (2006). Towards predictive ligand design with free-energy based computational methods? *Current Medicinal Chemistry*, *13*(29), 3583–3608. doi:10.2174/092986706779026165 PMID:17168725

Gangwal, R. P., Damre, M. V., Das, N. R., Dhoke, G. V., Bhadauriya, A., Varikoti, R. A., ... Sangamwar, A. T. (2015). Structure based virtual screening to identify selective phosphodiesterase 4B inhibitors. *Journal of Molecular Graphics & Modelling*, *57*, 89–98. doi:10.1016/j.jmgm.2015.01.007 PMID:25687765

Garg, P., & Verma, J. (2006). *In silico* prediction of blood brain barrier permeability: An artificial neural network model. *Journal of Chemical Information and Modeling*, *46*(1), 289–297. doi:10.1021/ci050303i PMID:16426064

Gleeson, M. P. (2008). Generation of a set of simple, interpretable ADMET rules of thumb. *Journal of Medicinal Chemistry*, *51*(4), 817–834. doi:10.1021/jm701122q PMID:18232648

Gohlke, H., Hendlich, M., & Klebe, G. (2000). Knowledge-based scoring function to predict protein-ligand interactions. *Journal of Molecular Biology*, *295*(2), 337–356. doi:10.1006/jmbi.1999.3371 PMID:10623530

Gorelik, B., & Goldblum, A. (2008). High quality binding modes in docking ligands to proteins. *Proteins*, *71*(3), 1373–1386. doi:10.1002/prot.21847 PMID:18058908

Green, D. V. (2003). Virtual screening of virtual libraries. *Progress in Medicinal Chemistry*, *41*, 61–97. doi:10.1016/S0079-6468(02)41002-8 PMID:12774691

Gupta, S. P., & Kumaran, S. (2005). A quantitative structure–activity relationship study on some aromatic/heterocyclic sulfonamides and their charged derivatives acting as carbonic anhydrase inhibitors. *Journal of Enzyme Inhibition and Medicinal Chemistry*, *20*(3), 251–259. doi:10.1080/14756360500067439 PMID:16119196

Hannu, R. (2011). *Insilico*toxicology–non-testingmethods. *Frontiers in Pharmacology*, *2*, 1–8. PMID:21779246

Harvey, M. J., & de Fabritiis, G. (2012). High-throughput molecular dynamics: The powerful new tool for drug discovery. *Drug Discovery Today*, *17*(19-20), 1059–1062. doi:10.1016/j.drudis.2012.03.017 PMID:22504137

He, W. (2013). Small molecular drug innovation & development. *Abstract: 2013 International bioeconomy conference, session 2: R&D in drug innovation*, 67–69.

Hohman, M., Gregory, K., Chibale, K., Smith, P. J., Ekins, S., & Bunin, B. (2009). Novel web-based tools combining chemistry informatics, biology and social networks for drug discovery. *Drug Discovery Today*, *14*(5-6), 261–270. doi:10.1016/j.drudis.2008.11.015 PMID:19231313

Huang, S. Y., Grinter, S. Z., & Zou, X. (2010). Scoring functions and their evaluation methods for protein-ligand docking: Recent advances and future directions. *Physical Chemistry Chemical Physics*, *12*(40), 12899–12908. doi:10.1039/c0cp00151a PMID:20730182

Huang, S. Y., & Zou, X. (2006). An iterative knowledge-based scoring function to predict protein-ligand interactions: I. Derivation of interaction potentials. *Journal of Computational Chemistry*, *27*(15), 1866–1875. doi:10.1002/jcc.20504 PMID:16983673

Ingles-Prieto, A., Ibarra-Molero, B., Delgado-Delgado, A., Perez-Jimenez, R., Fernandez, J. M., & Gaucher, E. A. (2013). 2YOI: Crystal Structure of Ancestral Thioredoxin Relative to Last Eukaryotes Common Ancestor (Leca) From the Precambrian Period. *Structure (London, England)*, *21*, 1690–1697. doi:10.1016/j.str.2013.06.020

Ish, K. (2012). Drug discovery in pharmaceutical Industry: Productivity challenges and trends. *Drug Discovery Today*, *17*(19/20), 1088–1102. PMID:22627006

Jain, A. N. (2004). Ligand-based structural hypotheses for virtual screening. *Journal of Medicinal Chemistry*, *47*(4), 947–961. doi:10.1021/jm030520f PMID:14761196

Jain, A. N. (2006). Scoring functions for protein-ligand docking. *Current Protein & Peptide Science*, *7*(5), 407–420. doi:10.2174/138920306778559395 PMID:17073693

Jain, N., & Yalkowsky, S. H. (2001). Estimation of the aqueous solubility I: Application to organic nonelectrolytes. *Journal of Pharmaceutical Sciences*, *90*(2), 234–252. doi:10.1002/1520-6017(200102)90:2<234::AID-JPS14>3.0.CO;2-V PMID:11169540

Jones, D. T. (1999). GenTHREADER: An efficient and reliable protein fold recognition method for genomic sequences. *Journal of Molecular Biology*, *287*(4), 797–815. doi:10.1006/jmbi.1999.2583 PMID:10191147

Jones, D. T., Taylort, W. R., & Thornton, J. M. (1992). A new approach to protein fold recognition. *Nature*, *358*(6381), 86–89. doi:10.1038/358086a0 PMID:1614539

Jorgensen, W. L. (2004). The many roles of computation in drug discovery. *Science*, *303*(5665), 1813–1818. doi:10.1126cience.1096361 PMID:15031495

Kapetanovic, I. M. (2008). Computer-aided drug discovery and development (CADDD): *In silico*-chemico-biological approach. *Chemico-Biological Interactions*, *171*(2), 165–176. doi:10.1016/j.cbi.2006.12.006 PMID:17229415

Kelder, J., Grootenhuis, P. D. J., Bayada, D. M., Delbressine, L. P. C., & Ploemen, J. P. (1999). Polar-molecular surface as a dominating determinant for oral absorption and brainpenetration of drugs. *Pharmaceutical Research*, *6*(10), 1514–1519. doi:10.1023/A:1015040217741 PMID:10554091

Kellogg, G. E., & Chen, D. L. (2004). The importance of being exhaustive. Optimization of bridging structural water molecules and water networks in models of biological systems. *Chemistry & Biodiversity*, *1*(1), 98–105. doi:10.1002/cbdv.200490016 PMID:17191777

Klebe, G. (2006). Virtual ligand screening: Strategies, perspectives and limitations. *Drug Discovery Today*, *11*(13-14), 580–594. doi:10.1016/j.drudis.2006.05.012 PMID:16793526

Klopman, G. (1992). MULTI-CASE. 1. A hierarchical computer automated structure evaluation program. *Molecular Informatics*, *11*, 176–184.

Klopman, G., Chakravarti, S. K., Harris, N., Ivanov, J., & Saiakhov, R. D. (2003). *In silico* screening of high production volume chemicals for mutagenicity using the MCASE QSAR expert system. *SAR and QSAR in Environmental Research*, *14*(2), 165–180. doi:10.1080/1062936031000073171 PMID:12747573

Koga, H., Itoh, A., Murayama, S., Suzue, S., & Irikura, T. (1980). Structure activity relationship of antibacterial 6,7 & 7,8 disubstituted 1-alkyl 1,4- dihydro 4-oxoquinolone, 3-carboxylic acid. *Journal of Medicinal Chemistry*, *23*(12), 1358–1363. doi:10.1021/jm00186a014 PMID:7452690

Koh, J. (2003). Making virtual screening a reality. *Proceedings of the National Academy of Science*, 6902–6903.

Kontogiorgis, C. A., & Hadjipavlou-Litina, D. (2003). Quantitative Structure - Activity Relationships (QSARs) of Thrombin Inhibitors: Review, Evaluation and Comparative Analysis. *Current Medicinal Chemistry*, *10*(7), 525–577. doi:10.2174/0929867033457935 PMID:12678789

Koppen, H. (2009). Virtual screening - what does it give us? *Current Opinion in Drug Discovery & Development*, *12*, 397–407. PMID:19396741

Kratochwil, N. A., Huber, W., Muller, F., Kansy, M., & Gerber, P. R. (2002). Predicting plasma protein binding of drugs: A new approach. *Biochemical Pharmacology*, *64*(9), 1355–1374. doi:10.1016/S0006-2952(02)01074-2 PMID:12392818

Kubinyi, H. (2006). Success stories of computer-aided design. In Computer Applications in Pharmaceutical Research and Development. Wiley-Interscience. doi:10.1002/0470037237.ch16

Kujawski, J., Bernard, M. K., Janusz, A., & Kuzma, W. (2012). Prediction of log P – ALOGPS Application in Medicinal Chemistry Education. *Journal of Chemical Education*, *89*(1), 64–67. doi:10.1021/ed100444h

Kujawski, J., Popielarska, H., Myka, A., Drabinska, B., & Bernard, M. K. (2012). The log *P* parameter as a molecular descriptor in the Computer-aided Drug Design – an overview. *Computational Methods in Science and Technology*, *18*(2), 81–88. doi:10.12921/cmst.2012.18.02.81-88

Kumalo, H. M., Bhakat, S., & Soliman, M. E. (2015). Theory and applications of covalent docking in drug discovery: Merits and pitfalls. *Molecules (Basel, Switzerland)*, *20*(2), 1984–2000. doi:10.3390/molecules20021984 PMID:25633330

Kumar, N., Hendriks, B. S., Janes, K. A., de Graaf, D., & Lauffenburger, D. A. (2006). Applying computational modeling to drug discovery and development. *Drug Discovery Today*, *11*(17–18), 806–811. doi:10.1016/j.drudis.2006.07.010 PMID:16935748

Kurup, A. (2003). C-QSAR: a database of 18,000 QSARs and associated biological and physical data. *Journal of Computer Aided Drug Design*, *17*, 187–196.

Lakings, D. B. (2009). Drug development teams. In R. Guarino (Ed.), *New drug approval process* (Vol. 139, pp. 1–15). Marcel Dekker.

Lakshmana Prabu, S., Thirumurugan, R., Mahesh Vijay, P. & Shanmugarathinam, A. (2016, October). Applications of computer in Health Profession: From Drug Discovery to Market. *International Journal of Research in Pharmacology & Pharmacotherapeutics,* 46-54.

Lakshmana Prabu, S., Thirumurugan, R., & Suriya Prakash, T. N. K. (2014). The role of the drug discovery, clinical and regulatory affairs teams in turning a potent agent into a registered product. In J. Reedijk (Ed.), *Elsevier Reference Module in Chemistry, Molecular Sciences and Chemical Engineering*. Waltham, MA: Elsevier; doi:10.1016/B978-0-12-409547-2.11400-3

Lanevskij, K., Dapkunas, J., Juska, L., Japertas, P., & Didziapetris, R. (2011). QSAR analysis of blood-brain distribution: The influence of plasma and brain tissue binding. *Journal of Pharmaceutical Sciences*, *100*(6), 2147–2160. doi:10.1002/jps.22442 PMID:21271563

Langer, T., & Krovat, E. M. (2003). Chemical features based pharmacophore and virtual library screening for discovery of new leads. *Current Opinion in Drug Discovery & Development*, *6*, 370–376. PMID:12833670

Launay-Vacher, V., Izzedine, H., Karie, S., Hulot, J. S., Baumelou, A., & Deray, G. (2006). Renal tubular drug transporters. *Nephron. Physiology*, *103*(3), 97–106. doi:10.1159/000092212 PMID:16554667

Laurie, A. T., & Jackson, R. M. (2005). Q-SiteFinder: An energy-based method for the prediction of protein-ligand binding sites. *Bioinformatics (Oxford, England)*, *21*(9), 1908–1916. doi:10.1093/bioinformatics/bti315 PMID:15701681

Le, A. V., Phan, T. C. Q., & Nguyen, T. H. (2015). *In silico* Drug Design: Prospective for Drug Lead Discovery. *International Journal of Engineering Science Invention*, *4*(10), 60–70.

Leach, A. R., Shoichet, B. K., & Peishoff, C. E. (2006). Prediction of protein–ligand interactions. Docking and scoring: Successes and gaps. *Journal of Medicinal Chemistry*, *49*(20), 5851–5855. doi:10.1021/jm060999m PMID:17004700

Lee, W., & Kim, R. B. (2004). Transporters and renal drug elimination. *Annual Review of Pharmacology and Toxicology*, *44*(1), 137–166. doi:10.1146/annurev.pharmtox.44.101802.121856 PMID:14744242

Lengauer, T. (2004). *Bioinformatics from genome to drugs*. Weinheim, Germany: Wiley- VCH.

Leonardo, G. F., Ricardo, N. S., Glaucius, O., & Adriano, D. A. (2015). Molecular Docking and Structure-Based Drug Design Strategies. *Molecules (Basel, Switzerland)*, *20*(7), 13384–13421. doi:10.3390/molecules200713384 PMID:26205061

Lewis, C. V. F., Ioannides, C., & Parke, D. V. (1998). An improved and updated version of the compact procedure for the evaluation of P450-mediated activation. *Drug Metabolism Reviews*, *30*(4), 709–737. doi:10.3109/03602539808996328 PMID:9844807

Lewis, D. F., Ioannides, C., & Parke, D. V. (1998). A combined COMPACT and HazardExpert study of 40 chemicals for which information on mutagenicity and carcinogenicity is known, including the results of human epidemiological studies. *Human & Experimental Pharmacology*, *17*, 577–586. PMID:9821022

Lewis, D. V. F. (2001). COMPACT: A structural approach to the modelling of cytochromes P450 and their interactions with xenobiotics. *Journal of Chemical Technology and Biotechnology (Oxford, Oxfordshire)*, *76*(3), 237–244. doi:10.1002/jctb.363

Lin, S. K. (2005). Pharmacophore Perception, Development and Use in Drug Design. *Molecules (Basel, Switzerland)*, *5*(12), 987–989. doi:10.3390/50700987

Lindert, S., Zhu, W., Liu, Y. L., Pang, R., Oldfield, E., & McCammon, J. A. (2013). Non-Bisphosphonate Inhibitors of Isoprenoid Biosynthesis Identified via Computer-Aided Drug Design. *Chemical Biology & Drug Design*, *81*, 742–748. doi:10.1111/cbdd.12121 PMID:23421555

Lionta, E., Spyrou, G., Vassilatis, D. K., & Cournia, Z. (2014). Structure-based virtual screening for drug discovery: Principles, applications and recent advances. *Current Topics in Medicinal Chemistry*, *14*(16), 1923–1938. doi:10.2174/1568026614666140929124445 PMID:25262799

Lipinski, C. A., Lombardo, F. M., Dominy, B. W., & Feeney, P. J. (2001). Experimental and computational approaches to estimate solubility and permeability in drug discovery and development settings. *Advanced Drug Delivery Reviews*, *46*(1-3), 3–26. doi:10.1016/S0169-409X(00)00129-0 PMID:11259830

Liu, C. X. (2013). Rethinking on research and development in innovation of biomedicines. *Drugs Clinic*, *28*, 469–475.

Liu, L. L., Lu, J., Lu, Y., Zheng, M. Y., Luo, X. M., Zhu, W. L., ... Chen, K. (2014). Novel Bayesian classification models for predicting compounds blocking hERG potassium channels. *Acta Pharmacologica Sinica*, *35*(8), 1093–1102. doi:10.1038/aps.2014.35 PMID:24976154

Loew, G. H., Villar, H. O., & Alkorta, I. (1993). Strategies for Indirect Computer-Aided Drug Design. *Pharmaceutical Research*, *10*(4), 475–486. doi:10.1023/A:1018977414572 PMID:8483829

Lombardino, J. G., & Lowe, J. A. (2004). The role of the medicinal chemist in drug discovery--then and now. *Nature Reviews. Drug Discovery*, *3*(10), 853–862. doi:10.1038/nrd1523 PMID:15459676

Mannhold, R., & van de Waterbeemd, H. (2001). Substructure and whole molecule approaches for calculating log P. *Journal of Computer-Aided Molecular Design*, *15*(4), 337–354. doi:10.1023/A:1011107422318 PMID:11349816

Mason, J. S., Good, A. C., & Martin, E. J. (2001). 3-D pharmacophores in drug discovery. *Current Pharmaceutical Design*, *7*(7), 567–597. doi:10.2174/1381612013397843 PMID:11375769

Mathieu, M. (Ed.). (2002). *New drug development: A regulatory overview* (6th ed.). Waltham: Parexel International Corporation.

McGann, M. (2012). FRED and HYBRID docking performance on standardized datasets. *Journal of Computer-Aided Molecular Design*, *26*(8), 897–906. doi:10.100710822-012-9584-8 PMID:22669221

McGuffin, L. J. (2008). Protein Fold Recognition and Threading. *Computational Structural Biology*, 37–60. doi:10.1142/9789812778789_0002

Meanwell, N. A. (2012). Synopsis of some recent tactical application of bioisosteres. *Journal of Medicinal Chemistry*, *54*(8), 2529–2591. doi:10.1021/jm1013693 PMID:21413808

Meireles, L. M., Domling, A. S., & Camacho, C. J. (2010). ANCHOR: A web server and database for analysis of protein-protein interaction binding pockets for drug discovery. *Nucleic Acids Research*, *38*(Web Server), W407–W411. doi:10.1093/nar/gkq502 PMID:20525787

Mendenhall, J. & Meiler, J. (2016). Improving quantitative structure-activity relationship models using Artificial Neural Networks trained with dropout. *Journal of Computer Aided Drug Design, 30*, 177–189.

Meng, X. Y., Zhang, H. X., Mezei, M., & Cui, M. (2011). Molecular docking: A powerful approach for structure-based drug discovery. *Current Computer-aided Drug Design*, *7*(2), 146–157. doi:10.2174/157340911795677602 PMID:21534921

Michael, D., & Jean, P. G. (2014). Key factors in the rising cost of new drug discovery and development. *Nature Reviews. Drug Discovery*, *3*, 417–429. PMID:15136789

Michael, H., David, W. T., Craighead, J. L., Economides, C., & Rosenthal, J. (2014). Clinical development success rates for investigational drugs. *Nature Biotechnology*, *32*(1), 40–51. doi:10.1038/nbt.2786 PMID:24406927

Michel, J., Tirado-Rives, J., & Jorgensen, W. L. (2009). Energetics of displacing water molecules from protein binding sites: Consequences for ligand optimization. *Journal of the American Chemical Society*, *131*(42), 15403–15411. doi:10.1021/ja906058w PMID:19778066

Moitessier, N., Englebienne, P., Lee, D., Lawandi, J., & Corbeil, C. (2008). Towards the development of universal, fast and highly accurate docking/scoring methods: A long way to go. *British Journal of Pharmacology*, *153*(S1), S7–S26. doi:10.1038j.bjp.0707515 PMID:18037925

Morgan, S., Grootendorst, P., Lexchin, J., Cunningham, C., & Greyson, D. (2011). The cost of drug development: A systematic review. *Health Policy (Amsterdam)*, *100*(1), 4–17. doi:10.1016/j.healthpol.2010.12.002 PMID:21256615

Morris, G. M., Goodsell, D. S., Huey, R., & Olson, A. J. (1996). Distributed automated docking of flexible ligands to proteins: Parallel applications of AutoDock 2.4. *Journal of Computer-Aided Molecular Design*, *10*(4), 293–304. doi:10.1007/BF00124499 PMID:8877701

Munos, B. (2009). Lessons from 60 years of pharmaceutical innovation. *Nature Reviews. Drug Discovery*, *8*(12), 959–968. doi:10.1038/nrd2961 PMID:19949401

Murray, C., Auton, T. R., & Eldridge, M. D. (1998). Empirical scoring functions. II. The testing of an empirical scoring function for the prediction of ligand-receptor binding affinities and the use of Bayesian regression to improve the quality of the model. *Journal of Computer-Aided Molecular Design*, *12*(5), 503–519. doi:10.1023/A:1008040323669 PMID:9834910

Nassar, A. E. F., Kamel, A. M., & Clarimont, C. (2004). Improving the decision-making process in structural modification of drug candidates: Reducing toxicity. *Drug Discovery Today*, *9*(24), 1055–1064. doi:10.1016/S1359-6446(04)03297-0 PMID:15582794

Nichols, S. E., Baron, R., Ivetac, A., & McCammon, J. A. (2011). Predictive power of molecular dynamics receptor structures in virtual screening. *Journal of Chemical Information and Modeling*, *51*(6), 1439–1446. doi:10.1021/ci200117n PMID:21534609

Nuez, A., & Rodriguez, R. (2008). Current methodology for the assessment of ADME-Tox properties on drug candidate molecules. *Biotecnología Aplicada*, *25*, 97–110.

Oh, W. S., Kim, D. N., Jung, J., Cho, K. H., & No, K. T. (2008). New combined model for the prediction of regioselectivity in cytochrome P450/3A4 mediated metabolism. *Journal of Chemical Information and Modeling*, *48*(3), 591–601. doi:10.1021/ci7003576 PMID:18290640

Oprea, T. I., & Matter, H. (2004). Integrating virtual screening in lead discovery. *Current Opinion in Chemical Biology*, *8*(4), 349–358. doi:10.1016/j.cbpa.2004.06.008 PMID:15288243

Ouyang, X., Zhou, S., Su, C. T. T., Ge, Z., Li, R., & Kwoh, C. K. (2013). Covalent Dock: Automated covalent docking with parameterized covalent linkage energy estimation and molecular geometry constraints. *Journal of Computational Chemistry*, *34*(4), 326–336. doi:10.1002/jcc.23136 PMID:23034731

Ouzounis, C. A. (2012). Rise and Demise of Bioinformatics? Promise and Progress. *PLoS Computational Biology*, *8*(4), e1002487. doi:10.1371/journal.pcbi.1002487 PMID:22570600

Palm, K., Stenberg, P., Luthman, K., & Artursson, P. I. (1997). Polar molecular surface properties predict the intestinal absorption of drugs in human. *Pharmaceutical Research*, *14*(5), 568–571. doi:10.1023/A:1012188625088 PMID:9165525

Pammolli, F., Magazzini, L. & Riccaboni, M. (2011). The productivity crisis in pharmaceutical R&D. *Nature Reviews Drug Discovery*, *10*, 428–38.

Patel, Y., Gillet, V. J., Bravi, G. & Leach, A. R. (2002). A comparison of the pharmacophore identification programme CATALYST, DISCO and GASP. *Journal of Computer Aided Drug Design, 16*, 653–681.

Prieto, P., Kinsner-Ovaskainen, A., Stanzel, S., Albella, B., Artursson, P., Campillo, N., ... Kopp-Schneider, A. (2013). The value of selected in vitro and in silico methods to predict acute oral toxicity in a regulatory context: Results from the European project ACuteTox. *Toxicology In Vitro*, *27*(4), 1357–1376. doi:10.1016/j.tiv.2012.07.013 PMID:22922246

Pritchard, J. F., Romet, M. J., Reimer, M. L. J., Mortimer, E., Rolfe, B., & Cayen, M. N. (2003). Making better drugs: Decision gates in non-clinical drug development. *Nature Reviews. Drug Discovery*, *2*(7), 542–553. doi:10.1038/nrd1131 PMID:12815380

Prival, M. J. (2001). Evaluation of the TOPKAT system for predicting the carcinogenicity of chemicals. *Environmental and Molecular Mutagenesis*, *37*(1), 55–69. doi:10.1002/1098-2280(2001)37:1<55::AID-EM1006>3.0.CO;2-5 PMID:11170242

Profile Biopharmaceutical Industry. (2016). Retrieved from http://phrma-docs.phrma.org/sites/default/files/pdf/biopharmaceutical-industry-profile.pdf

Raies, A. B., & Bajic, V. B. (2016). *In silico* toxicology: Computational methods for the prediction of chemical toxicity. *WIREs Computational Molecular Science.*, *6*(2), 147–172. doi:10.1002/wcms.1240 PMID:27066112

Ranganatha, N., & Kuppast, I. J. (2012). A review on alternatives to animal testing methods in drug development. *International Journal of Pharmacy and Pharmaceutical Sciences*, *4*(5), 28–32.

R&D Organizational Structure. (n.d.). Retrieved from https://www.slideshare.net/teresatreasures/drug-development-biotechnology

Regulatory control of active pharmaceutical ingredients. Version 1, Appendix 14. (n.d.). Retrieved from https://npra.moh.gov.my/images/Announcement/2011/Regulatory-Control-of-Active-Pharmaceutical-Ingredients/API_Guideline_VERSION_1_-_PBKD.pdf

Rester, U. (2008). From virtuality to reality - virtual screening in lead discovery and lead optimization: A medicinal chemistry perspective. *Current Opinion in Drug Discovery & Development*, *11*, 559–568. PMID:18600572

Roche, O., & Guba, W. (2005). Computational chemistry as an integral component of lead generation. *Mini-Reviews in Medicinal Chemistry*, *7*(7), 677–683. doi:10.2174/1389557054368826 PMID:16026314

Roncaglioni, A., Toropov, A. A., Toropova, A. P., & Benfenati, E. (2013). *In silico* methods to predict drug toxicity. *Current Opinion in Pharmacology*, *13*(5), 802–806. doi:10.1016/j.coph.2013.06.001 PMID:23797035

Rydberg, P., Gloriam, D. E., Zaretzki, J., Breneman, C., & Olsen, L. (2010). SMARTCyp: A 2D method for prediction of Cytochrome P450-mediated drug metabolism. *ACS Medicinal Chemistry Letters*, *1*(3), 96–100. doi:10.1021/ml100016x PMID:24936230

Salsbury, F. R. Jr. (2010). Molecular dynamics simulations of protein dynamics and their relevance to drug discovery. *Current Opinion in Pharmacology*, *10*(6), 738–744. doi:10.1016/j.coph.2010.09.016 PMID:20971684

Sanderson, D. M., & Earnshaw, C. G. (1991). Computer prediction of possible toxic action from chemical structure; the DEREK system. *Human and Experimental Toxicology*, *10*(4), 261–273. doi:10.1177/096032719101000405 PMID:1679649

Satya, P. G. (2003). Quantitative structure activity relationships of renin inhibitors. *Mini-Reviews in Medicinal Chemistry*, *3*(4), 315–321. doi:10.2174/1389557033488051 PMID:12678825

Scannell, J. W., Alex, B., Helen, B., & Brian, W. (2012). Diagnosing the decline in pharmaceutical R&D efficiency. *Nature Reviews. Drug Discovery*, *11*(3), 191–200. doi:10.1038/nrd3681 PMID:22378269

Schwede, T., Kopp, J., Guex, N., & Peitsch, M. C. (2003). SWISS-MODEL: An automated protein homology-modeling server. *Nucleic Acids Research*, *31*(13), 3381–3385. doi:10.1093/nar/gkg520 PMID:12824332

Scior, T., Bender, A., Tresadern, G., Medina-Franco, J. L., Martínez-Mayorga, K., Langer, T., ... Agrafiotis, D. K. (2012). Recognizing pitfalls in virtual screening: A critical review. *Journal of Chemical Information and Modeling*, *52*(4), 867–881. doi:10.1021/ci200528d PMID:22435959

Seierstad, M., & Agrafiotis, D. K. (2006). A QSAR model of hERG binding using a large, diverse, and internally consistent training set. *Chemical Biology & Drug Design*, *67*(4), 284–296. doi:10.1111/j.1747-0285.2006.00379.x PMID:16629826

Singh, S. B., Shen, L. Q., Walker, M. J., & Sheridan, R. P. (2003). A model for predicting likely sites of CYP3A4-mediated metabolism on drug like molecules. *Journal of Medicinal Chemistry*, *46*(8), 1330–1336. doi:10.1021/jm020400s PMID:12672233

Sippl, W. (2002). Development of biologically active compounds by combining 3D QSAR and structure-based design methods. *Journal of Computer Aided Drug Design*, *16*, 825–830.

Smith, P. A., Sorich, M. J., McKinnon, R. A., & Miners, J. O. (2002). Pharmacophore and quantitative structure activity relationship (QSAR) modelling: Complemetary approaches to the rationalization and prediction of UDP gluconosyltransferase 1A4 (UGT1A4) substrate selectivity. *Journal of Medicinal Chemistry*, *46*(9), 1617–1626. doi:10.1021/jm020397c PMID:12699380

Soding, J., Biegert, A., & Lupas, A. N. (2005). The HHpred interactive server for protein homology detection and structure prediction. *Nucleic Acids Research*, *33*(Web Server), W244–W248. doi:10.1093/nar/gki408 PMID:15980461

Sorich, M. J., Smith, P. A., McKinnon, R. A., & Miners, J. O. (2002). Pharmacophore and quantitative structure activity relationship modelling of UDP-glucuronosyl transferase 1A1 (UGT1A1) substrates. *Pharmacogenetics*, *12*(8), 635–645. doi:10.1097/00008571-200211000-00008 PMID:12439224

Sousa, S. F., Fernandes, P. A., & Ramos, M. J. (2006). Protein-ligand docking: Current status and future challenges. *Proteins*, *65*(1), 15–26. doi:10.1002/prot.21082 PMID:16862531

Stahura, F. L., & Bajorath, J. (2004). Virtual screening methods that complement HTS. *Combinatorial Chemistry & High Throughput Screening*, *7*(4), 259–269. doi:10.2174/1386207043328706 PMID:15200375

Steven, M. P., Daniel, S. M., Christopher, T. D., Charles, C. P., Bernard, H. M., Stacy, R. L., & … . (2010). How to improve R&D productivity: The pharmaceutical industry's grand challenge. *Nature Reviews. Drug Discovery*, *9*(3), 203–214. doi:10.1038/nrd3078 PMID:20168317

Subramaniam, S., Mehrotra, M., & Gupta, D. (2008). Virtual high throughput screening (vhts) - a perspective. *Bioinformation*, *3*(1), 14–17. doi:10.6026/97320630003014 PMID:19052660

Sumudu, P. L., & Steffen, L. (2016). Computational methods in drug discovery. *Beilstein Journal of Organic Chemistry*, *12*, 2694–2718. doi:10.3762/bjoc.12.267 PMID:28144341

Sun, H. (2006). An accurate and interpretable Bayesian classification model for prediction of hERG liability. *ChemMedChem*, *1*(3), 315–322. doi:10.1002/cmdc.200500047 PMID:16892366

Sushko, I., Salmina, E., Potemkin, V. A., Poda, G., & Tetko, I. V. (2012). ToxAlerts: A web server of structural alerts for toxfic chemicals and compounds with potential adverse reactions. *Journal of Chemical Information and Modeling*, *52*(8), 2310–2316. doi:10.1021/ci300245q PMID:22876798

Swaan, P. W., Szoka, F. C. Jr, & Oie, S. (1997). Molecular modeling of the intestinal bile acid carrier: A comparative molecular field analysis study. *Journal of Computer Aided Drug Design*, *11*(6), 581–588. doi:10.1023/A:1007919704457 PMID:9491350

Tang, L. D. (2013). Drug discovery & development: strategies and management. *Abstract: 2013 International Bioeconomy Conference, session 2: R&D in drug innovation*, 59–60.

Tetko, I. V. (n.d.). *Associative Neural Network, CogPrints archive code: cog00001441*. Retrieved from http://www.vcclab.org/lab/alogps/library.html

Tetko, I. V., Gasteiger, J., Todeschini, R., Mauri, A., Livingstone, D., Ertl, P., ... Prokopenko, V. V. (2005). Virtual Computational Chemistry Laboratory – Design and Description. *Journal of Computer-Aided Molecular Design*, *19*(6), 453–463. doi:10.100710822-005-8694-y PMID:16231203

Thayer, A. M. (2011). Emerging strategies. *Chemical and Engineering News*, *89*(42), 15–20. doi:10.1021/cen-v089n042.p015

The Pharmaceutical Innovation Platform. (2004). International Federation of Pharmaceutical Manufacturers Associations.

Thomas, M. T., Roger, M., Larry, S., & David, K. (2006). *R&D structure in a changing world*. Industrial Research Institute, Inc.

Thomas, S., Brightman, F., Gill, H., Lee, S., & Pufong, B. (2008). Simulation modelling of human intestinal absorption using Caco-2 permeability and kinetic solubility data for early drug discovery. *Journal of Pharmaceutical Sciences*, *97*(10), 4557–4574. doi:10.1002/jps.21305 PMID:18300298

Tollman, P. (2001). *A Revolution in R&D: How Genomics and Genetics are Transforming the Biopharmaceutical Industry*. Academic Press.

Trainor, G. L. (2007). The importance of plasma protein binding in drug discovery. *Expert Opinion on Drug Discovery*, *2*(1), 51–64. doi:10.1517/17460441.2.1.51 PMID:23496037

Tushman, M., & O'Reilly, C. III. (1996). Ambidextrous Organizations: Managing Evolutionary and Revolutionary Change. *California Management Review*, *38*(4), 8–30. doi:10.2307/41165852

Valerio, L. G. Jr. (2009). *In silico* toxicology for the pharmaceutical sciences. *Toxicology and Applied Pharmacology*, *241*(3), 356–370. doi:10.1016/j.taap.2009.08.022 PMID:19716836

Venkatapathy, R., & Wang, N. C. Y. (2013). Developmental toxicity prediction. In B. Reisfeld & A. N. Mayeno (Eds.), *Computational Toxicology* (pp. 305–340). New York: Humana Press.

Verma, J., Khedkar, V. M., & Coutinho, E. C. (2010). 3D-QSAR in drug design – A review. *Current Topics in Medicinal Chemistry*, *10*(1), 95–115. doi:10.2174/156802610790232260 PMID:19929826

Verma, R. P., & Hansch, C. (2009). Camptothecins: A SAR/QSAR Study. *Chemical Reviews*, *109*(1), 213–235. doi:10.1021/cr0780210 PMID:19099450

Vernon, J. A., Golec, J. H., & Dimasi, J. A. (2010). Drug development costs when financial risk is measured using the Fama-French three-factor model. *Health Economics*, *19*(8), 1002–1005. doi:10.1002/hec.1538 PMID:19655335

Vogt, M., & Bajorath, J. (2011). Predicting the performance of fingerprint similarity searching. In J. Bajorath (Ed.), *Chemoinformatics and Computational Chemical Biology* (pp. 159–173). Totowa, NJ: Humana Press.

Voronkov, A., Holsworth, D. D., Waaler, J., Wilson, S. R., Ekblad, B., Perdreau-dahl, H., ... Krauss, S. (2013). Structural basis and SAR for G007-LK, a lead stage 1,2,4-triazole based specific tankyrase 1/2 inhibitor. *Journal of Medicinal Chemistry*, *56*(7), 3012–3023. doi:10.1021/jm4000566 PMID:23473363

Wang, S. C., Li, Y. Y., Wang, J. M., Chen, L., Zhang, L. L., Yu, H. D., & Hou, T. (2012). ADMET evaluation in drug discovery. 12. Development of binary classification models for prediction of hERG potassium channel blockage. *Molecular Pharmaceutics*, *9*(4), 996–1010. doi:10.1021/mp300023x PMID:22380484

Wang, S. C., Li, Y. Y., Xu, L., Li, D., & Hou, T. J. (2013). Recent developments in computational prediction of hERG blockage. *Current Topics in Medicinal Chemistry*, *13*(11), 1317–1326. doi:10.2174/15680266113139990036 PMID:23675938

Wang, Y., Xing, J., Xu, Y., Zhou, N., Peng, J., Xiong, Z., ... Jiang, H. (2015). *In silico* ADME/T modelling for rational drug design. *Quarterly Reviews of Biophysics*, *48*(4), 488–515. doi:10.1017/S0033583515000190 PMID:26328949

Wells, J. A., & McClendon, C. L. (2007). Reaching for high-hanging fruit in drug discovery at protein-protein interfaces. *Nature*, *450*(7172), 1001–1009. doi:10.1038/nature06526 PMID:18075579

Wichmann, K., Diedenhofen, M., & Klamt, A. (2007). Prediction of blood-brain partitioning and human serum albumin binding based on COSMO-RS sigma-moments. *Journal of Chemical Information and Modeling*, *47*(1), 228–233. doi:10.1021/ci600385w PMID:17238268

Wiggins, S. N. (1987). *The Cost of Developing a New Drug*. Washington, DC: Pharmaceutical Manufacturers Association.

Williams, J. A., Hyland, R., Jones, B. C., Smith, D. A., Hurst, S., & Goosen, T. C. (2004). Drug-drug interactions for UDP-glucuronosyl transferase substrates: A pharmacokinetic explanation for typically observed low exposure (AUCi/ AUC) ratios. *Drug Metabolism and Disposition: the Biological Fate of Chemicals*, *32*(11), 1201–1208. doi:10.1124/dmd.104.000794 PMID:15304429

Xiang, Z. (2006). Advances in homology protein structure modeling. *Current Protein & Peptide Science*, *7*(3), 217–227. doi:10.2174/138920306777452312 PMID:16787261

Yamashita, F., & Hashida, M. (2004). *In silico* approaches for predicting ADME properties of drugs. *Drug Metabolism and Pharmacokinetics*, *19*(5), 327–338. doi:10.2133/dmpk.19.327 PMID:15548844

Young, D. (2009). *Computational drug design*. John Wiley & Sons. doi:10.1002/9780470451854

Yuriev, E., Agostino, M., & Ramsland, P. A. (2011). Challenges and advances in computational docking: 2009 in review. *Journal of Molecular Recognition*, *24*(2), 149–164. doi:10.1002/jmr.1077 PMID:21360606

Zhu, H. (2013). From QSAR to QSIIR: searching for enhanced computational toxicology models. In B. Reisfeld & A. N. Mayeno (Eds.), *Computational Toxicology* (pp. 53–65). New York: Humana Press. doi:10.1007/978-1-62703-059-5_3

Zhu, W., Zhang, Y., Sinko, W., Hensler, M. E., Olson, J., Molohon, K. J., ... Oldfield, E. (2013). Antibacterial drug leads targeting isoprenoid biosynthesis. *Proceedings of the National Academy of Sciences of the United States of America*, *110*(1), 123–128. doi:10.1073/pnas.1219899110 PMID:23248302

Zsila, F., Bikadi, Z., Malik, D., Hari, P., Pechan, I., Berces, A., & Hazai, E. (2011). Evaluation of drug-human serum albumin binding interactions with support vector machine aided online automated docking. *Bioinformatics (Oxford, England)*, *27*(13), 1806–1813. doi:10.1093/bioinformatics/btr284 PMID:21593135

Zsoldos, Z., Reid, D., Simon, A., Sadjad, S. B., & Johnson, A. P. (2007). eHiTS: A new fast, exhaustive flexible ligand docking system. *Journal of Molecular Graphics & Modelling*, *26*(1), 198–212. doi:10.1016/j.jmgm.2006.06.002 PMID:16860582

Chapter 2
Chemical Structure Databases in Drug Discovery

Pramodkumar Pyarelal Gupta
D. Y. Patil University (Deemed), India

Virupaksha Ajit Bastikar
Amity University Mumbai, India

Santosh Subhash Chhajed
MET Bhujbal Knowledge City, India

ABSTRACT

Biologically active and approved molecules have attracted great interest from scientists working in the therapeutic area. This has greatly increased the pressure on the pharma and life science industry in fueling new molecules to the market. Chemical structure database, the backbone of cheminformatics and the bioinformatics industry, has warehoused millions of active and non-active molecules/ligands/derivatives of drug compounds. Numerous public and private chemical databases support the drug discovery projects by contributing their data source in terms of 2D, 3D structure, and annotation reports in development of effective therapeutic projects. In this chapter, the authors discuss important chemical structure databases and their diverse dataset utilization in drug discovery projects.

INTRODUCTION

In last few decades, chemical resources and structural databases are major support and exhibit a numerous contribution in the development of drug designing and discovery projects, whether it is bioinformatics, cheminformatics, clinical informatics, pharmacoinformatics. The data from these resources and setup provides information that can be employed to build or predict the models for designing and discovering of new potent lead or drug molecules. Taking into account the vast number of experimental and computational data currently generated from past and ongoing drug discovery projects, the use of storage, manage and analytic cheminformatics tools have become increasingly necessary.

DOI: 10.4018/978-1-5225-7326-5.ch002

Running out of patent drug from the existing market has increased the pressure on pharmaceutical industry to develop newer and safer drugs. To achieve the therapeutic applicable molecule with high efficacy and low toxicity that desires prescribers to show value of money, in last one decade the industry has changed the view of design and development process such that the early phase of drug discovery is being taken up by SMEs and academic research groups (Hersey et al., 2015). As the small research groups do not have enough resource and big data repositories of chemical database unlike the giant pharma companies, they mainly rely on the public available chemical database (Hersey et al., 2015).

In last 2-3 decades, chemical databases have progressed from few thousand compound entries to a numerous million compounds. Exponential exploration of chemical structure and related dataset into the database is directly proportional to the growth of chemical database in the drug discovery research that has fueled a growth in commercial software too (Miller, 2002).

Cheminformatics projects are the source to easily mine the data from the large datasets. The ability to identify the compound equivalence between databases, InChI, Smile and related line notations have made easier to the users. Advancement in the methods to identify the compounds on the basis of similar substructure, connectivity, parent connectivity or same connectivity are now enabling to mine the compounds from the similar group or not (Hersey et al., 2015).

ChEMBL

ChEMBL is an open source large scale bioactivity database and is publicly available at (https://www.ebi.ac.uk/chembl) ("ChEMBL," n.d.-a), reported in Nucleic Acid Research Database Issue in the year 2012 Figure 1. The database largely consists of manually extracted datasets from the medicinal chemistry literature. In-depth data such as compounds structure, biological or physiochemical assays performed for these compounds, the targets from the related assays and other drug discovery related question are addressed. Application of the ChEMBL data includes the suitable chemical tools for target identification, investigation of the off-target drug effects, data mining, construction of predictive modeling for target identification, Identification of bioisostere replacement. In association to literature sources and databases, ChEMBL assimilates bioactivity data and deposited screening results from other public database such as PubChem Bioassay, whereas Dailymed and U.S. Food and Drug Administration (FDA) Orange Book adds a data for the approved drug (Bento et al., 2014). The user can retrieve the data from ChEMBL using Ligand search, target search, browse target, browse drug,browse drug targets and browse drug indications that are listed onto the home page of ChEMBL database Figure 1. In the ligand search option, the user can sketch the drug/ligand structures per their requirement as web based sketching tool is facilitated Figure 1. As well as can search for targets Figure 2 ("ChEMBL," n.d.-a). It has 2,101,843 compound records, 1,735,442 compounds (of which 1,727,112 have mol files), 14,675,320 activities, 1,302,147 assays, 11,538 targets and 67,722 documents Table 1 ("ChEMBL," n.d.-b)

PubChem

PubChem is a huge public repository by the National Institute of Health in the field of bioactivity, and chemical information (https://pubchem.ncbi.nlm.nih.gov) was launched in 2004 Figure 3. Serving as a chemical information repository to the open scientific community, PubChem has grown into a giant repository of chemical and bioactivity data too. It has grown very fast and hold the vital chemical in-

Figure 1. Home page ChEMBL database, https://www.ebi.ac.uk/chembl/

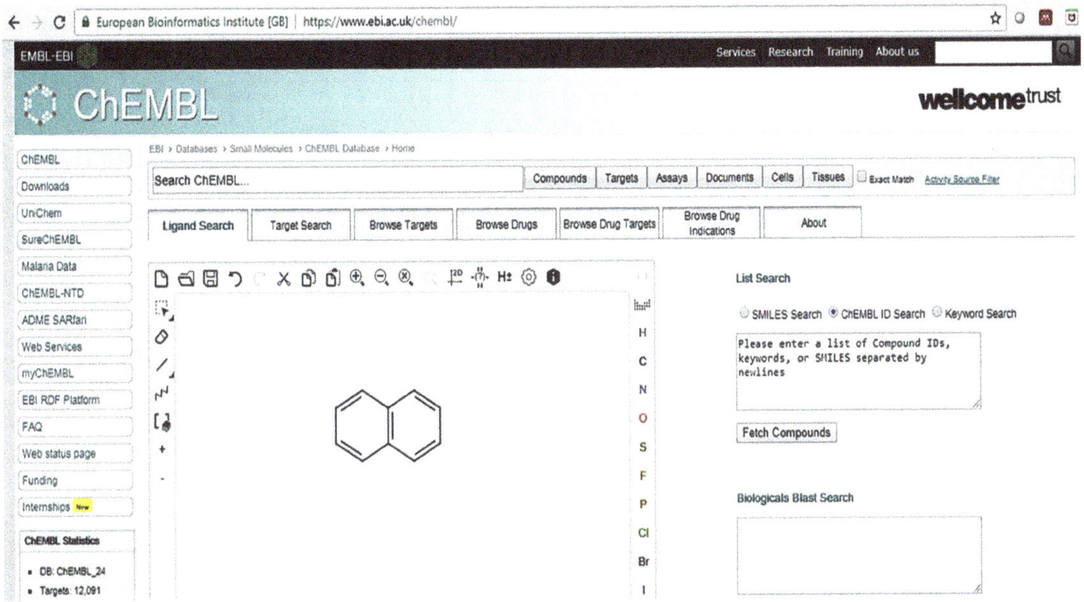

Figure 2. Target report card for Mitogen-activated protein kinase 4

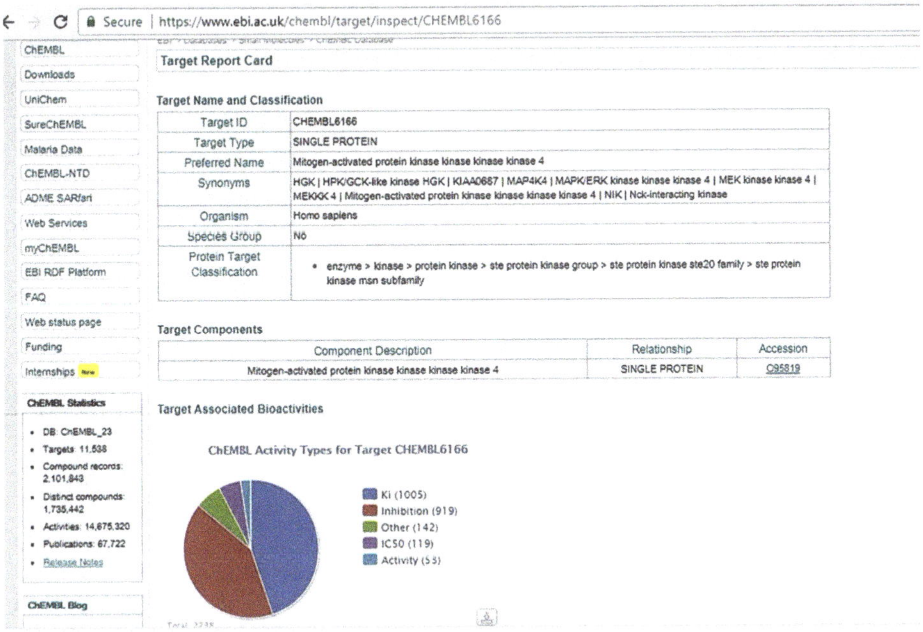

formation resources that provided the route map in many fields of chemical biology, cheminformatics, drug discovery and medicinal chemistry (Kim et al., 2016).

The three interlinked components of PubChem database are Substance, Compound and BioAssay database.

Table 1. List of data sources to ChEMBLdatabase ("ChEMBL," n.d.-b)

BioAssay Data Sources:	Number Assays:	Number Compound Records:	Number Activities:
Scientific Literature	1016903	1255440	5913066
Open TG-GATEs	158199	633	158199
DrugMatrix	113678	2706	350929
TP-search Transporter database	3592	4383	6765
PubChem bioassay	3076	531694	7559601
BindingDB database	1868	69421	99039
FDA Approval packages	1386	80	1387
Patent Bioactivity Data	1134	11358	20941
Sanger Institute Genomics of drug sensitivity in cancer	714	139	73169
Curated Drug Pharmacokinetic data	521	98	1163
GSK Published Kinase inhibitor	456	1101	169451
Drugs for Neglected Diseases Initiative (DNDi)	233	7070	14452
MMV Malaria Box	138	8438	45158
MMV Pathogen Box	82	774	3857
Open TG-GATEs Source malaria Screening	22	211	344
CO-ADD antimicrobial screening data	22	20	180
St Jude Malaria screening	16	1524	5456
WHO-TDR Malaria screening	16	740	5853
AstraZeneca Deposited Data	15	5799	11687
GSK Tuberculosis Screening	15	826	1814
Deposited Supplementary Bioactivity Data	13	1786	4817
GSK Kinetoplastid Screening	13	592	7235
Curated Metabolism Pathways	11	867	11
St Jude Leishmania Screening	6	13643	42105
GSK Malaria Screening	6	13533	81198
Novartis Malaria Screening	6	10119	27888
Harvard Malaria Screening	4	37	111
Gates library compound	2	137238	69444

PubChem Substance Database

PubChem Substance database: Individual scientist and data contributors deposit data into the PubChem Substance database. The data containing annotation and optional structures, each record from each data source will be assigned with a unique Substance Identifier (SID), for, eg: Ten organisation submit a record of information for anticancer drug, Lapatinib, then ten substance Identifier (SID) will be created ("PubChem Docs," n.d.) Figure 4.

Figure 3. PubChem homepage

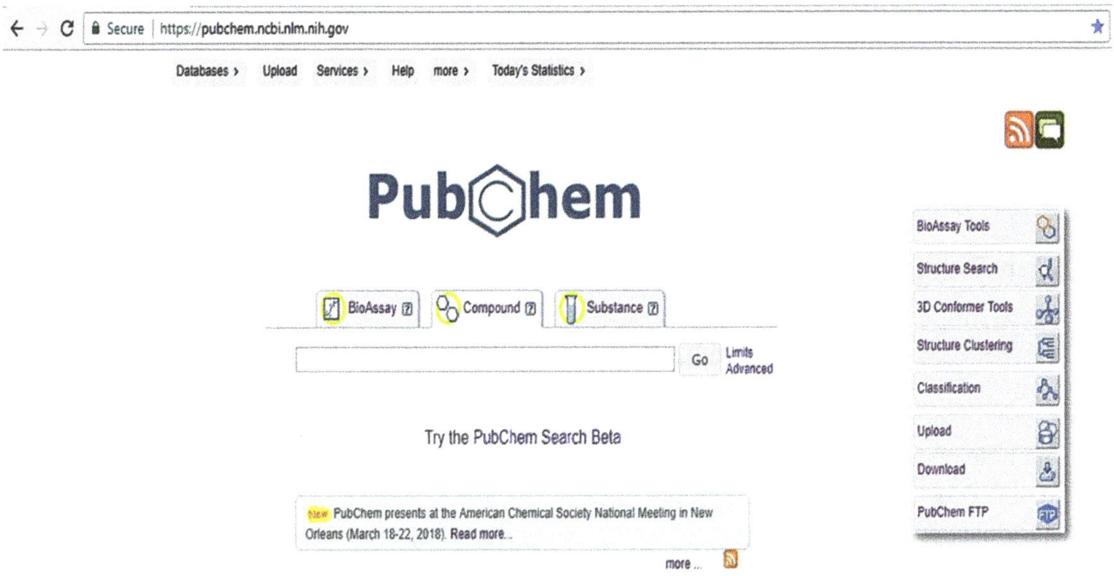

Figure 4. PubChem Substance database

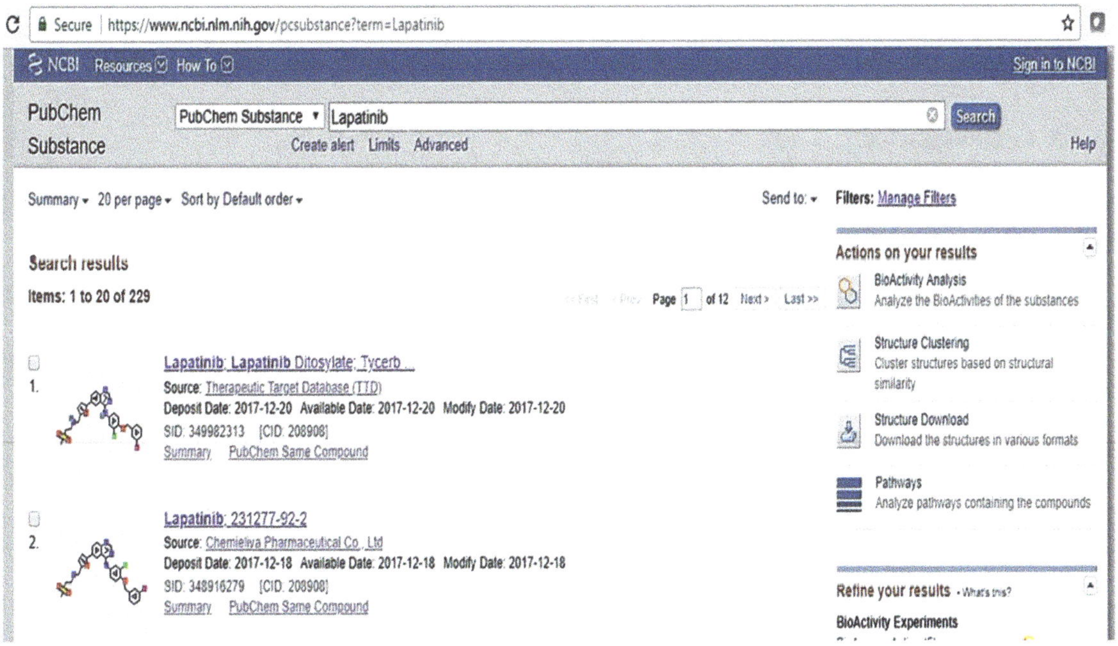

PubChem Compound Database

PubChem Compound database: The unique chemical structures extracted from the PubChem substance database are stored in PubChem database. If multiple identical substance records are available then, that can be standardized into one chemical structure and finally a single compound record (CID) will be automatically generated. For example, many chemical substance records containing the same structure of lapatinib will be aggregated into a single compound record (CID) ("PubChem Docs," n.d.) Figure 5.

PubChem BioAssay Database

PubChem BioAssay database: Annotated information of biological evaluated or assay experimental tested substances are stored and can be retrieved from BioAssay database.

Here, each experiment from each data source is assigned a unique Bioassay identifier (AID) the records include researcher defined active/inactive determinations of bioactivity of substances with an explanation ("PubChem Docs," n.d.) Figure 6.

The current statistics of the data can be found on the PubChem home page under the tab of "Today's Statistics" at https://pubchem.ncbi.nlm.nih.gov/#. It has more than 94 million compounds, 2.5 million tested compounds, 200 million chemical Substance, 04 million tested substances, 01 million BioAssays, 170 RNAi BioAssays, 234 million BioActivities, 10,000 protein targets and 22,000 gene targets ("PubChem," n.d.)

Figure 5. PubChem Compound database

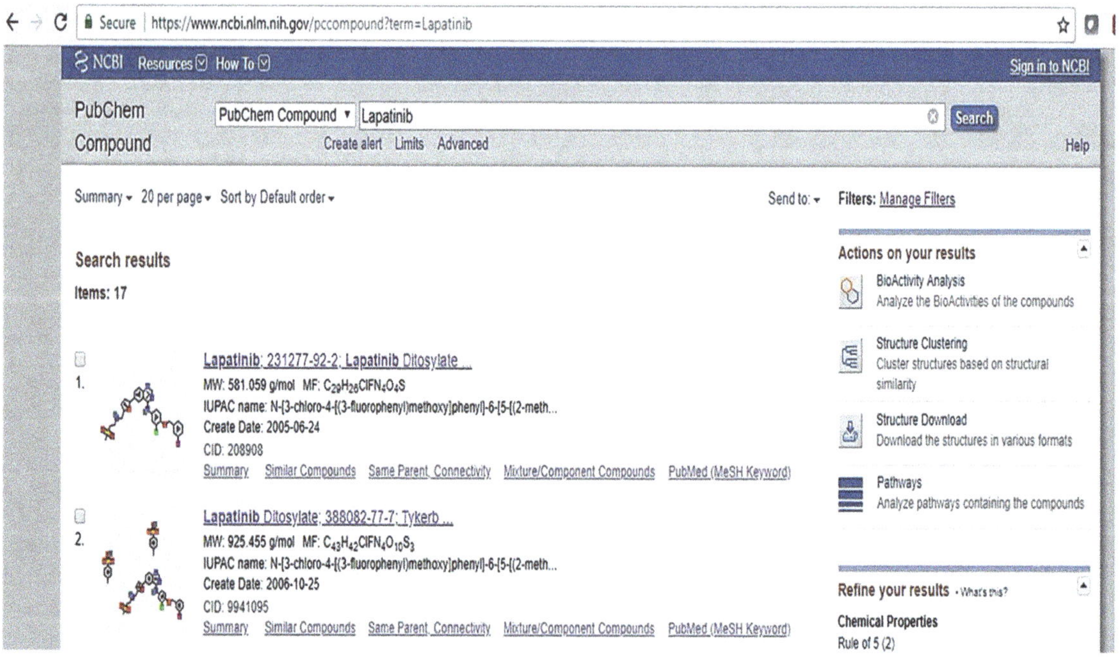

Figure 6. PubChem BioAssay database

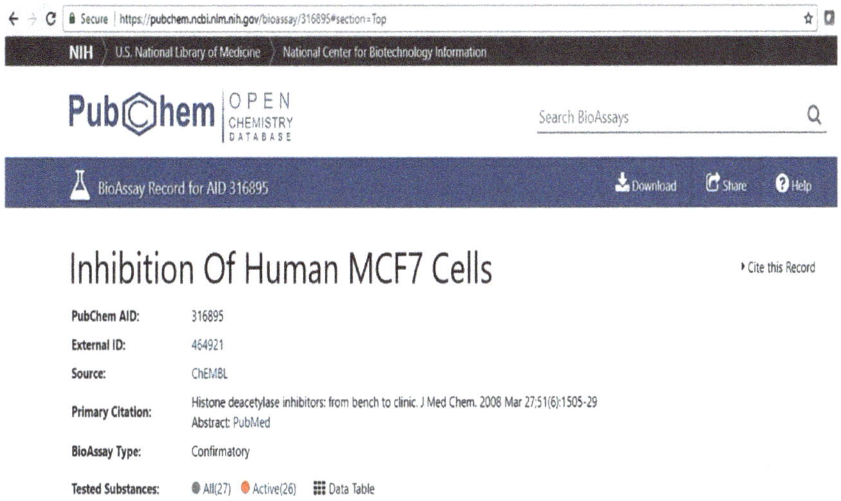
Secure https://pubchem.ncbi.nlm.nih.gov/bioassay/316895#section=Top
NIH U.S. National Library of Medicine National Center for Biotechnology Information
PubChem OPEN CHEMISTRY DATABASE
Search BioAssays
BioAssay Record for AID 316895
Download
Share
Help
Inhibition Of Human MCF7 Cells
Cite this Record
PubChem AID: 316895
External ID: 464921
Source: ChEMBL
Primary Citation: Histone deacetylase inhibitors: from bench to clinic. J Med Chem. 2008 Mar 27;51(6):1505-29
Abstract: PubMed
BioAssay Type: Confirmatory
Tested Substances: All(27) Active(26) Data Table

SureChEMBL

SureChEMBL is a large publicly available large-scale database containing compounds extracted from full text literature, images and relevant data from patent documents and can be accessed via a web-based interface at https://www.surechembl.org/, Figure 7.

SureChEMBL was built by Digital Science Ltd, in late 2013. The whole system was donated to EMBL-EBI and further termed as SureChEMBL. From 15 million patent documents, more than 17 mil-

Figure 7. SureChEMBL database web page

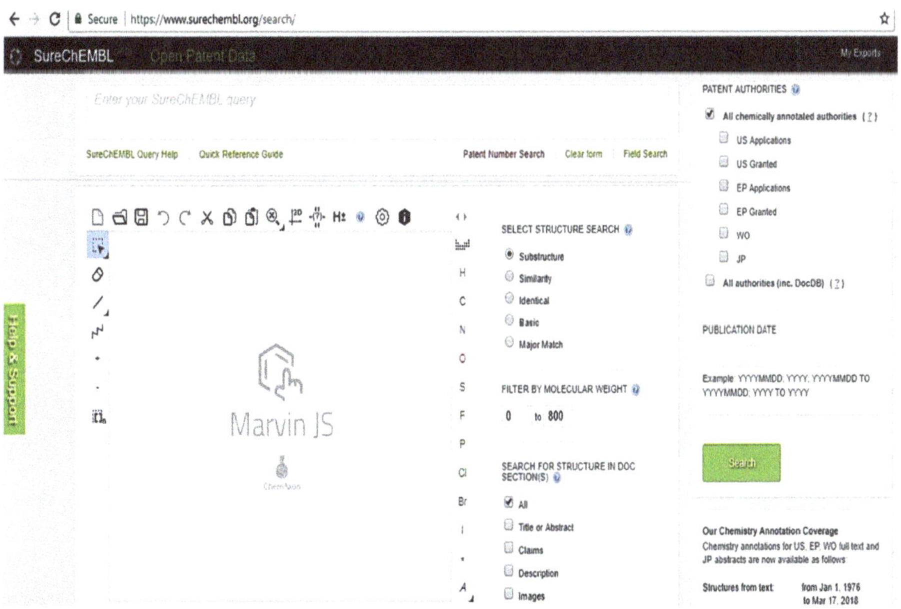

lion compounds were extracted and accommodated in the database. In the early release of the database, from 4.7 million full- text patents including (EPO, WIPO and USPTO) more than 2.3 million chemical structures were extracted. In addition, 11 million biomedical journal abstracts from 1976 to 2000 were also extracted (Papadatos et al., 2016) The classification and retrieval of data from the patent literature resources are conceded out using an automated text and image mining algorithm on a daily basis (Papadatos et al., 2016).

The database gives access to the formerly unavailable, open and annotated patent compounds. SureChEMBL is harmonized with combined search and key based search against the compound repository and patent documents that provides the user with an enormous wealth of compound based information buried deep in the patent documents. This database has led the computational chemist and medicinal chemist to utilize its application in the field of drug discovery and development Table 2 (Papadatos et al., 2016). Undeniably, worldwide persistent growth in the numerous published patent applications and automated data mining techniques have opened new opportunities and challenges and patent information management system and mining techniques, especially in the context of chemical and pharmaceutical patents where accurate and exceptionally annotated datasets acquire notable changes in the research (Papadatos et al., 2016).

In SureChEMBL, the user can search and retrieve the data from major patent authorities such as the European Patent Office (EPO, https://www.epo.org), the United States Patent and Trademark Office (USPTO, http://www.uspto.gov), the Japanese Patent Office (JPO, https://www.jpo.go.jp) and the World Intellectual Property Organization (WIPO, http://www.wipo.int) provide web resources which can be accessed and queried online (Papadatos et al., 2016).

Table 2. Patent content and datasets coverage of SureChEMBL database (Papadatos et al., 2016)

	Data	Description and languages	Years
EP applications	Bib. data	DocDB + Original	From 1978
	Full text	Original (EN, DE, FR)	
EP granted	Bib. data	DocDB + Original	From 1980
	Full text	Original (EN, DE, FR)	
WO applications	Bib. data	DocDB + Original	From 1978
	Full text	Original (EN, DE, FR, ES, RU)	From 1978
US applications	Bib. data	DocDB + Original	From 2001
	Full text	Original (EN)	From 2001
US granted	Bib. data	DocDB + Original	From 1920
	Full text	Original (EN)	From 1976
JP applications	Bib. data	DocDB	From 1973
		English abstracts/titles	From 1976
JP granted	Bib. data	DocDB	From 1994
90+ countries	Bib. data	DocDB	From 1920

DrugBank

DrugBank is a massive and comprehensive publicly available online database flooded with biochemical and pharmacological information, mechanism and targets about drugs and can easily be accessed at (http://www.drugbank.ca). It is also known as unique bioinformatics and cheminformatics wealth that supplies the user with extensive detailed information on drug and their target Figure 8.0 ("DRUGBANK," n.d.).

As most of the DrugBank data are expertly curated from literature sources, it has turned out to be the reference to the well known database such as PharmGKB (Thorn, Klein, & Altman, 2013), ChEBI (Hastings et al., 2013), KEGG (Kanehisa, Goto, Sato, Furumichi, & Tanabe, 2012), GeneCards (Stelzer et al., 2011), PDB (Rose et al., 2013), PubChem (NCBI Resource Coordinators, 2013), UniProt (UniProt Consortium, 2013) and Wikipedia. DrugBank was first described in 2006, and have been widely used to facilitate drug and *In silico* drug target discovery (Law et al., 2014).

DrugBank first version was limited to providing data on selected Food and Drug Administration (FDA)-approved drugs and their drug targets (Wishart et al., 2006). Pharmacological, pharmacogenomic and molecular biological data were added to DrugBank 2.0, along with a substantial increase in the number of approved and experimental drugs (Wishart et al., 2008). DrugBank 3.0, released in 2010, was expanded to incorporate data on drug-drug and drug-food interactions, metabolic enzymes and transporters as well as pharmacokinetic and pharmacoeconomic information (Knox et al., 2011). ADMET, pharmacometabolomics, pharmacogenomics and a variety of QSAR data fields were added to the DrugBank 4.0 (Law et al., 2014).

The latest release DrugBank version 5.0.11 released on 2017-12-20 holds about 11,002 drug entries including 2503 approved small drugs, 943 approved biotech (protein/peptide) drugs, 109 nutraceuticals and over 5,110 experimental drugs. Additionally, 4,910 non-redundant protein (i.e. drug target/enzyme/transporter/carrier) sequences are linked to these drug entries ("DRUGBANK," n.d.).

Figure 8. Home page https://www.drugbank.ca/

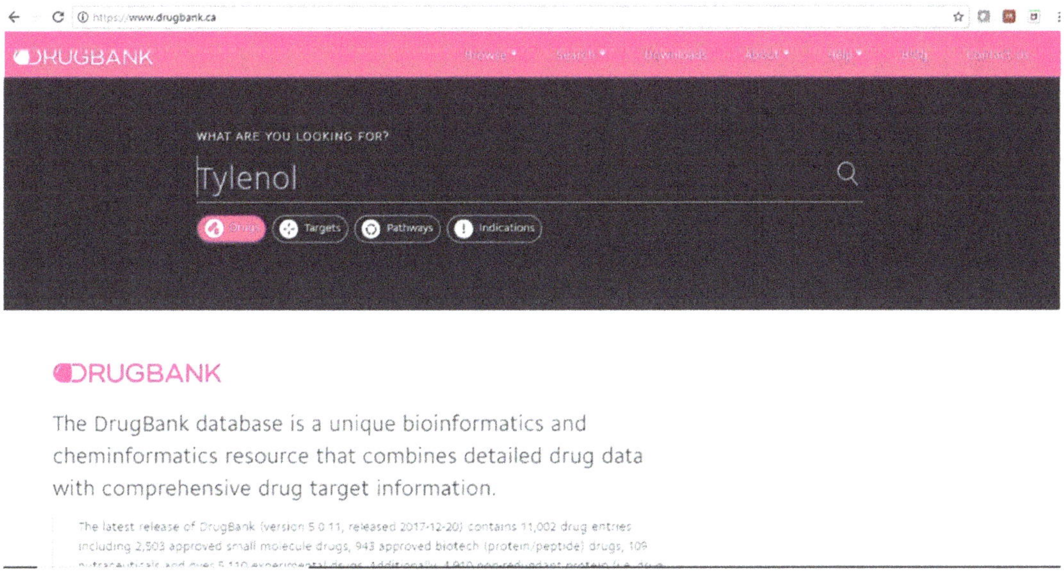

The information page of each drug is called DrugCard. Each DrugCard entry contains more than 200 data fields dedicated, the first half with drug/chemical data and other half with drug target or protein data (Law et al., 2014), the drug statistics holds the count of per day data Table 3.

ZINC

ZINC (ZINC Is Not Commercial) is a publicly accessible database that can be accessed at http://zinc.docking.org/ and ready to use compounds for virtual screening, ligand discovery, pharmacophore screens, benchmarking and force fields development (Sterling & Irwin, 2015).

About 35 million compounds are present in the ZINC12 database for docking and purchasable Figure 9, ("ZINC12," n.d.) and over 230 million compounds are ready to dock and over 120 million to purchasable in the ZINC15 (Sterling & Irwin, 2015; "ZINC15," n.d.). User can search the compounds

Table 3. Drug statistics in DrugBank

Total Number of Small Molecule Drugs	9335
Total Number of Biotech Drugs	1227
Total Number of Approved Drugs	3254
Total Number of Approved Small Molecule Drugs	2337
Total Number of Nutraceutical Drugs	106
Total Number of Experimental Drugs	5030
Total Number of Illicit Drugs	202
Total Number of Withdrawn Drugs	218
Total Number of Drugs	10562

Figure 9. ZINC12 database homepage

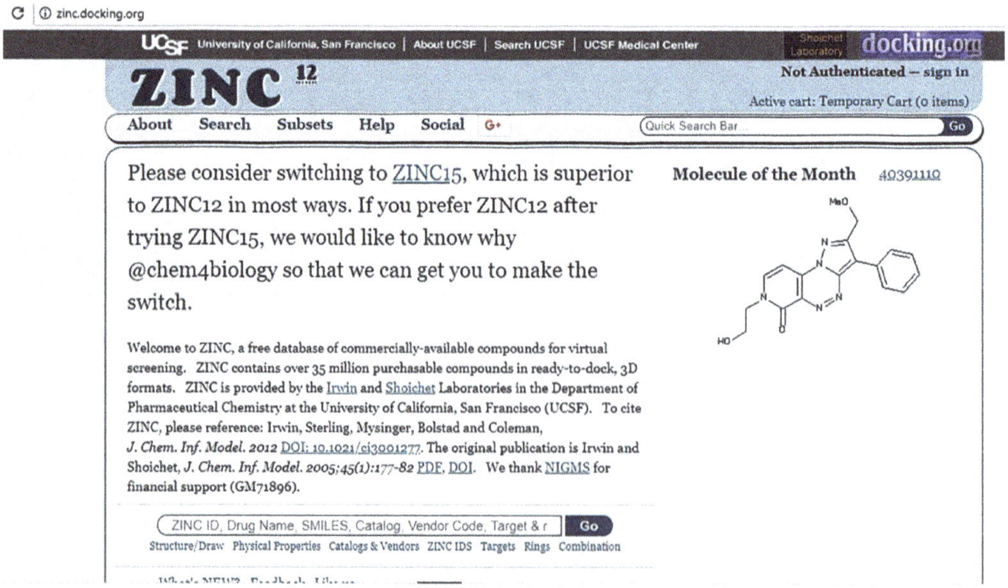

and retrieve it from ZINC database by target by focused libraries, activities by organism class, Chemical search such as: Chemical similarity, compound substructure, Multiple compounds look up (SMILES, CAS number, name, ZINC ID, or an original catalog ID, such as CHEMBL ID) and Chemical Patterns (Sterling & Irwin, 2015) Figure 10.

In ZINC15, there are 70539 metabolites that have been annotated, 15006 of which may be purchased from vendors. Restricting this to endogenous human metabolites, there are 46941 molecules, of which 8271 are for sale (Sterling & Irwin, 2015). The database is free in numerous structural file formats including 3D SDF, Dock, mol2 and SMILES, Canonical SMILES, InChi and InChiKey (Irwin & Shoichet, 2005; Sterling & Irwin, 2015). One can search the database by drawing a molecule using web-based query tool and molecular drawing interface (Irwin & Shoichet, 2005; Sterling & Irwin, 2015). Users can process their molecules by uploading them into the ZINC database (Irwin & Shoichet, 2005).

eMolecule

In eMolecules database, over 8 million compounds are available from their trusted suppliers and global networks ("eMolecule," n.d.-a). eMolecules empowers researchers to explore uncharted chemical and biological spaces and deliver more efficient drug-discovery programs Figure 11. Over the years, carefully understanding the needs of the chemist and users, eMolecules have created a free search engine to facilitate the users in the drug discovery process. The eMolecule database is trusted by the leading biotechnology, pharmaceutical as well as academic research organizations to be their optimum tool for searching and purchasing the chemicals and therapeutic molecules.

The user can mine the data using substructure search, exact search, similarity search in the sketching tool draw can find on https://www.emolecules.com/#?click=building-blocks, and list search (where a user can make a multiple query set) under the building block options against 1.5 million compounds. In the screening compound option, the user can screen the desired structure against 7 million compounds,

Figure 10. Search of anti-cancer drug lapatinib in ZINC12 database

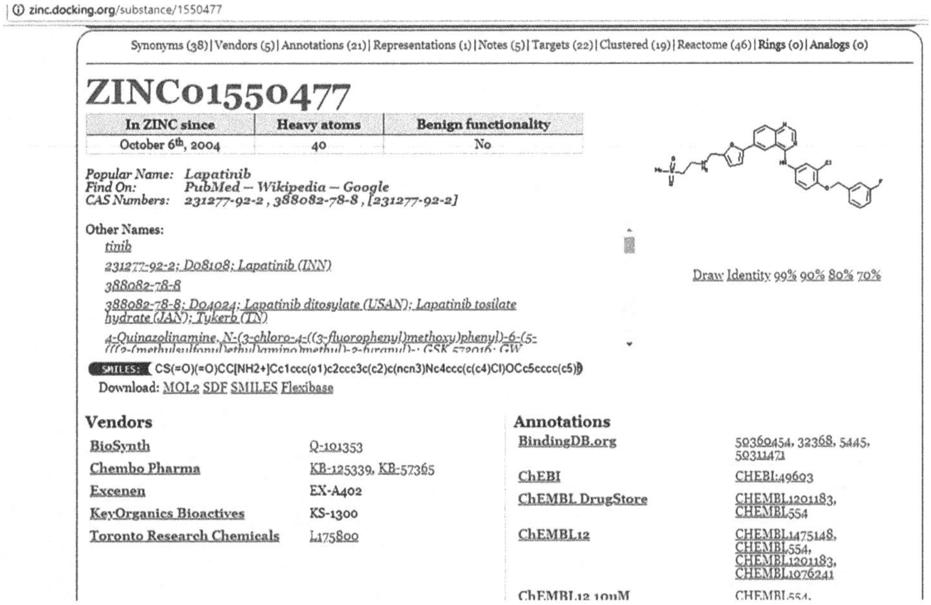

Figure 11. eMolecule database home page

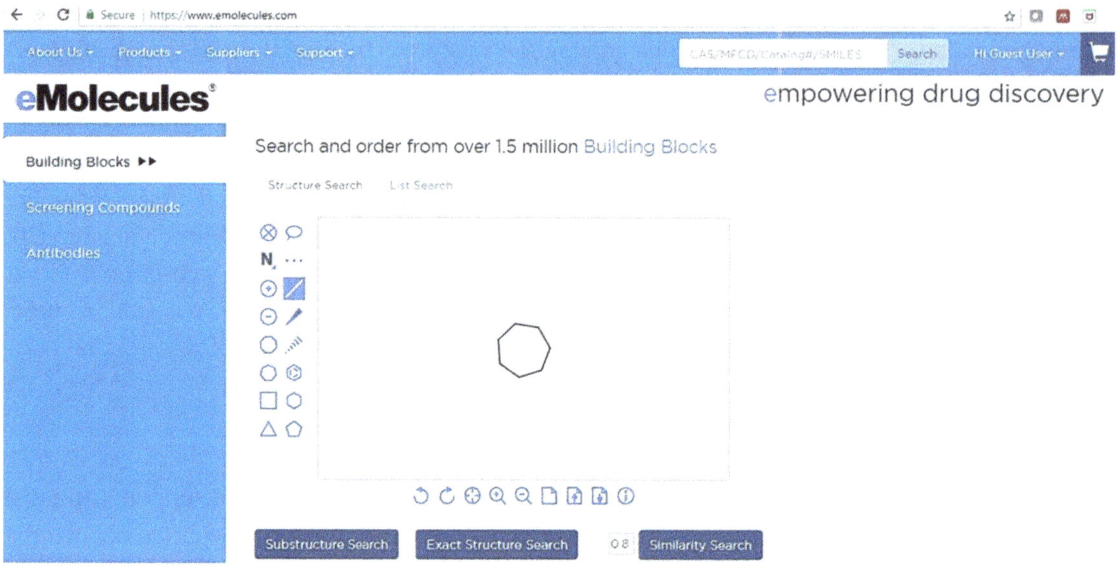

https://www.emolecules.com/#?click=screening-compounds, whereas one can search and order for antibodies from over 600,000 antibodies entries Figure 11 ("eMolecule," n.d.-b).

The eMolecule, chemical search engine uses CAS number, chemical name, catalogue number, eMolecule ID number, SD files or SMILES. Dedicated eMolecules purchasing manager supports all procurement lists and exports each supplier's details, the order in multiple formats: CSV, Excel, SDF or TSV. The free version of eMolecules offers to get your projects moving and a full version is available with annual subscription rate which contains enhanced data sets ("eMolecule," n.d.-c). Table 4.

Table 4. Free and commercial data

Sr no	Data	Free Download	Full Plus License
1	Monthly Updates	Yes	Yes
2	SMILES	Yes	Yes
3	2D SDF	Yes	Yes
4	eMolecules ID	Yes	Yes
5	Chemical Name	No	Yes
6	Supplier Details	No	Yes
7	SKU/Supplier Catalog Number	No	Yes
8	Pack Size	No	Yes
9	CAS Number	No	Yes
10	MFCD Number	No	Yes
11	Price	No	Yes
12	Availability	No	Yes
13	Lead Time	No	Yes

CONCLUSION

Online, off-line, Public and private chemical information sources in the form of structural data and text data are the vital resources of the drug discovery projects. Currently numerous on-line databases hold millions of curated and annotated datasets for free and open. The data from these databases are used to build knowledge based model to predict the enhanced or reduced toxicity activity. Here we have listed few freely available chemical databases in Table 5.

Table 5. Other list of the database

Sr no	Database name	Web Url	description
1	BindingDB	http://www.bindingdb.org/bind/index.jsp	web-accessible database of measured binding affinities
2	ChEBI	http://www.ebi.ac.uk/chebi/	Chemical Entities of Biological Interest (ChEBI) is a freely available dictionary of molecular entities focused on 'small' chemical compounds.
3	ChemExper	http://www.chemexper.com/	Chemical Directory
4	ChemSpider	http://www.chemspider.com/	Chemical database
5	Compendium of Common Pesticide Names	http://www.alanwood.net/pesticides/	ISO-approved standard names of chemical pesticides
6	ChemBank	http://chembank.broadinstitute.org/	Small molecule database
7	Computational Chemistry Comparison and Benchmark DataBase	https://cccbdb.nist.gov/	Experimental and computational thermochemical data for a selected set of 1420 gas-phase atoms and molecules
8	The Cambridge Structural Database (CSD)	https://www.ccdc.cam.ac.uk/solutions/csd-system/components/csd/	The Cambridge Structural Database (CSD) is a highly curated and comprehensive resource.
9	IUPAC-NIST Solubility Database	https://srdata.nist.gov/solubility/	Data compiled and evaluated by IUPAC (International Union of Pure and Applied Chemistry)
10	KEGG DRUG Database	http://www.genome.jp/kegg/drug/	KEGG DRUG is a comprehensive drug information resource for approved drugs in Japan, USA, and Europe
11	National Institute of Allergy and Infectious Diseases Database	https://chemdb.niaid.nih.gov/	This database contains information extracted from the scientific literature on the structure and activity of compounds that have been tested against HIV, HIV enzymes or opportunistic pathogens.
12	NIST Chemistry WebBook	https://webbook.nist.gov/chemistry/	provides thermochemical, thermophysical, and ion energetics data compiled by NIST under the Standard Reference Data Program.
13	NIST Chemical Kinetics Database	https://kinetics.nist.gov/kinetics/index.jsp	compilation of kinetics data on gas-phase reactions
14	Organic Syntheses	http://www.orgsyn.org/	Organic Compounds
15	NMRShiftDB	http://nmrshiftdb.nmr.uni-koeln.de/	NMR database (web database) for organic structures and their nuclear magnetic resonance (NMR) spectra.
16	Spectral Database for Organic Compounds	http://sdbs.db.aist.go.jp/sdbs/cgi-bin/cre_index.cgi?lang=eng	spectral database system for organic compounds
17	Wikipedia	https://www.wikipedia.org/	All chemical information and other.
18	WebReactions	http://webreactions.net/	synthetic and medicinal chemistry

REFERENCES

Bento, A. P., Gaulton, A., Hersey, A., Bellis, L. J., Chambers, J., Davies, M., ... Overington, J. P. (2014). The ChEMBL bioactivity database: An update. *Nucleic Acids Research*, *42*(Database issue), D1083–D1090. doi:10.1093/nar/gkt1031 PMID:24214965

ChEMBL. (n.d.a). Retrieved February 10, 2018, from https://www.ebi.ac.uk/chembl/

ChEMBL. (n.d.b). Retrieved February 15, 2018, from ftp://ftp.ebi.ac.uk/pub/databases/chembl/ChEMBLdb/releases/chembl_23/chembl_23_release_notes.txt

DRUGBANK. (n.d.). Retrieved from https://www.drugbank.ca/

eMolecule. (n.d.a). Retrieved February 25, 2018, from https://www.emolecules.com/

eMolecule. (n.d.b). Retrieved February 25, 2018, from https://www.emolecules.com/info/support-intro-to-searching.html

eMolecule. (n.d.c). Retrieved February 25, 2018, from https://www.emolecules.com/info/products-data-downloads.html

Hastings, J., de Matos, P., Dekker, A., Ennis, M., Harsha, B., Kale, N., ... Steinbeck, C. (2013). The ChEBI reference database and ontology for biologically relevant chemistry: Enhancements for 2013. *Nucleic Acids Research*, *41*(Database issue), D456–D463. doi:10.1093/nar/gks1146 PMID:23180789

Hersey, A., Chambers, J., Bellis, L., Patrícia Bento, A., Gaulton, A., & Overington, J. P. (2015). Chemical databases: Curation or integration by user-defined equivalence? *Drug Discovery Today. Technologies*, *14*, 17–24. doi:10.1016/j.ddtec.2015.01.005 PMID:26194583

Irwin, J. J., & Shoichet, B. K. (2005). ZINC--a free database of commercially available compounds for virtual screening. *Journal of Chemical Information and Modeling*, *45*(1), 177–182. doi:10.1021/ci049714+ PMID:15667143

Kanehisa, M., Goto, S., Sato, Y., Furumichi, M., & Tanabe, M. (2012). KEGG for integration and interpretation of large-scale molecular data sets. *Nucleic Acids Research*, *40*(Database issue), D109–D114. doi:10.1093/nar/gkr988 PMID:22080510

Kim, S., Thiessen, P. A., Bolton, E. E., Chen, J., Fu, G., Gindulyte, A., ... Bryant, S. H. (2016). PubChem Substance and Compound databases. *Nucleic Acids Research*, *44*(D1), D1202–D1213. doi:10.1093/nar/gkv951 PMID:26400175

Knox, C., Law, V., Jewison, T., Liu, P., Ly, S., Frolkis, A., ... Wishart, D. S. (2011). DrugBank 3.0: A comprehensive resource for "omics" research on drugs. *Nucleic Acids Research*, *39*(Database issue), D1035–D1041. doi:10.1093/nar/gkq1126 PMID:21059682

Law, V., Knox, C., Djoumbou, Y., Jewison, T., Guo, A. C., Liu, Y., ... Wishart, D. S. (2014). DrugBank 4.0: Shedding new light on drug metabolism. *Nucleic Acids Research*, *42*(D1), D1091–D1097. doi:10.1093/nar/gkt1068 PMID:24203711

Miller, M. A. (2002). Chemical database techniques in drug discovery. *Nature Reviews. Drug Discovery*, *1*(3), 220–227. doi:10.1038/nrd745 PMID:12120506

NCBI Resource Coordinators. (2013). Database resources of the National Center for Biotechnology Information. *Nucleic Acids Research*, *41*(Database issue), D8–D20. doi:10.1093/nar/gks1189 PMID:23193264

Papadatos, G., Davies, M., Dedman, N., Chambers, J., Gaulton, A., Siddle, J., ... Overington, J. P. (2016). SureChEMBL: A large-scale, chemically annotated patent document database. *Nucleic Acids Research*, *44*(D1), D1220–D1228. doi:10.1093/nar/gkv1253 PMID:26582922

PubChem. (n.d.). Retrieved from https://pubchem.ncbi.nlm.nih.gov/#

PubChem Docs. (n.d.). Retrieved March 10, 2018, from https://pubchemdocs.ncbi.nlm.nih.gov/data-organization

Rose, P. W., Bi, C., Bluhm, W. F., Christie, C. H., Dimitropoulos, D., Dutta, S., ... Bourne, P. E. (2013). The RCSB Protein Data Bank: New resources for research and education. *Nucleic Acids Research*, *41*(Database issue), D475–D482. doi:10.1093/nar/gks1200 PMID:23193259

Stelzer, G., Dalah, I., Stein, T. I., Satanower, Y., Rosen, N., & Nativ, N. … Lancet, D. (2011). In-silico human genomics with GeneCards. *Human Genomics, 5*(6), 709–17. Retrieved from http://www.ncbi.nlm.nih.gov/pubmed/22155609

Sterling, T., & Irwin, J. J. (2015). ZINC 15--Ligand Discovery for Everyone. *Journal of Chemical Information and Modeling*, *55*(11), 2324–2337. doi:10.1021/acs.jcim.5b00559 PMID:26479676

Thorn, C. F., Klein, T. E., & Altman, R. B. (2013). PharmGKB: The Pharmacogenomics Knowledge Base. *Methods in Molecular Biology (Clifton, N.J.)*, *1015*, 311–320. doi:10.1007/978-1-62703-435-7_20 PMID:23824865

UniProt Consortium. (2013). Update on activities at the Universal Protein Resource (UniProt) in 2013. *Nucleic Acids Research*, *41*(Database issue), D43–D47. doi:10.1093/nar/gks1068 PMID:23161681

Wishart, D. S., Knox, C., Guo, A. C., Cheng, D., Shrivastava, S., Tzur, D., ... Hassanali, M. (2008). DrugBank: A knowledgebase for drugs, drug actions and drug targets. *Nucleic Acids Research*, *36*(Database issuesuppl_1), D901–D906. doi:10.1093/nar/gkm958 PMID:18048412

Wishart, D. S., Knox, C., Guo, A. C., Shrivastava, S., Hassanali, M., Stothard, P., ... Woolsey, J. (2006). DrugBank: A comprehensive resource for in silico drug discovery and exploration. *Nucleic Acids Research*, *34*(Database issue), D668–D672. doi:10.1093/nar/gkj067 PMID:16381955

ZINC12. (n.d.). Retrieved from http://zinc.docking.org/

ZINC15. (n.d.). Retrieved from http://zinc15.docking.org/

Chapter 3
Lead Optimization in the Drug Discovery Process

S. Lakshmana Prabu
Anna University, India

Rathinasabapathy Thirumurugan
Plants for Human Health Institute, USA

ABSTRACT

Discovering a new drug molecule against disease is the main objective of drug discovery. Lead optimization is one of the important steps and acts as a starting point. Over the years, it has significantly changed the drug discovery process. Its main focus is the development of preclinical candidates from "Hit" or "Lead." Lead optimization comprises lead selection and optimization, drug candidate confirmation, and preclinical drug characterization. Lead optimization process can improve the effectiveness towards its target potency, selectivity, protein binding, pharmacokinetic parameters, and to develop a good preclinical candidate. Lead optimization from high-throughput screening to identification of clinical drug candidate is a seamless process that draws new techniques for accelerated synthesis, purification, screening from iterative compound libraries, validation, and to deliver clinical drug candidate with limited human resources. In conclusion, lead optimization phase is done under the suggestion that the optimized lead molecule will have activity against a particular disease.

INTRODUCTION

To develop a new drug molecule about a decade to reach the market with an average cost of around $1 billion. Today pharmaceutical industry faced steady turn down in R&D efficiency and approval of fewer drugs to the market regardless of the increased investments (Adams & Brantner, 2006; DiMasi *et al.*, 2003). Withdrawn of the drugs from the market due to its adverse drug reactions and failures in clinical phase III are the other problems faced by the Pharmaceutical industries (Congressional Budget Office (CBO) study, Research and Development in the Pharmaceutical Industry, 2016). Major reasons for the failure of the drug candidate in the final stage are due to its safety issues or side effects which are undiscovered in the initial stage of drug discovery process.

DOI: 10.4018/978-1-5225-7326-5.ch003

Failures of the new drug molecule in the drug discovery and development process are

1. Inability to configure a reliable assay
2. Unable to get a developable hits through HTS
3. Drug molecule may not have a desired assay or activity
4. Drug molecule might to toxic *in vitro* or *in vivo*
5. Undesirable side effects
6. Unable to get good PK or PD profile
7. Unable to get good permeation to the desired target site (Hughes *et al.,* 2011).

Today developing a new drug molecule for many health issues through drug discovery process is a challenging and complex because it includes different phases such as analysis, modelling and experimentation on the data. An ideal new drug molecule must have therapeutic effect in a defined pathway towards its biological target with minimal effects on other pathways and to have fewer side effects. Success towards the drug discovery for a particular disease is depends on the selection of the target interest and its validation. Two key issues in the drug discovery and development of new drug molecules are

1. Selection of biological target
2. Appropriate therapeutic agent towards the activity of the target (Hajduk & Greer, 2007)

BIOLOGICAL TARGET IDENTIFICATION

Biological target is a collective term for a macromolecule includes protein, genes, RNA and DNA. Generation of protein function modulators are the key process in the biological target identification. A good target must be safe, meet the clinical needs and it should be druggable one. Druggable target is an accessible by drug molecule upon binding and produces its biological activity, which can be determined by *in vitro* and *in vivo* methods (Keseru & Makara 2006; Yang *et al.,* 2009).

Approaches in Target Identification

If the target is identified, examine the certain protein role in disease onset and its biological consequences. Approaches in the target identification are

1. Screening of genome wide forward and reverse genetics
2. small-interfering RNAs (siRNAs)
3. Gene expression profiling
4. Examination of mRNA/protein levels
5. Genetic associations
6. Phenotypic screening (Hajduk & Greer, 2007; Butcher 2005; Van der Greef & McBurney 2005; Hardy & Peet 2004; Betz *et al.,* 2005)

Target Validation

After determination of the target, the target macromolecule should be fully validated. Target validation by the drug target of interest is an important and crucial process which is needed to be performed in the drug discovery at the early stage. Target validation can be performed in different biological methods utilizing animal models or isolated cell line (Lakshmana Prabu *et al.*, 2014). Comparison of phenotypic screening and molecular target-based screening in drug discovery and development is shown in Figure 1 (Zheng *et al.*, 2013). Some examples of cell and assay types used in phenotypic screening are given in Table 1.

HIT DISCOVERY PROCESS

Identification of hit and generation of lead are the other crucial process in the drug discovery. A "hit" is defined as the drug molecule which has the desired activity on the target. Hit or lead can be identified based on the similarity of the marketed drugs (Lakshmana Prabu *et al.*, 2014). Both quality and quantity lead classes are available for the identification of hit from the compound library. Important characteristics of an ideal hit-lead molecule include physical, chemical, biological and pharmacological properties (potency, selectivity, in vitro ADME features – hepatocyte clearance and permeability). Other important and necessary requirements of the lead compound include synthetic accessibility, potential optimization and patentability.

In hit identification, affinity screening approach is a technique based on the interaction between the target and drug molecule.

Affinity screening approaches are

1. NMR spectroscopy
2. X-ray crystallography

Figure 1. Comparison of phenotypic-based screening and molecular target-based screening in drug discovery and development

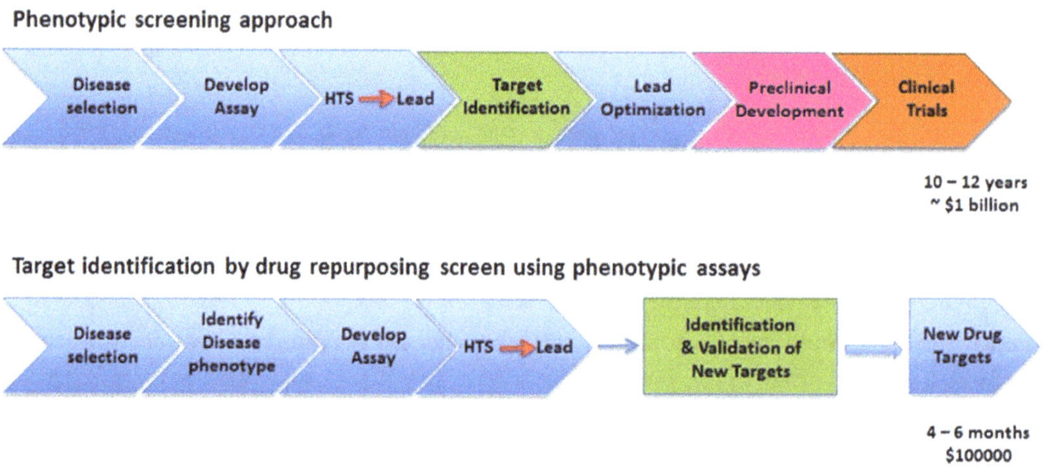

Table 1. Examples of cell types used in phenotypic screening

Disease	Cell type	Assay type	References
Primary cells			
Thyroid cancer	Thyrocytes	TSH responsive proteins	Neumann, *et al.*, 2009
Cystic fibrosis	Bronchial epithelial cells	Electrophysiology	Neuberger *et al.*, 2011
Immortalized primary cells			
Respiratory papillomatosis	Tumor cells	Cell viability (ATP content)	Yuan *et al.*, 2012
Cystic fibrosis	Bronchial epithelial cells	Electrophysiology	Fulcher *et al.*, 2009
Engineered cell lines			
Huntington disease	PC12 expressing HTT Q103-GFP	Protein aggregates (GFP)	Titus *et al.*, 2012
SMA	U2OS expressing SM2-luciferase reporter	RNA splicing (luciferase)	Xiao *et al.*, 2011
Human cells derived from stem cells			
Familial dysautonomia	Neural crest precursors	RT-PCR	Lee *et al.*, 2012
NSC proliferation/differentiation	Neuroepithelial-like stem cell line	Cell viability (ATP content)	McLaren *et al.*, 2013

3. Mass spectroscopy (MS)
4. Surface Plasmon Resonance (SPR) (Keseru & Makara 2006; Proudfoot 2002; Comes, & Schurdak, 2004; Yang *et Al.*, 2012).

Screening Strategies - Hit discovery

1. High throughput
2. Focused screen
3. Fragment
4. Structural aided drug design
5. Virtual screen
6. Physiological screen

1. **High-Throughput Screening (HTS):** Is a technique extensively used in the identification of hit or lead discovery process. Large number of compounds from library is screened against the target by cell based assay in plates.
2. **Focused Screen:** Compounds which has similar structures and compounds which are previously identified as hit for a particular target are screened for its activity.
3. **Fragment Screen:** It is an alternative approach to HTS. In fragment screen process low mM activity compounds are obtained by soaking small compounds into crystals, which are used to build the larger molecules.

4. **Structural Aided Drug Design:** Drug molecules are designed from the crystal structures. **Virtual Screen:** By docking models, virtual screen is performed by examine the simulated compound from the library with the X-ray structure of protein.
5. **Physiological Screen:** It is a tissue based approach, performed by assessing the efficacy of the drug with the tissue.
6. **NMR Screen:** Assessed by soaking small fragments from the compound into known crystal structure of protein targets (Hughes *et al.,* 2011).

False Positive and False Negative Mechanisms in Hit Discovery Process

In the hit discovery process different false positive and false negative interpretation are predicted which may mislead the hit discovery process.

False positive interpretations are

- Nonspecific hydrophobic binding
- Poor solubility
- Tendency to aggregation of small molecules
- Reactive functional groups
- Low purity
- Incorrect structural assignment
- Compound concentration
- Interference with the assay
- Experimental errors (Barnash *et al.,* 2017)

False Negative interpretations are

- Poor solubility
- Chemical instability
- Low purity
- Lower than expected compound concentration
- Interference with the assay
- Experimental errors (Hann & Oprea, 2004).

Assay Development

After the identification of the hit-lead, it has been analyzed for its efficacy. There are two assay procedures are performed to assess its efficacy.

1. **Cell Based Assay:** In this method the compound activity is assess by applying the compound to target which includes membrane receptors, ion channels and nuclear receptors.
2. **Biochemical Assay:** This method is used to assess the compound efficacy in target as receptor and enzyme.

Factors in the Assay Development

1. **Pharmacological Relevance of the Assay:** Performed to verify whether the compound has desired efficacy and mechanism of action by using known ligands against the target.
2. **Reproducibility of the Assay:**The assay procedure should be reproducible across screening day, assay plates and duration of the entire drug discovery development programme.
3. **Assay Costs:** Cost for the compound screening is based on the assay volume and the assay reagents.
4. **Assay Quality:** Quality of the assay is assessed by a statistical parameter (Z factor). The Z factor has the value range between 0 and 1 and the Z factor value greater than 0.4 is considered appropriately robust.
5. **Effects of Compounds in the Assay:** In general DMSO and ethanol are used as organic solvents for chemical compounds. Thus, the solvent should not have any sensitive or interference in the assay (Hughes et al., 2011; Popa-Burke et al., 2004; Dunne et al., 2009; Michelini et al., 2010).

In Vitro Assay Parameters

1. **Aqueous Solubility:** Aqueous solubility is important to perform in vitro assays and for in vivo delivery of drug.
2. **Log $D_{7.4}$:** Measurement of lipophilicity, which is important for movement across membranes.
3. **Microsomal Stability Cl_{int}:** Measure the clearance of compound, it can provide information regarding the in vivo clearance.
4. **CYP450 Inhibition:** CYP450 is a main enzyme in the human being, which metabolizes many drugs.
5. **Caco-2 Permeability:** Measure the permeability across the intestinal epithelium and asses the drug absorption from gut.
6. **MDR1-MDCK:** MDK cells are transfected with the MDRI gene, which translates the efflux P glycoprotein.
7. **Hep G2 Hepatotoxicity:** Human HepG2 cells from liver can be used as an alternative cell to assess the hepatotoxicity.
8. **Cytotoxicity in Suitable Cell Line:** Reduce the likelihood of cellular toxicity in in vivo (Hughes et al., 2011)

Hit-to-Lead Phase

In this phase modifications are made in the hit series to produce desired properties such as potent, pharmacokinetic parameters and its efficacy through *in vivo* methods. Structural activity relationship is used to examine the chemical structure along with its activity and selectivity against the target. X-ray crystallography and NMR techniques are utilized to assess the activity and selectivity of the compound and to make SAR modification in a focused way to determine the lead compound faster. Fragment based lead discovery is an additional source if HTS hits are insufficient to provide lead compound. Compound is ruled out based on the assessment of its solubility and permeability which plays a critical role in identification of lead molecule. Steps in the identification of lead are shown in figure 2. Once the compound meets the desired properties cell based assays and biochemical assays are performed to assess its activity.

The significant requirement of hit-to-lead process is

Figure 2. Steps in the identification of lead molecule from HTS assay

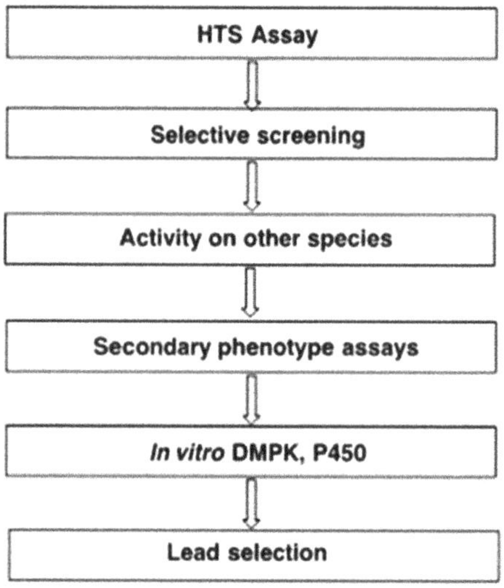

1. Determination of hit-to-lead compound by validating the promising hit by dedicated medicinal chemistry group.
2. Ensuring the activity of the chosen hit molecule by cell based assays, biochemical assays and secondary screening.
3. ADME characterization by in vitro and in vivo methods and determine the toxicological parameter profile of the chosen hit molecule (Baxter *et al.,* 2003; Jahnke *et al.,* 2003; Nienaber *et al.,* 2000; Congreve 2003; Golebiowski *et al.,* 2003; Mestres & Veeneman, 2003; Villar *et al.,* 2004; Hartshorn *et al.,* 2005; Hajduk *et al.,* 2005; Bleicher *et al.,* 2003; Deprez & Deprez-Poulain 2006; Wunberg *et al.,* 2006).

LEAD OPTIMIZATION

The main aim of the lead optimization phase is first rank the chemotypes from previous hit-to-lead phase study and then optimizes the lead compound with suitable drug molecule properties such as physicochemical properties, desired activity, pharmacokinetic and toxicological properties. After the hit-to-lead phase, selected/identified lead molecule has been considered as a starting point for new drug molecule. The chosen lead molecule may not have the desired attributes like absorption, distribution, metabolism and excretion.

These attributes enable the molecule to be dosed suitably by further chemical modification in the structure to improve and focus the drug molecule selectivity, specificity, pharmacokinetic and safety profile by maintaining its optimistic properties through lead optimization process. Optimizing the lead compound into a drug candidate is longest and very much expensive phase in the drug discovery process. Key step of this process is to optimize the pharmacological and mechanism of action of the drug molecule. This phase has a significant role in the success or failure of a new drug molecule in its efficacy, pharmacokinetic and safety profile of the drug molecule in the clinical studies.

In this process, optimization of the new drug molecule is done by medicinal chemist by synthesis, characterization of the drug through advanced organic synthesis methods like Structure activity relationship (SAR) and quantitative structure activity relationships (QSAR). If the chemical structure of the drug target is known, *in silico* techniques can be used to develop or modify the structure of the compound and assess the role of chemical structures towards the activity with its target and metabolism through *in vitro* and *in vivo* models. Chemical structure modification and its activity towards the target are assessed; optimization cycle is continued until to get a new drug molecule with desired properties.

Making Go/No-Go decisions are made in all the phases of drug discovery and development process, but it is very crucial during lead optimization to provide valuable information in optimizing the drug molecule for "Fit-for-purpose". A model of lead optimization process is shown in Figure 3 (Compound profile optimization – For preclinical candidate in identification-http://www.riken.jp/dmp/english/kagaku_en.html).

Different techniques are used to assess the biological activity of the drug molecule. Assessing the activity is based on the efficacy, interaction between compound-target, detection of adverse effects and safety profile. This decision can help to predict the later outcome based on the scientific parameters which will save considerable amount of money and time invested by pharmaceutical industry in the drug discovery and development.

Most of the drug molecule exhibits its biological effect through binding with specific receptor sites. Biological effect of the drug molecule is based concentration of the drug-receptor complex and the fractional occupancy of the receptor. The interaction of drug-receptor complex and binding kinetics is based on the drug ligand association and dissociation, with the ratio between these two factors as a metric (KD). The potent lead molecule should have higher KD value.

Figure 3. Lead optimization Process

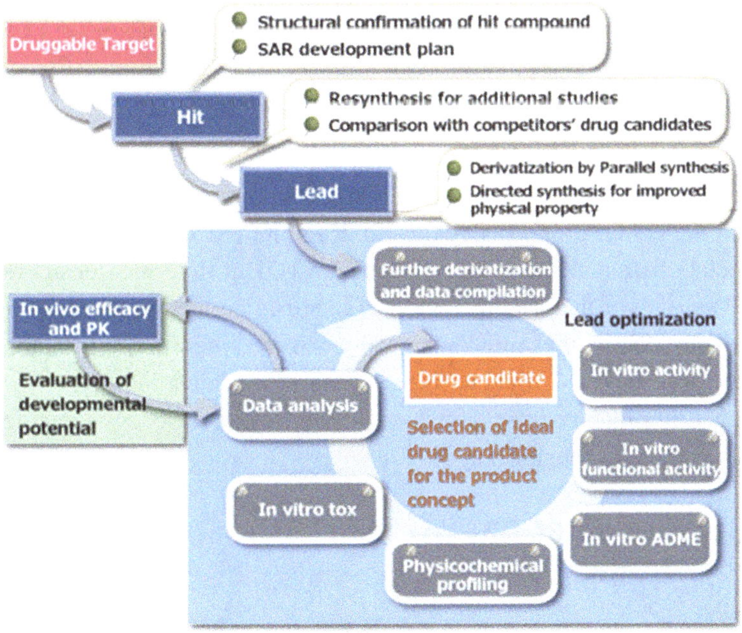

If the new drug molecule has been considered for oral route of administration, then the drug molecule should have the ability to stay long duration of time in the site of action of the body and to produce its therapeutic effect without any side effects. Oral bioavailability has been considered as one of the important properties for the new drug molecule in the lead optimization. Before performing the clinical trials the optimized lead molecule is need to be evaluated for its oral bioavailability. If the new drug has low drug uptake leads to low oral bioavailability it can cause variation among the inter-individual which increases the risk of adverse effects and toxicity. A best and ideal new drug molecule should have highest oral bioavailability and it can be considered for further process when compare to the other compounds. If any new drug molecule doesn't shows sufficient oral bioavailability in human being during clinical trials then the drug development process is stopped (Hughes *et al.,* 2011; Cooper, K.A. Cramer http://www.iptonline.com/articles/public/iptfive46np.pdf; Cole & Pfund 2000; Li 2005; Borrotti *et al.,* 2013; Oprea *et al.,* 2007; Keseru & Makara, 2003; Patodar *et al.,* 2011; Jorgensen, 2009).

Druglikeness

It is defined as a balance of various molecular properties and structural features of the drug molecule. The drug molecule property includes hydrophobicity, hydrogen bonding characteristics, electronic distribution, molecule size and flexibility; pharmacophoric features influence bioavailability, transport properties, affinity to proteins, reactivity, metabolic stability, toxicity and many others (Copeland *et al.,* 2006; Leeson & Springthorpe, 2006; Dhivyan & Anroop, https://arxiv.org/abs/1209.2793).

Physicochemical Properties Optimization

Physicochemical properties of the drug molecule are optimized based on Lipinski's rule of five. The rule states the drug molecule should have

1. logP <= 5
2. Molecular weight <= 500
3. Number of hydrogen bond acceptors <= 10
4. Number of hydrogen bond donors <= 5.

The rule is called "Rule of 5", because the border values are 5, 500, 2*5, and 5. The rule also describes the important molecular properties relates to drug pharmacokinetic parameters such as absorption, distribution, metabolism and excretion in human body. But this rule doesn't describe or calculate the pharmacological activity of the drug molecule. If the drug molecules are deviating from these rules by modification leads to have higher molecular weight, more rings, more rotatable bonds and higher lipophilicity; then the drug molecule may have problem in the bioavailability.

Poor solubility, absorption and permeation are exhibited when the drug molecule have the following properties (Leeson & Springthorpe, 2007).

1. Number of H-bond donors (NH, OH) > 5
2. Number of H-bond acceptors >10
3. Molecular weight > 500
4. clogP >5

Polar Surface Area

Polar surface area is another property of drug molecule contributed by polar groups like oxygen and nitrogen. These polar groups can help to determine the number of hydrogen bond donors or acceptor of the drug molecule.

Lipophilicity

Lipophilicity is a key physical property of drug molecule for predicting its biological activity. Human body is made up of cell membrane as fatty compartments and aqueous compartment. To produce the therapeutic effect, drug molecule must pass through between these compartments. Lipophilic compounds have poor aqueous solubility leads to poor absorption. Enzyme CYPs metabolise lipophilic compounds leads to poor bioavailability. So, drug molecule must have a suitable balance between the hydrophilicity and lipophilicity.

Drug molecule will be too lipophilic when few NH/OH/N/O groups are present in the molecular structure; whereas drug molecule can't desolvate when lots of NH/OH/N/O groups are present in the molecular structure. If the drug molecule has many H-bond donors/acceptors desolvation of the drug molecule will be difficult leads to prevent the absorption across the gut wall. H-bond donors (NH, OH) are poorer than H-bond acceptor (O, N).

Also, if the molecular weight of the drug molecule increases, site of metabolism will get increased whereas the membrane penetration will be decreased.

Other Properties Related to Drug Molecule

1. **Neutral Compound:** Neutral compounds are not ionized and protonated at physiologically relevant pH (7.4).
2. **Basic compounds:** Basic compounds are protonated at physiological pHs.
3. **Acidic Compounds:** Acidic compounds are deprotonated and ionized at physiological pH.
4. Unionized drug only can cross the membrane.
5. Ionized drug must first lose its charge.

Metabolism

Most of the drugs are metabolized by CYPs.

1. Acidic compounds metabolized by CYP2C9
2. Basic drugs are metabolized by CYP2C6
3. Acidic, basic and neutral compounds are metabolized by CYP3A

Typical drug profiles of drug molecule are

1. clogP < 5
2. 0 < logD < 2.5
3. Molecular weight < 500
4. Low H-bond Donor/ Acceptor count (<5, 10 respectively)

Pharmacokinetic Optimization

After optimizing the physicochemical properties, pharmacokinetic parameters will be optimized by *in vitro* or suitable animal models. Optimization of pharmacokinetic parameters includes assessment of concentration of the drug enters into the systemic circulation after drug administration, apparent volume of distribution, clearance of the drug from the body, transport of the drug molecule towards the specific

Table 2. Prediction of Pharmacokinetic properties based on Nature of molecule

Nature of molecule	Parameters	Molecular weight less than 400 and clogP<4	Molecular weight more than 400 and clogP>4
Neutral Molecules	Solubility	Average	Lower
	Permeability	Higher	Averagae/higher
	Bioavailability	Average	Lower
	Volume of distribution	Average	Average
	Plasma protein binging	Average	Higher
	CNS penetration	Higher/ Average	Averagae/higher
	Brain tissue binding	Lower	Higher
	P-gp efflux	Average	Higher/ Average
	In vivo clearance	Average	Average
	hERG inhibition	Lower	Lower
	P450 inhibition	Lower 2C9, 2C19, 2D6 and 3A4 inhibition	Higher 2C9, 2C19 and 3A4 inhibition
	P450 inhibition	Higher 1A2 inhibition	Lower 1A2 inhibition
	P450 inhibition		Average 2D6 inhibition
Basic molecules	Solubility	Higher/Average	Higher/Average
	Permeability	Higher/Average	Average
	Bioavailability	Average	Lwer
	Volume of distribution	Higher/Average	Higher
	Plasma protein binging	Lower	Average
	CNS penetration	Higher/Average	Average/Lower
	Brain tissue binding	Lower	Higher
	P-gp efflux	Average	Higher/Average
	In vivo clearance	Average	Higher/Average
	hERG inhibition	Average/Higher	Higher
	P450 inhibition	Lower 1A2, 2C9, 2C19 inhibition	Lower 1A2 inhibition
	P450 inhibition	Average 2D6 and 3A4 inhibition	Average 2C9, 2C19 inhibition
	P450 inhibition		Higher 2D6 and 3A4 inhibition

continued on following page

Table 2. Continued

Nature of molecule	Parameters	Molecular weight less than 400 and clogP<4	Molecular weight more than 400 and clogP>4
Acidic substances	Solubility	Higher	Average/Higher
	Permeability	Lower	Average/Higher
	Bioavailability	Average	Average
	Volume of distribution	Lower	Lower
	Plasma protein binging	Average/Higher	Higher
	CNS penetration	Lower	Lower
	Brain tissue binding	Lower	Higher
	P-gp efflux	Lower	Lower
	In vivo clearance	Lower/Average	Average
	hERG inhibition	Lower	Lower
	P450 inhibition	Lower 1A2, 2C9, 2C19, 2D6 and 3A4 inhibition	Lower 1A2, 2C19, 2D6 and 3A4 inhibition
	P450 inhibition		Higher 2C9 inhibition
Zwitterionic molecules	Solubility	Higher	Average/higher
	Permeability	Lower	Lower/Average
	Bioavailability	Lower	Lower
	Volume of distribution	Lower	Lower/Average
	Plasma protein binging	Average/Lower	Higher
	CNS penetration	Average/Lower	Lower
	Brain tissue binding	Lower	Higher
	P-gp efflux	Average	Average
	In vivo clearance	Average	Average
	hERG inhibition	Lower	Average/Lower
	P450 inhibition	Lower 1A2, 2C9, 2C19, 2D6 and 3A4 inhibition	Lower 1A2, 2C9 and 3A4 inhibition
	P450 inhibition		Average 2C9 and 2D6 inhibition

target, side effects, no toxic effect dose, toxicology, ED_{50} and therapeutic benefit to produce the desired activity. Safety of the lead molecule also assessed to ensure the side effects through safety optimization. The side effects caused by drug molecule are classified as undesired expected, desired excessive effects, undesired unexpected, poor predictability effects and drug-drug interactions. Before performing the clinical trial, required dose in human being is determined based on the pharmacokinetic parameters observed in the animal model. Medicinal chemist can make the structural modification to improve the potency of the lead molecule towards the given target based on the pharmacokinetic parameter observed results. Overall the different stage of drug discovery and development is shown in Figure 4.

Figure 4. Drug discovery and development process from bench to market

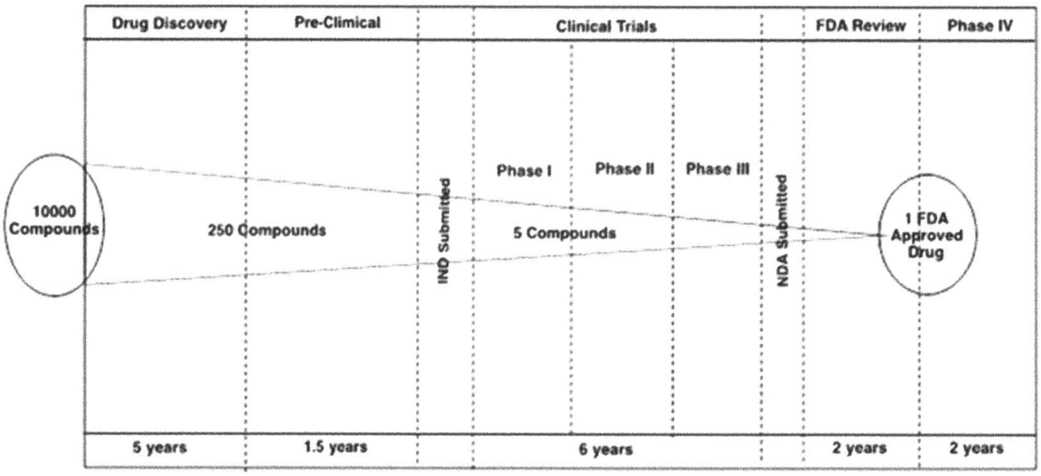

Tactics in Lead Optimization

1. Start the drug discovery and development with a good lead which includes low molecular weight, logP, potent, selective, novel and functionally active.
2. Look before you leap
3. Chemistry should allow rapid diversification (multiple site of variation for parallel follow-up)
4. Optimize lipophilic interaction.
5. Optimize polar interaction
6. Insertion of hetero atom (aryl/heterocycle group)
7. Bioisoters
8. Dipole optimization
9. Conformational control
10. Change the hypotheses and invest in alternative templates (Gleeson. 2008; Lipinski *et al.,* 1997; Hit-to-lead (H2L) and Lead Optimization in Medicinal Chemistry. https://sk.ru/cfs.../Lead-Optimization-_2D00_-Ivan-Efre_7E00_.pdf; Waring, 2010; Gleeson *et al.,* 2011)

CONCLUSION

The scientific community specifically pharmaceutical industries are struggling to find a new chemical molecule to treat any specific disease efficiently in low cost. Identification of hit (ligand) and lead generation are the key process in the development of new chemical molecule. Nowadays cheminformatics an affordable and fast technique, encompassed as a standard method to facilitate the lead generation and optimization in the drug discovery and development process. Active compounds (hits), which are identified from a compound library based on the interaction between known ligand and target binding site. Ability of the molecule, ease of synthesis, its transport within the body and patentability are the parameters need to be taken into the consideration when identification and development of hits. Hits, which satisfy the above criteria, can be promoted to lead molecule. After the hit-to-lead phase, the lead molecule undergoes some structural modification, assessed for its physicochemical properties, pharmacokinetic properties and its efficacy through *in vivo* methods. NMR and X-ray crystallography techniques are used to access the lead molecules activity and selectivity. Several other techniques can also be utilized to assess the lead molecules properties to deliver a good therapeutic drug molecule with safety into the clinical study. These lead discovery and lead optimization process comprise the properties of various lead compounds which will help to identify a suitable lead molecule with greatest potential and can be developed into a safe, effective and high quality medicine into the market. However, the addition of new techniques, checkpoints and validation are the key process which increasing the cost in getting the new drug molecule into the market.

REFERENCES

Adams, C. P., & Brantner, V. V. (2006). Estimating the cost of new drug development: Is it really 802 million dollars? *Health Affairs*, *25*(2), 420–428. doi:10.1377/hlthaff.25.2.420 PMID:16522582

Barnash, K. D., James, L. I., & Frye, S. V. (2017). Target class drug discovery. *Nature Chemical Biology*, *13*(10), 1053–1056. doi:10.1038/nchembio.2473 PMID:28926557

Baxter, A., Bennion, C., Bent, J., Boden, K., Brough, S., Cooper, A., ... Unitt, J. (2003). Hit-to-lead studies: The discovery of potent, orally bioavailable triazolethiol CXCR2 receptor antagonists. *Bioorganic & Medicinal Chemistry Letters*, *13*(16), 2625–2628. doi:10.1016/S0960-894X(03)00561-4 PMID:12873480

Betz, U. A., Farquhar, R., & Ziegelbauer, K. (2005). Genomics: Success or failure to deliver drug targets? *Current Opinion in Chemical Biology*, 9, 387–391. PMID:15990354

Bleicher, K. H., Bohm, H. J., Muller, K., & Alanine, A. I. (2003). Hit and lead generation: Beyond high-throughput screening. *Nature Reviews. Drug Discovery*, *2*(5), 369–378. doi:10.1038/nrd1086 PMID:12750740

Borrotti, M., De March, D., Slanzi, D., & Poli, I. (2013). Designing Lead Optimization of MMP-12 Inhibitors. Computational and Mathematical Methods in Medicine. *Article ID, 258627*. doi:10.1155/2014/258627

Butcher, E. C. (2005). Can cell systems biology rescue drug discovery? *Nature Reviews. Drug Discovery*, *4*(6), 461–467. doi:10.1038/nrd1754 PMID:15915152

Cole, C. J., & Pfund, W. P. (2000). Permeability Assays. *Modern Drug Discovery*, *3*, 73–76.

Comes, K. M., & Schurdak, M. E. (2004). Affinity-based screening techniques for enhancing lead discovery. *Current Opinion in Drug Discovery & Development*, *7*, 411–416. PMID:15338950

Congressional Budget Office (CBO) study. (n.d.). *Research and Development in the Pharmaceutical Industry*. Retrieved from https://www.cbo.gov/sites/default/files/109th-congress-2005-2006/reports/10-02-drugr-d.pdf

Congreve, M. S. (2003). Detection of ligands from a dynamic combinatorial library by X-ray crystallography. Angewandate Chemie (International Ed. in English), 42, 4479–4482.

Cooper, T., & Cramer, K. A. (n.d.). Designed chemical libraries for hit/lead optimization. *Innovations in Pharmaceutical Technology*, 46-53. Retrieved from http://www.iptonline.com/articles/public/iptfive46np.pdf

Copeland, R. A., Pompliano, D. L., & Meek, T. D. (2006). Drug–target residence time and its implications for lead optimization. *Perspectives*, *5*, 730–740. PMID:16888652

Deprez, B., & Deprez-Poulain, R. (2006). Trends in hit-to-lead:an update. *Frontiers in Medicinal Chemistry*, *3*, 653–673.

Dhivyan, M. A. J. E., & Anoop, M. N. (n.d.). *Virtual screening and lead optimization to identify novel inhibitors for HDAC-8*. Retrieved from https://arxiv.org/abs/1209.2793

DiMasi, J. A., Hansen, R. W., & Grabowski, H. G. (2003). The price of innovation: New estimates of drug development costs. *Journal of Health Economics*, *22*(2), 151–185. doi:10.1016/S0167-6296(02)00126-1 PMID:12606142

Dunne, A., Jowett, M., & Rees, S. (2009). Use of primary cells in high throughput screens. *Methods in Molecular Biology (Clifton, N.J.)*, *565*, 239–257. doi:10.1007/978-1-60327-258-2_12 PMID:19551366

Fulcher, M. L., Gabriel, S. E., Olsen, J. C., Tatreau, J. R., Gentzsch, M., Livanos, E., ... Randell, S. H. (2009). Novel human bronchial epithelial cell lines for cystic fibrosis research. *American Journal of Physiology. Lung Cellular and Molecular Physiology*, *296*(1), L82–L91. doi:10.1152/ajplung.90314.2008 PMID:18978040

Gleeson, M. P. (2008). Generation of a Set of Simple, Interpretable ADMET Rules of Thumb. *Journal of Medicinal Chemistry*, *51*(4), 817–834. doi:10.1021/jm701122q PMID:18232648

Gleeson, M. P., Hersey, A., Montanari, D., & Overington, J. (2011). Probing the links between in vitro potency, ADMET and physicochemical parameters. *Nature Reviews. Drug Discovery*, *10*(3), 197–208. doi:10.1038/nrd3367 PMID:21358739

Golebiowski, A., Klopfenstein, S. R., & Portlock, D. E. (2003). Lead compounds discovered from libraries: Part 2. *Current Opinion in Chemical Biology*, *7*(3), 308–325. doi:10.1016/S1367-5931(03)00059-0 PMID:12826118

Hajduk, P. (2005). *NMR-based screening in drug discovery and design. 230th ACS National Meeting*, Washington, DC.

Hajduk, P. J., & Greer, J. (2007). A decade of fragment-based drug design: Strategic advances and lessons learned. *Nature Reviews. Drug Discovery*, *6*(3), 211–219. doi:10.1038/nrd2220 PMID:17290284

Hann, M. M., & Oprea, T. I. (2004). Pursuing the leadlikeness concept in pharmaceutical research. *Current Opinion in Chemical Biology*, *8*(3), 255–263. doi:10.1016/j.cbpa.2004.04.003 PMID:15183323

Hardy, L. W., & Peet, N. P. (2004). The multiple orthogonal tools approach to define molecular causation in the validation of druggable targets. *Drug Discovery Today*, *9*(3), 117–126. doi:10.1016/S1359-6446(03)02969-6 PMID:14960389

Hartshorn, M. J., Murray, C. W., Cleasby, A., Frederickson, M., Tickle, I. J., & Jhoti, H. (2005). Fragment-based lead discovery using X-ray crystallography. *Journal of Medicinal Chemistry*, *48*(2), 403–413. doi:10.1021/jm0495778 PMID:15658854

Hit-to-lead (H2L) and Lead Optimization in Medicinal Chemistry. (n.d.). Retrieved from https://sk.ru/cfs.../Lead-Optimization-_2D00_-Ivan-Efre_7E00_.pdf

Hughes, J. P., Rees, S., Kalindjian, S. B., & Philpott, K. L. (2011). Principles of early drug Discovery. *British Journal of Pharmacology*, *162*(6), 1239–1249. doi:10.1111/j.1476-5381.2010.01127.x PMID:21091654

Jahnke, W., Florsheimer, A., Blommers, M. J., Paris, C. G., Heim, J., Nalin, C. M., & Perez, L. (2003). Second-site NMR screening and linker design. *Current Tropical Medicinal Chemistry*, *3*(1), 69–80. doi:10.2174/1568026033392778

Jorgensen, W. L. (2009). Efficient Drug Lead Discovery and Optimization. *Accounts of Chemical Research*, *42*(6), 724–733. doi:10.1021/ar800236t PMID:19317443

Keseru, G. M., & Makara, G. M. (2003). The influence of lead discovery strategies on the properties of drug candidates. *Nature Reviews. Drug Discovery*, *8*(3), 203–212. doi:10.1038/nrd2796 PMID:19247303

Keseru, G. M., & Makara, G. M. (2006). Hit discovery and hit-to-lead approaches. *Drug Discovery Today*, *11*(15/16), 741–748. doi:10.1016/j.drudis.2006.06.016 PMID:16846802

Lakshmana Prabu, S., Thirumurugan, R., & Suriya Prakash, T. N. K. (2014). The role of the drug discovery, clinical and regulatory affairs teams in turning a potent agent into a registered product. In J. Reedijk (Ed.), *Elsevier Reference Module in Chemistry, Molecular Sciences and Chemical Engineering*. Waltham, MA: Elsevier. doi:10.1016/B978-0-12-409547-2.11400-3

Lee, G., Ramirez, C. N., Kim, H., Liu, N. Z. B., & Radu, C. (2012). Large-scale screening using familial dysautonomia induced pluripotent stem cells identifies compounds that rescue IKBKAP expression. *Nature Biotechnology*, *30*(12), 1244–1248. doi:10.1038/nbt.2435 PMID:23159879

Leeson, P. D., & Springthorpe, B. (2007). The influence of drug-like concepts on decision-making in medicinal chemistry. *Nature Reviews. Drug Discovery*, *6*(11), 881–890. doi:10.1038/nrd2445 PMID:17971784

Li, A. P. (2005). Preclinical in Vitro Screening Assays for Drug- Like Properties. *Drug Discovery Today*, *2*(2), 179–185. doi:10.1016/j.ddtec.2005.05.024 PMID:24981846

Lipinski, C. A., Lombardo, F., Dominy, B. W., & Feeney, P. J. (1997). Experimental and Computational Approaches to Estimate Solubility and Permeability in Drug Discovery and Development Settings. *Advanced Drug Delivery Reviews*, *23*(1-3), 3–25. doi:10.1016/S0169-409X(96)00423-1 PMID:11259830

McLaren, D., Gorba, T., Rotrou, A. M., Pillai, G., Chappell, C., Stacey, A., & … . (2013). Automated large-scale culture and medium-throughput chemical screen for modulators of proliferation and viability of human induced pluripotent stem cell-derived neuroepithelial-like stem cells. *Journal of Biomolecular Screening*, *18*(3), 258–268. doi:10.1177/1087057112461446 PMID:23042076

Mestres, J., & Veeneman, G. H. (2003). Identification of "latent hits" in compound screening collections. *Journal of Medicinal Chemistry. Medicinal Chemistry (New York)*, *46*, 3441–3444. PMID:12877579

Michelini, E., Cevenini, L., Mezzanotte, L., Coppa, A., & Roda, A. (2010). Cell Based Assays: Fuelling drug discovery. *Analytical Biochemistry*, *397*, 1–10. PMID:19761747

Neuberger, T., Burton, B., Clark, H., & Van Goor, F. (2011). Use of primary cultures of human bronchial epithelial cells isolated from cystic fibrosis patients for the pre-clinical testing of CFTR modulators. *Methods in Molecular Biology (Clifton, N.J.)*, *741*, 39–54. doi:10.1007/978-1-61779-117-8_4 PMID:21594777

Neumann, S., Huang, W., Titus, S., Krause, G., Kleinau, G., Alberobello, A. T., ... Gershengorn, M. C. (2009). Small-molecule agonists for the thyrotropin receptor stimulate thyroid function in human thyrocytes and mice. *Proceedings of the National Academy of Sciences of the United States of America*, *106*(30), 12471–12476. doi:10.1073/pnas.0904506106 PMID:19592511

Nienaber, V. L., Richardson, P. L., Klighofer, V., Bouska, J. J., Giranda, V. L., & Greer, J. (2000). Discovering novel ligands for macromolecules using Xray crystallographic screening. *Nature Biotechnology*, *18*(10), 1105–1108. doi:10.1038/80319 PMID:11017052

Oprea, T. I., Allu, T. K., Fara, D. C., Rad, R. F., Ostopovici, L., & Bologa, C. G. (2007). Lead-like, drug-like or "pub-like": How different are they? *Journal of Computer-Aided Molecular Design*, *21*(1-3), 113–119. doi:10.100710822-007-9105-3 PMID:17333482

Patodar, A.A., Selvam, G., Jayakandan, M., Mobiya, A.K., Bagherwal, A. & Sanadya, G. *et al.*, (2011). Lead discovery and lead optimization: A useful strategy in molecular modification of lead compound in analog design. *International Journal of Drug Design and Discovery, 2*(2), 458-463.

Popa-Burke, I. G., Issakova, O., Arroway, J. D., Bernasconi, P., Chen, M., Coudurier, L., ... Hodge, C. N. (2004). Streamlined system for purifying and quantifying a diverse library of compounds and the effect of compound concentration measurements on the accurate interpretation of biological assay results. *Analytical Chemistry*, *76*(24), 7278–7287. doi:10.1021/ac0491859 PMID:15595870

Proudfoot, J. R. (2002). Drugs, leads, and drug-likeness: An analysis of some recently launched drugs. *Bioorganic & Medicinal Chemistry Letters*, *12*(12), 1647–1650. doi:10.1016/S0960-894X(02)00244-5 PMID:12039582

Titus, S. A., Southall, N., Marugan, J., Austin, C. P., & Zheng, W. (2012). High-throughput multiplexed quantitation of protein aggregation and cytotoxicity in a Huntington's disease model. *Current Chemical Genomics*, *6*, 79–86. doi:10.2174/1875397301206010079 PMID:23346268

Van der Greef, J., & McBurney, R. N. (2005). Innovation: Rescuing drug discovery: *in vivo* systems pathology and systems pharmacology. *Nature Reviews. Drug Discovery*, *4*(12), 961–967. doi:10.1038/nrd1904 PMID:16341061

Villar, H. O., Yan, J., & Hansen, M. R. (2004). Using NMR for ligand discovery and optimization. *Current Opinion in Chemical Biology*, *8*(4), 387–391. doi:10.1016/j.cbpa.2004.05.002 PMID:15288248

Waring, M. J. (2010). Lipophilicity in drug discovery. *Expert Opinion on Drug Discovery*, *5*(3), 235–248. doi:10.1517/17460441003605098 PMID:22823020

Wunberg, T., Hendrix, M., Hillisch, A., Lobell, M., Meier, H., Schmeck, C., ... Hinzen, B. (2006). Improving the Hit-to-Lead Process: Data-Driven Assessment of Drug-Like and Lead-Like Screening Hits. *Drug Discovery Today*, *11*(3-4), 175–180. doi:10.1016/S1359-6446(05)03700-1 PMID:16533716

Xiao, J., Marugan, J. J., Zheng, W., Titus, S., Southall, N., Cherry, J. J., ... Austin, C. P. (2011). Discovery, synthesis, and biological evaluation of novel SMN protein modulators. *Journal of Medicinal Chemistry*, *54*(18), 6215–6233. doi:10.1021/jm200497t PMID:21819082

Yang, S. S. O., Lu, J. Y., Kong, X. Q., Ling, Z. J., Luo, C., & Jiang, H. (2012). Computational drug discovery. *Acta Pharmacologica Sinica*, *33*(9), 1131–1140. doi:10.1038/aps.2012.109 PMID:22922346

Yang, Y., Adelstein, S. J., & Kassis, A. I. (2009). Target discovery from data mining approaches. *Drug Discovery Today*, *14*(3-4), 147–154. doi:10.1016/j.drudis.2008.12.005 PMID:19135549

Yuan, H., Myers, S., Wang, J., Zhou, D., Woo, J. A., Kallakury, B., ... Schlegel, R. (2012). Use of reprogrammed cells to identify therapy for respiratory papillomatosis. *The New England Journal of Medicine*, *367*(13), 1220–1227. doi:10.1056/NEJMoa1203055 PMID:23013073

Zheng, W., Thorne, N., & McKew, J. C. (2013). Phenotypic screens as a renewed approach for drug discovery. *Drug Discovery Today*, *18*(21-22), 1067–1073. doi:10.1016/j.drudis.2013.07.001 PMID:23850704

Chapter 4
QSAR and Lead Optimization

N. Ramalakshmi
C. L. Baid Metha College of Pharmacy, India

S. Arunkumar
Gulf Medical University, UAE

Sakthivel Balasubramaniyan
Anna University, India

ABSTRACT

There are many diseases for which suitable drugs have not been identified. As the population increases and the environment gets polluted, new infections are reported. Random screening of synthesized compounds for biological activity is time consuming. QSAR has a prominent role in drug design and optimization. It is derived from the correlation between the physicochemical properties and biological activity. QSAR equations are generated using statistical methods like regression analysis and genetic function approximation. Both 2D parameters and 3D parameters are involved in generating the equation. Among several QSAR equations generated, the best ones are selected based on statistical parameters. Validation techniques usually verify the predictive power of generated QSAR equations. Once the developed QSAR model is validated to be good, the results of that model may be applied to predict the biological activity of newer analogues. This chapter illustrates the various steps in QSAR and describes the significance of statistical parameters and software used in QSAR.

INTRODUCTION

Introduction to Drug Design

The cost involved in the drug discovery process is very high. It is also time consuming because of extensive clinical testing. Drug design is the process of inventing drugs depending on their ability to bind with biological targets. The process of drug design consists of various stages.

DOI: 10.4018/978-1-5225-7326-5.ch004

Choosing a Disease

Drug design begins by choosing a disease. There are many ailments which can affect human body. Infections by pathogens or due to faulty function of organs may be the cause for the disease. Genetic or congenital factor may also cause disease. Overproduction or under production of some metabolites is also the reason for disease. Thus, the medicinal chemist must be very careful in choosing the disease for drug design. The pathology of the disease must be studied thoroughly before designing a drug.

Choosing a Drug Target

Biochemical processes are important for functioning of human body. This biochemical process produces many chemicals necessary for normal body functioning. Enzymes regulate these biochemical processes. Therefore, the most common biological target for drug design is enzyme which catalyzes the biochemical process. Many drugs available in the market are enzyme inhibitors. The mode of action of anti-inflammatory drugs involves the inhibition of the enzyme cyclooxygenase. It produces prostaglandins. The prostaglandin causes pain, fever and inflammation. The other important biological target is receptors. Receptors produce their effect through hormones. Some of the antihypertensive drugs like atenolol act by blocking beta adrenergic receptors. Another biological target is nucleic acid. The mechanism of anti-tubercular antibiotic rifampin is inhibition of RNA synthesis. Hence, the study of structure of biological target is very important step in drug design.

Validating the Target

After selection of biological target, it becomes necessary to confirm that correct target has been identified. The validation of biological target may use *in vitro* tools which involves the use of whole animals. Antisense technology which uses RNA like chemical oligonucleotides is another method of target validation. Transgenic animals are powerful validation tools. Other validation tools include monoclonal antibodies, chemical genomics etc.

Lead Identification

"Lead compound" is the structure that has some activity against the biological target, but not yet good enough to be the drug itself (Franz, 2008). The lead molecule has various structural features for further development of the structure to a complete drug. Lead molecule can be identified from natural and synthetic products viz random screening, high throughput screening, pharmacophore mapping, virtual screening; NMR based screening, chemical genetics etc.

Lead Optimization

Once the lead structure is identified, the next step is to optimize the lead structure. In this stage, the medicinal chemist utilizes Structure Activity Relationships (SAR) to improve certain features of lead compound. These features include increasing activity against the biological target, reducing the biological activity against unrelated targets, and improve the drug likeness and ADME properties. The various ways in lead optimization are Structure Based Drug Design (SBDD), Quantitative Structure Activity Relationship (QSAR) etc.

This process takes many years. A typical development time from a chemical to drug is estimated to be 10-15 years.

Introduction to Computer Aided Drug Design (CADD)

With the development of *in silico* methods in all fields, CADD greatly reduced the time and cost involved in the process of designing a new drug. In CADD, the ligand or drug molecule is represented as small molecule and protein or target is represented as macromolecule. The designing of new drug molecules is based on the following methods (Wenbo & Alexander, 2017).

1. Small molecule based drug design (Ligand based CADD)
2. Macromolecule based drug design (Structure based CADD)

In ligand based CADD (LBDD), information about the biological target is not known. It is based on the structure of small molecule that binds to biological target. From the results of binding, the structure of pharmacophore (molecular features in the target molecule that are needed for pharmacological action) may be designed. When the structure of the target protein is not known, the drug design can be initiated with structure and known potency of the parent molecule and their analogues using QSAR. Since, QSAR determines the relationship between the structure of the compounds and their activities, it provides a scope for improving the efficacy of the compounds thus aiding the medical chemists.

In structure based drug design (SBDD), information about 3D structure of the biological target is well established by NMR studies, crystallography etc. As the structure of the biological target is known it is possible to design drugs which fit to the binding site with high affinity and selectivity using docking method. The 3D structure of protein or the target structure can be downloaded from the protein data bank. The proposed ligand molecule is checked for binding with the active site of receptor molecule.

Figure 1. Drug discovery pipeline. (Aarthi et al 2015)

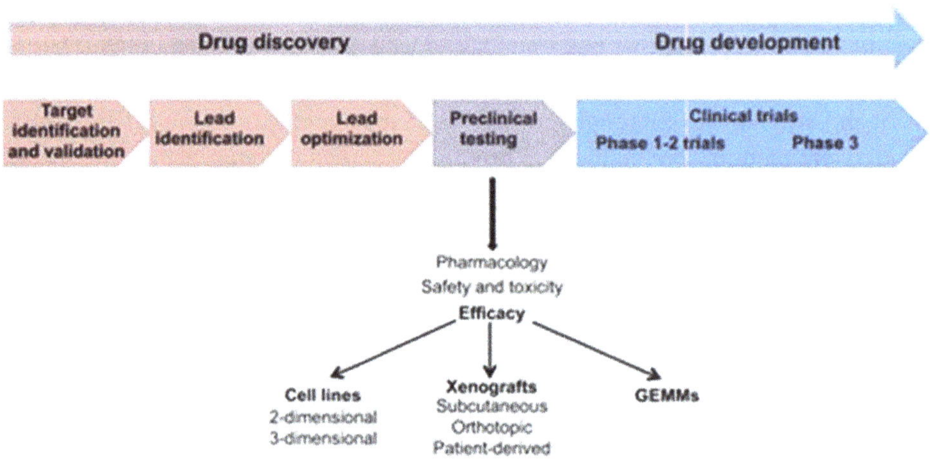

Figure 2. Types of CADD (Gregory et al 2014)

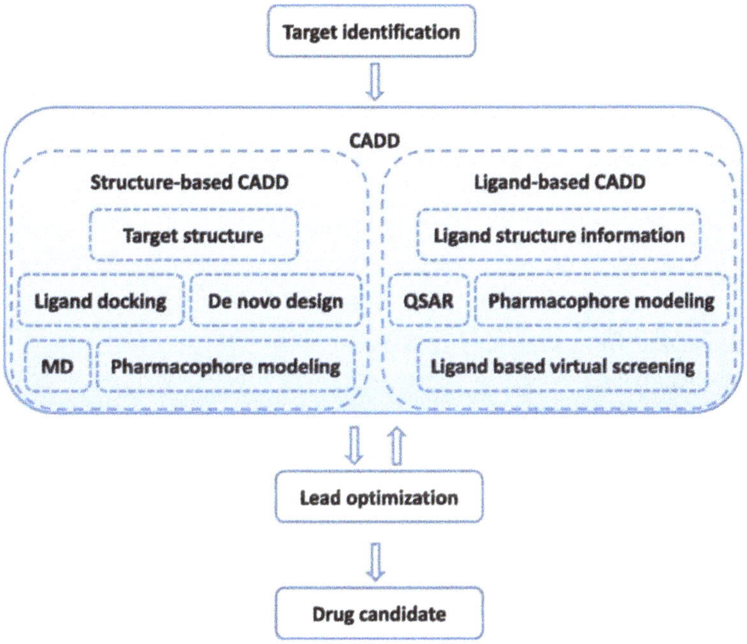

In CADD, Structure based drug design is the one where molecules are designed according to the target (Polamarasetty et al 2012). The designed molecules are then docked with the downloaded target protein to identify the best fit on the active site.

QSAR

Drug receptor interactions mainly depend upon the physicochemical parameters of the drug molecule. A number of researchers in the field drug discovery made an attempt to quantitate these parameters and correlate these with biological activity (Ishikawa et al 2012) that resulted in the development of QSAR. The development of QSAR model has several purposes and applications. Mechanisms of binding affinity between compounds and biological systems can be predicted by this method. This provides structural feature necessary for binding to produce biological effect. They are used to predict activity of new chemical compounds even before synthesis. When many conformations are available for a new structure, QSAR predicts best pharmacophoric features that fit the QSAR model (Scott 2002). QSAR tries to discover relationship between biological activity and molecular properties viz hydrophobic, steric and hydrophilic etc to evaluate which property provides activity and which reduces the activity (Ravichandran et al 2011). QSAR includes statistical methods where biological activities (expressed as logarthims molar activities) are related with structural element (Free Wilson analysis), physicochemical properties (Hanch analysis) or fields (3D-QSAR). There are certain basic requirements for selecting a series for QSAR. All analogues must belong to a congeneric series and exert similar mechanism of action. The effect of isosteric replacement must be predictable and binding energies are to be correlated to interaction energies. Eventually, this correlation depicts the corresponding biological activities.

QSAR METHODOLOGIES

Basically, the QSAR methodologies are divided into two classes

Classical QSAR

1. Free-Wilson analysis model
2. Hansch analysis

3D-QSAR

1. Comparative molecular field analysis (COMFA)
2. Molecular Shape Analysis
3. Molecular similarity matrices
4. Pharmacophoric Modelling.
5. Receptor Surface Analysis

Classical QSAR

Free-Wilson Analysis Model

This regression technique describes the contribution of substitution and the parent ring to the biological activity in the form of mathematical equation.

Hansch Analysis

1. Hansch model is one of the most successfully applied methods in the field of QSAR (Vikramjeet et al 2011). It was developed, based on the following postulates: Drug reaches near the receptor site by crossing various lipid barriers through passive diffusion process
2. Drug binds with the receptor forming a complex.
3. The drug -receptor complex undergoes chemical reaction or conformational changes for obtaining the desired biological activity.
4. The drugs in a congeneric series act through same mechanism of action. $\log 1/c = k1\pi - k2\pi2 + k3\sigma + k4Es + k5$.

Hydrophobicity

Lipids are constituents of all kinds of membranes. Absorption of a drug from the site of administration and its partitioning to different compartments of the body depends on hydrophobicity. Receptor site naturally possess lipophilic pockets that binds hydrophobic portion of small molecules (Helen, 2015). However, optimum lipophilicity is required to maintain sufficient concentration of drug in extracellular fluid. Hydrophobicity plays a pivotal role in the determination of biological half life of a drug and the process of elimination of a drug from the body. The hydrophobic nature of small molecules is expressed in terms of partition coefficient (log P) between n-octanol-water systems. It is emphasized that Log P is one of the most important parameters in the quantitative analysis of structure-activity-relationships Various chromatographic parameters like R_M, log K, log D etc., also have been used instead of log P.

Electronic Influence

Various electronic influences like dispersion forces, charge transfer interactions, electrostatic interactions, hydrogen bonding, polarization effects and acid base catalysis influence biological activity (Pengyu et al 2012).

Steric Influence

The binding of a drug to receptor rely on various steric factors like bulk and spatial arrangements of the substituent, conformational influence, and receptor requirement for specific influence.

3D-QSAR

COMFA

This 3D-QSAR technique can be used when 3D structure of molecule and their biological activity values are known even if the 3D structure of receptor is unknown (Sharma et al, 2008). This technique derives correlation between the biological activity of a set of molecules and their 3D shape, electrostatic, hydrogen bonding features etc. This relationship is established by superimposing the series of the biologically active conformations in their common binding mode.

Molecular Shape Analysis

Molecular shape is essentially a key molecular descriptor necessary for outlining ligands interaction with receptors, ion channels, enzymes and transporters and a range of other proteins and complex biological processes. This technique generates quantitative measurements of molecular shape properties and correlates them with biological activity in terms of molecular interactions (Verma et al 2010). This analysis helps in identifying the reactive site of molecule, ligand-protein interaction indirectly and be used for elucidation of conformational rearrangements to acquire reinforced active compounds. The basic concept of molecular analysis is that shape of molecule is related to binding site and thus shape affects the biological activity.

Molecular complementarity can be achieved either using the shape of the receptor binding site or the conformation of ligands crystal structure in the PDB as a shape-based search query (Sandhya et al, 2008).

Molecular Similarity

This technique aims to give quantitative results while comparing similar two given molecules. This tool is used as molecular feature to configure quantitative structure activity / property relationship and as a descriptor for finding molecular alignments. It is based on the fact that structurally more similar molecules are more likely to exhibit similar properties than structurally less similar molecules (Benigni,

1995). Molecular similarity calculations are used for both generating parameters in structure activity relationship and optimizing structure superposition.

Receptor Surface Analysis

This technique is used when the structure of receptor is not known. A hypothetical model of receptor is built based on information from the commonalities of the compounds that bind to the receptor (Hirashima et al, 2004). A receptor surface model is generated from series of aligned molecule with associated binding activities. This involves the generation of a steric surface to enclose the aggregate aligned molecules. This model provides interactive and qualitative feedback for evaluating and testing new structures.

Pharmacophoric Modeling

Pharmacophore is an essential molecular feature which is necessary for recognition of ligand by the biological macromolecule. A pharmacophore model describes about the chemical functionalities required for a ligand to bind with the receptor (Khedkar 2007). In pharmacophoric modeling is designed to explain the observed binding data of series of ligands. The model is then tested by assaying the ligands that fit to the model.

Figure 3.Various Steps Involved in QSAR

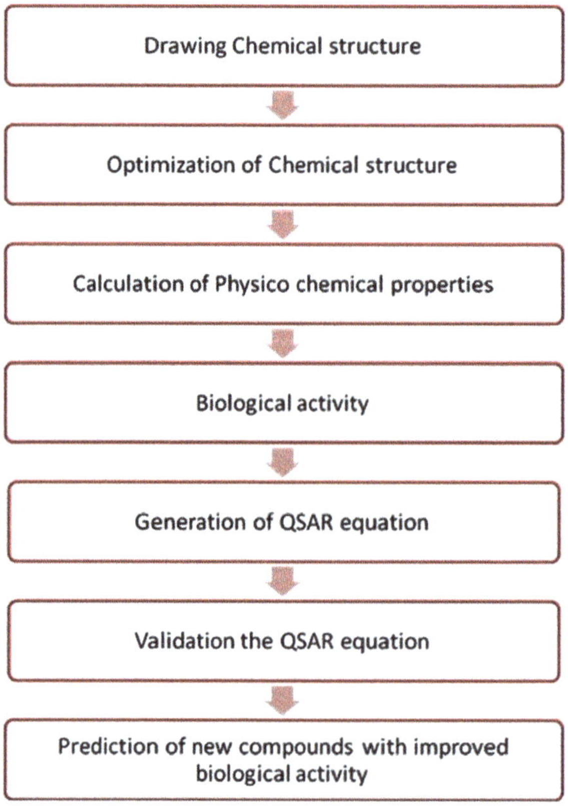

Various Steps Involved in QSAR

Drawing Chemical Structure

The first step in carrying out QSAR studies is drawing the chemical structures of compounds that we want to do QSAR. ACD/ CHEMSKETCH 11 freeware, ACD/3DViewer, Biomer, MOLKEL, Hyperchem 7.0 (Hypercube Inc., USA) etc (Prija et al 2013).

ACD/ CHEMSKETCH 11 Freeware

It is used to draw various chemical structures like organics, organometallics, polymers, and Markush structures. It includes a number of features for calculation of physicochemical parameters like molecular weight, density, parachor, surface tension, polarizability, partition co-efficient etc. Besides, it exhibits IUPAC name for the structure, SMILES, stereochemical descriptors etc. It allows holding and moving round 3D models, manipulating viewpoints, zooming in and out, recording frames, in wide array of ways

Biomer (B)

This online biomolecular modelling is renamed as B to avoid copyright issues. B is a Java-based, is written using the Java 1.0 and Java 1.1 APIs and used as model builders for initial structures of poly-nucleotides (DNA/RNA), polysaccharides, proteins and small organic molecules. It is used for AMBER force field geometry optimization, molecular dynamics etc and it has the ability to save the structures as gif, jpeg and ppm images.

MOLKEL

It is an open source (GPL) multiplatform molecular visualization program, it is operated in windows, Linux, Mac OS X. Visualization of orbitals, Iso-surface from density matrix, vanderWaals forces etc can be performed with MOLKEL. Animation of molecular surfaces and vibrational modes may also be performed. The structure can be exported to post script and PDF.

Hyperchem

HyperChem is a sophisticated molecular modeling environment. It has high quality, flexibility, and it is very easy to use. 3D visualization and animation with quantum chemical calculations, molecular mechanics, and dynamics can be performed.

Optimization of Chemical structure

Conformation of the structures plays pivotal role in the determination of physiochemical properties of molecules (Xin et al, 2017). There are several tools to generate 2D/3D structure/conformer. The geometry of each conformer should be optimized using semi quantum mechanics modules.

List of Software Used for Structural Optimization of Molecules

- **Openbabel:** Openbabel is free software, used in the inter-conversion of chemical structure/conformers (2D/3D) and different chemical file formats, substructure search, force field calculation, extraction of stereochemical information and fingerprint calculation. Open Babel is a chemical toolbox designed to handle many languages of chemical data. Anyone can search, convert, analyze, or store data from molecular modeling, chemistry, solid-state materials, biochemistry, or related areas using open babel.
- **SMI23D:** SMI 23D program converts one or more SMILIES strings into 3D. This is a 3D-coordinate generator. SMI 23D uses a two-stage process to generate 3D coordinates, an initial pass with smi2sdf generates rough coordinates and subsequent refinement results in the final coordinates.
- **FROG:** The web tool FROG (Free Online drug) builds conformation ensembles of small molecules 1 D/2D or 3D descriptors. It allows input in three formats as SMILES, Mol 2 and sdf format. This conformation ensemble generation engine, allows the input coordinates as a starting point for the conformation ensemble generation. Parameters related to the generation of ensembles correspond to a maximal number of conformations, and energy thresholds to define the allowed energy window referred to the lowest energy conformation generated.
- **TINKER:** TINKER is molecular modeling software having many features such as molecular dynamics, minimization and conformational sampling. It exhibits a range of algorithams viz flexible implementation of atomic multipole-based electrostatics with explicit dipole polarizability, various continuum solvation treatments including several generalized Born (GB/SA) models, generalized Kirkwood implicit solvation for AMOEBA, an interface to APBS for Poisson-Boltzmann calculations, efficient truncated Newton (TNCG) local optimization etc. TINKER 8 is a product of Ponder Lab for molecular mechanical and dynamics calculation.
- **MOPAC:** Molecular Orbital PACkage (MOPAC) is an open source semi-empirical quantum chemistry program. Semi-empirical quantum chemistry algorithms are implemented through this technique, and it runs on Windows, Mac, and Linux. It generates descriptors for QSAR very quickly and gives information about molecular structures and reactions. This tool was designed to perform calculations on small molecules, enzyme as well.
- **Balloon:** 3D atomic coordinates may be generated using molecular connectivity via distance geometry using balloon software. The input must be in the form of SMILES, SDF or MOL2 format. Output is SDF or MOL2. This multi-objective genetic algorithm runs on Linux, Mac OS X, and Microsoft Windows platforms for the generation of conformer ensembles.. Balloon software handle flexibility of aliphatic rings and and tetrahedral chiral atoms. This technique provides information about aliphatic ring's flexibility, stereochemistry of double bonded compounds and tetrahedral chiral atoms.
- **Cyndi:** It is capable of performing multiobjective evolution algorithm. This high speed technique generates geometrically diverse conformers at the large scale. It is a powerful alternative method for extensive conformational sampling and large-scale conformer database. It builds conformers in nearly constant time disregarding the molecular flexibility, and therefore, can be utilized to prepare conformational database for large-scale molecular database used in virtual screening.
- **DG-AMMOS:** This new open source program generates conformers of small molecules using distance geometry and minimizes the energy of the molecules. The ChemBridge Diversity database, Astex dataset was used to validate the programme on known crystal structures of several

small molecules. The crystal structures can be obtained from Cambridge Structural Database. The validation of DG-AMMOS on several different datasets proves that generated structures are generally of equal quality or sometimes better than structures obtained by other tested methods.

Physico Chemical Parameters

Calculation of Physico Chemical Properties

Calculation of Physico chemical properties is an important step in carrying out QSAR. A number of software is available for the calculation descriptors (Yap 2011).

List of Software Available for Calculation of Physicochemical Descriptors

- **PaDEL:** Uses both graphical user interface and command line interfaces. Molecular descriptors and fingerprints can be calculated using PaDEL software. This free and open source software currently calculates 1875 descriptors (1444 1D, 2D descriptors and 431 3D descriptors) and 12 types of fingerprints. It consists of both graphical user interface and command line interfaces. This tool works on all major platforms viz Windows, Linux, MacOS and supports more than 90 different molecular file formats, and is multithreaded. PaDEL-Descriptor is a useful addition to the currently available molecular descriptor calculation software.
- **Power MV:** Statistical analysis, molecular viewing, descriptor generation and similarity search can be calculated using PowerMV software. It supports MDL, SDF format. This programme displays molecules in multiple coloumn and calculates drug-likeness properties such as LogP, PSA, MW, HBAs, HBDs, etc. It exhibits anti-alias technology for best picture quality.
- **JOELib/JOELib2:** This programme calculates different descriptor types and the two main types are native value descriptors and atom property descriptors. As part of cheminformatics library, it supports SMARTS substructure search descriptor calculation, processing pipes, conversion of file formats, 100% pure Java, and interfaces to external programs (e.g. Ghemical).
- **CDK:** This technique calculates topological, geometrical charge based and constitutional descriptors. This free software is a java based descriptor tool read and write file formats via SMILES, SDF, InChl, CML and others. Apart from that ring finding, kekulisation and aromaticity are the main characters of CDK.
- **ODDescriptors:** This java based tool calculates molecular descriptor to develop the model for QSAR/QSPR. This tool converts an MDL SD file into ARFF and LIBSVM format for machine learning and data mining purposes using CDK and JOELib2.
- **MODEL:** MODEL calculates 3778 descriptors from following categories: constitutional descriptor, electronic descriptor, physico chemical properties, topological indices geometrical molecular descriptors and quantum chemistry.
- **Filter-it:** This tool filter out molecules with unwanted properties and identifies drug like molecules. It is built along with OpenBabel open source C++ API for rapid calculation of molecular properties. This programme consists of a range of molecular properties that is used to remove the unwanted properties of the molecules viz Physicochemical parameters include logP, topological polar surface area criteria, number of hydrogen bond acceptors and donors, and Lipinski's rule-of-

five. In addition, graph-based properties comprise ring-based parameters and rotatable bond criteria. Apart from that it exhibits selection criteria by means of smarts patterns, Similarity criteria, three-dimensional distances between user-definable fragments.

- **AFGen:** This tool analyse the properties based on graph. It includes paths, acyclic subgraphs and orbitary topograph subgraphs. Input is given as set of chemical compounds. This software generates vector space representation depending on the descriptors of the fragments. These descriptors describe the structural characteristics of chemical compounds.
- **ISIDA-Fragmentor:** The input for this tool is given as SDF. It calculates the properties based on substructure fragment.
- **Dragon:** It calculates 4885 molecular descriptors viz Structure activity relationship, structure property relationship, similarity analysis and high throughput screening using the descriptors generated.
- **VLife:** Vlife is a well-known software tool which evaluates a wide variety of descriptors as high as 1000 descriptors at a time. Residue ligand interactions can be performed on Vlife software. This is a novel approach for lead optimization.
- **PreADMET:** Molecular descriptors calculation, drug-likeness prediction, ADME and toxicity prediction can be performed in latest version PreADMETver 2.0. This web-based application gives information about whether the given structure passes the CMC like rule, Lead like rule, Rule of 5 etc to identify drug likeness properteis. Besides, this ADME tool predicts Caucasian adeno carcinoma cell-2 permeability, Madin-Darby canine kidney cell (MDCK) permeability, blood brain barrier permeability, human intestinal absorption (HIA) permeability, plasma protein binding and skin permeability data. Various toxicity prediction tests like Ames test, carcinogenicity prediction assay can also be performed using this software.
- **MOE:** SAR analysis molecular visualization can be performed using MOE software tool. Topological, physical and structural descriptors can be generated for a given structure using this software tool. Structure based design, fragment based design, and pharmacophore mapping can be performed using this tool. It is also used for protein and antibody modeling. The latest version of this software can build RNA and DNA structures.
- **MOLGENQSPR:** 708 descriptors are calculated using MOLGENQSPAR tool. It includes arithmetical, topological and geometrical descriptors. Structural elucidation of a novel compound can be performed using this tool. In combinatorial chemistry structure generation, descriptor calculation and regression analysis can be performed using this software.
- **Sybyl:** This programme evaluates 3D QSAR, ligand based virtual screening and docking. Tripos is the force field used in Sybyl. This module includes Advanced Computation, BioPolymer, Composer, Triad, Dynamics, GeneFold, HQSAR, Receptor, StereoPlex, Advanced CoMFA, Distill, Ampac, Concord, FlexX, ProTable, CScore, LeapFrog, MM3, MOLCAD, UNITY, DISCO, FlexS, GASP, Selector, SiteID, CLogP/CMR, and QSAR w/CoMFA.

QSAR Parameters

The QSAR Parameters are Discussed Under Three Types:

- Hydrophobic descriptors
- Spatial descriptors

- Electronic descriptors.

Hydrophobic Descriptors

Solubility

Solubility has a prominent contribution in selection of compounds for drug screening (Gozalbes, & Pineda-Lucena 2010). Hundred years ago Crum Brown and Fraser correlated that biological activity is depended on aqueous solubility. Some softwares for finding solubility are ChemAxons solubility predictor, OPERA, PaDEL, MATLAB etc.

Partition Coefficient

Hansch established the correlation between partition coefficient and biological activity. Log P influences binding of ligand molecule to enzyme/receptor, aqueous solubilty of ligand, absorption through membrane, binding to blood/tissue protein.

$$\log P = \log (\text{drug})_{\text{octanol}} - \log (\text{drug})_{\text{water.}}$$

Partition coefficient determines how and what extent the drug dissociates and crosses the cellular barrier. In short, the partition coefficient determines the absorption ability of a drug. For good absorption the log P values lies between 1 and 3. A log p value greater than 6 or less than 1, indicates poor transport characters. Softwares for calculating partition coefficient such as molinspiration, Osiris property predictor, PROLOGP- atomic, MOLCAD, Chemdraw etc. LogP is a component of Lipinski rule of 5.

Retardation Factor Rf

The amount that each component of a mixture travels can be quantified using retention factors (Rf). The retention factor of a particular material is the ratio of the distance travelled by component to the distance travelled by the solvent front. It is characteristic for drug molecule. So it is used in identification of drug molecule. CORAL is the software used to calculate Rf value for a given structure.

Distribution Coefficient log D

Log P describes the partition coefficient of neutral molecule whereas log D is the distribution constant descriptor of lipophilicity of a molecule that is ionisable at physiological pH (Małgorzata et al 2012). It is a pH dependent value. The determination of log D is similar to LogP but instead of using water, the aqueous phase is adjusted to a specific pH using a buffer. The pH at which log D is measured must be indicated. Some software used for solubility prediction are ChemAxons, Medchem Designer 3.0 etc.

Hydrophobic Constant π

The hydrophobicity of a molecule is measured in terms of hydrophobic constant. A positive value indicates that molecule is more hydrophobic and negative value indicates that molecule is less hydrophobic. This value indicates which region of the molecule might interact with hydrophobic regions in the binding site. **π** identifies specific region in a molecule which may interact with hydrophobic regions in the binding site. Some software for **π** determination is ACD/Labs Percepta Predictors—Software Modules, PLATINUM (**P**rotein **L**igand **AT**ractions **I**nvestigation **NUM**merically) etc.

Hydrophobic Fragment Constant

This parameter describes the absolute configuration of substituents and substructure contribution to total lipophilicity. It indicates constituent part of a structure to the total lipophilicity. Examples of software for calculating Hydrophobic fragment constant are ACD/Labs, PLATINUM, MULTICASE etc.

Electronic Parameters

Hammet Constant

This constant describes the effect of aromatic substitution on benzoic acid ionization. Hammet constant is determined by measuring contribution of substitution on acid dissociation constants of benzoic acid. The electron withdrawing or electron donating ability of substituent on aromatic benzene is described by this constant. The inductive and resonance effect, meta or para substituent affects the Hammet constant. Ortho values do not affect the hammet constant due to steric factors.

Taft Inductive Effect

The electrical effect of a substituent X bonded to SP^2 hybridized atom is best represented by this constant. It is a measure of inductive effect in an aliphatic series in direct comparison with aromatic σ value.

$\sigma 1 = 0.45 \times \sigma^*$

Dipole Moment

Dipole moment is equal to the distance between the charges multiplied by the charge. Dipole moment is measure of polarity. Its unit is Debye.

$\mu = \sum q_i r_i$
μ=Dipole moment
q_i=magnitude of charge
r_i=position of charge.

Dielectric Constant

The dielectric constant is the ratio of the permittivity of a substance to the permittivity of free space. It is an expression of the extent to which a material concentrates electric flux, and is the electrical equivalent of relative magnetic permeability.

Ionization Constant

An acid dissociation constant, K_a, (also known as acidity constant, or acid-ionization constant) indicates the strength of an acid in solution. It is the equilibrium constant for a chemical reaction known as dissociation in the context of acid–base reactions.

Electronic Field Effect

The electron withdrawing and electron releasing effect of substituent on biological activity is described by electronic field effect. This para meter unlike Hammet constant is not dependent on position of substituent group.

Resonance Effect

Resonance effect is a significant parameter in chemical compounds which contain double bond. Resonance effect plays a pivotal role in molecules interaction with binding site.

NMR Chemical Shift

The chemical shift in absolute terms is defined by the frequency of the resonance expressed with reference to a standard compound which is *defined* to be at 0 ppm. The scale is expressed in parts per million (ppm) and is indepedent of the spectrometer frequency.

Steric Parameters

Molecular Weight

Lipinski rule states that molecular weight should be less than 500 for a molecule to be active as a drug. Molecular weight greatly influences the oral bioavailability. Increase in molecular weight may increase lipophilicity. This greatly increases target protein binding but it affects aqueous solubility of the molecule.

Taft Steric Constant

It is important for those substituents which interact sterically with the tetrahedral transition state for the reaction. But for substituents which interact with the transition state by resonance or hydrogen bonding this parameter cannot be used. It may undervalue the steric effect of groups in an intermolecular process (i.e. a drug binding to a receptor). It is measured by rate of hydrolysis of substituted aliphatic ester against standard ester.

Es=log Kx-log ko

Kx=rate of hydrolysis of substituted ester.

Ko= rate of hydrolysis of parent ester.

Molecular Surface Area

It describes the vanderWalls area of molecule and determines the extent to which a molecule exposes itself to experimental environment (Anderson & Yuji 1992). It is related to binding, transport and solubility.

Sterimol Parameter

It gives dimensions of substituents from standard bond angle, vanderWaals radii, bond length and possible conformations for the substituent. Unlike Taft steric parameter, this descriptor may be used for any substituent (Jo-Lena et al, 2007). This parameter defines the dimension of a molecule in five directions.

Charton Steric Parameter

vanderWaals radius of any symmetrical substituent can be calculate from this parameter. Chaton introduced a corrected vanderWaals radius U, in which minimum value of vanderWaals radius of the substituent (r(v min) is corrected for corresponding radius for hydrogen (rvH). (Marvin, 1978)

U=r v(min)- rvH= r v(min)- 1.20

VanderWaals Volume

The vanderWaals volume, V_w, also called atomic volume or molecular volume (Yuan et al 2003), is the atomic property most directly related to the vanderWaals radius. It is the volume occupied by an individual atom (or molecule).

Other Parameters

Molar Refractivity, MR

According to Lorentz-Lorentz equation: MR = $(n^2 - 1)$ M/$(n^2 + 2)$ Q (Pacák, 1989) Where n is the index of refraction, M is the molecular weight, and Q is the density. For QSAR studies, the value of MR is usually divided by 10 so that the range of typical MR values is similar to the range of logP and other typical descriptors. Molar refractivity of a compound can be measured using an Abbe' refractometer. It is related not only to volume but also to London dispersive forces of molecule that act in drug receptor interaction.

Zagreb Index (Zagreb)

The Zagreb Indices is calculated simply as the sum of the squares of the number of non-hydrogen bonds formed by each heavy atom (Muhuo & Bolian 2010). This parameter is reported in QSAR and QSPR studies.

The Balaban J Index

The Balaban index (Hanyuan, 2011), also called the average distance sum connectivity index, and is computed as follows: the numbers of edges from atom i to all other atoms in a molecule are summed, and this procedure are repeated for all other atoms. The sums for adjacent atoms are then multiplied together, and the reciprocal square roots taken and summed. This number is then multiplied by (B/(C + 1)), where B = number of bonds in the molecule and C = number of rings, to give the Balaban index J. Unlike other topological indices, it does not increase rapidly with molecular size. J did not correlate well with a range of physicochemical properties or with acute toxicity of ethers.

Kappa

Kier (Kunal, 2017) devised a numerical index (kappa, κ) of molecular shape from the hydrogen-suppressed graph of a molecule. It is based on the count of 2-bond fragments in a graph relative to the maximum number possible (if the molecule is star-shaped) and the minimum number in the isomeric linear graph.

Radius of Gyration

It is a two dimensional descriptor. Radius of gyration is the distance of a point from the axis of rotation. (Gharaghani et al 2013).

Radius of gyration= $\sqrt{\sum (x_i^2+y_i^2+ z_i^2)/N}$.

It is mainly used to determine diffusion coefficient of different macro molecules. In addition, it determines the compactness of the structure. A steady value of Rg indicates that protein folding is stable. If a protein unfolds, its Rg will change over time."

E-State Parameter

This parameter combines both the electronic character and the topological environment of individual atom in a molecule (Roy & Mitra, 2012). It is a descriptor for an atom within a covalently bonded molecule. It describes the electronegativity, pi and lone pair electron content, topological status and the environment of an atom within the molecule.

Biological Activity

QSAR can be performed on any kind of biological value. The only requirement is a numerical value for biological activity. QSAR cannot be a qualitative results like Yes or No type answers for biological data. The values obtained in biological activity must be converted into logarithmic form for generating QSAR equation.

Generation of QSAR Equation

QSAR/QSPR is basically a statistical approach correlating the response property or activity data with descriptors encoding chemical information. Such correlation may be derived either in a regression-based approach (in cases where the response property is quantitative and available in a continuous scale) or a classification-based approach (in cases where the response property is graded or semi-quantitative). The most commonly used regression-based approaches are as follows:

- Multiple linear regression (MLR)
- Partial least squares (PLS)
- Linear discriminant analysis (LDA)
- Cluster analysis

Multiple Linear Regression

Multiple linear regression (MLR) is a statistical technique that uses several explanatory variables to predict the outcome of a response variable. The goal of multiple linear regression (MLR) is to model the relationship between the explanatory and response variables. The model for MLR, given in observations, is

$y_i = B_0 + B_1x_{i1} + B_2x_{i2} + ... + B_px_{ip} + E_i$ where i = 1,2, ..., n

This method requires at least as many molecules as independent variables. To produce reliable results, typically need 5 times as many molecules as independent variables.

Partial Least Squares (PLS)

Partial least square is a recent technique. It combines features from principal component analysis and multiple regressions. It is particularly useful to predict a set of dependent variables from a (very) large set of independent variables (i.e., predictors). It originated in the social sciences but became popular first in chemometrics (i.e., computational chemistry). PLS is a multivariate technique for non-experimental and experimental data alike.

Linear Discriminant Analysis (LDA)

This technique is used in the pre-processing step for pattern-classification and machine learning applications. The objective of LDA is to perform dimensionality reduction while getting as much of the class discriminatory information as possible. This statistical method maximizes the separation between multiple classes which cannot be performed in partial least square analysis.

Cluster Analysis

Cluster analysis is an exploratory data analysis tool for organizing observed data or cases into two more groups. Unlike LDA cluster analysis, requires no prior knowledge of which elements belong to which clusters. Cluster analysis maximizes the similarity of cases within each cluster while maximizing dissimilarity between the groups that are initially unknown.

Validation of the QSAR Equation

QSAR model can lead to false prediction of biological activity if the developed QSAR model is not validated. So validation of QSAR models, after model development, is most important part in QSAR studies.

Two types of validation

1. Internal validation.
2. External validation

Least Square Fit (R^2)

Determination coefficient (R^2) is defined in the following manner:

$$R^2 = 1 - \Sigma(Yobs - Ycal)^2 / \Sigma(Yobs - Y\ obs)^2$$

In the above equation, Yobs stands for the observed response value, while Ycalc is the model-derived calculated response and Yobs is the average of the observed response values. For the ideal model, the sum of squared residuals being 0, the value of R2 is 1. As the value of R2 deviates from 1, the fitting quality of the model deteriorates.

Leave-One-Out (LOO) and Leave-Many-Out (LMO)

Some of the most popular validation techniques are the well-known Leave-one-out (LOO) and Leave-many-out (LMO) cross-validation (CV) procedures.In its basic formulation, the LOO-CV procedure can be applied when a fixed set of descriptors is considered for a set of *n* molecules. For each molecule, a model is built considering the experimental property value of the *n*-1 remaining compounds and the respective descriptors. Then, this model is used to make a prediction for the molecule left out. The above primary algorithm is named here the *kernel* of the standard LOO-CV method.

To determine the LOO cross-validation, the training set is primarily modified by eliminating one compound from the set. The QSAR model is then rebuilt based on the remaining molecules of the training set using the descriptor combination originally selected, and the activity of the deleted compound is computed based on the resulting QSAR equation. This cycle is repeated until all the molecules of the training set have been deleted once, and the predicted activity data obtained for all the training set compounds are used for the calculation of various internal validation parameters. Finally, the model predictivity is judged using the predicted residual sum of squares (PRESS) and cross-validated R^2 (Q^2) for the model while the value of standard deviation of error of prediction (SDEP) is calculated from PRESS.

Leave-Many-Out (LMO) Cross-Validation

The fundamental principle of the LMO technique is that a specific section of the training set is held out and eliminated in each cycle. For each cycle, the model is constructed based on the remaining molecules (and using the originally selected descriptors) and then the activity of the deleted compounds is predicted using the developed model. After all the cycles have been completed, the predicted activity values of the compounds are used for the calculation of the LMO-Q2

When Can One Accept the Developed QSAR Model as Reliable and Predictive One?

- If correlation coefficient $R \geq 0.8$ (for *in vivo* data).
- If coefficient of determination $R^2 \geq 0.6$
- If the standard deviations is not much larger than standard deviation of the biological data.
- If its F value indicate that overall significance level is better than 95%.
- If its confidence interval of all individual regression coefficients proves that they are justified at the 95% significance level.
- If cross-validated $R^2(Q^2) \geq 0.5$
- If R^2 for external test set, $R^2pred \geq 0.6$
- Randomized R^2 value should be as low as to R^2.
- Randomized Q^2 value should be as low as to Q^2 .
- $(R^2 - R^20)/R^2 < 0.1$and $0.85 <= k <= 1.15$, or $(R^2 - r'^2 0) / R^2 < 0.1$ and $0.85 <= k' <= 1.15$ (for test set).
- r^2 m (overall) and Rp^2 are ≥ 0.5 (or at least near 0.5).
- In addition, the biological data should cover a range of at least one, two or even more logarithmic units: they should be well distributed over whole distance. Also, physicochemical parameter should be spread over a certain range and should be more or less evenly distributed.

Equation Has to Be Rejected

- If the above mentioned statistical measures are not satisfied
- If the number of the variables in the regression equation is unreasonably large.
- If standard deviation is smaller than error in the biological data.

Disadvantages of QSAR

- False correlation due to error in biological data
- Retro specific method. That is QSAR can be carried out only for those compounds reported with biological value.

Prediction of New Molecules

Based on the results of QSAR equation, new molecules can be developed by varying substituent groups which may increase or decrease a particular physicochemical property. The biological activity of the newly designed molecules may be predicted by substituting the parameters value in QSAR equation. The compounds can be synthesized and their actual biological value may be determined. It will have a better biological activity than the series of compounds which were taken for QSAR.

CONCLUSION

Insilco methods are highly advantageous in reducing time and cost involved in drug design process. Though QSAR is a retro specific methodology, it is an important tool in drug design. QSAR has come a long way from classical Hansch analysis to latest COMFA techniques. QSAR is an important tool in lead optimization. Apart from lead optimization, QSAR can be applied in understanding mechanism of action, virtual screening, combinatorial library generation, database searches etc.

REFERENCES

Aarthi, G., Jennifer, P. M., Duncan, I. J., & Owen, J. S. (2015). GEMMs as preclinical models for testing pancreatic cancer therapies. *Disease Models & Mechanisms*, *8*(10), 1185–1200. doi:10.1242/dmm.021055 PMID:26438692

Anderson, C. G., & Yuji, T. (1992). Calculation of molecular surface area with numerical factors. *Computers & Chemistry*, *16*(4), 277–284. doi:10.1016/0097-8485(92)80047-4

Benigni, R., Cotta-Ramusino, M., Giorgi, F. & Gallo, G. (1995). Molecular similarity matrices and quantitative structure-activity relationships: a case study with methodological implications. *Journal of Medicinal Chemistry*, *38*(4), 629-635.

Franz, F. H. (2008). Requirements for a lead compound to become a clinical candidate. *BMC Neuroscience*, *9*(3), S7. PMID:19091004

Gharaghani, S., Khayamian, T., & Ebrahimi, M. (2013). Molecular dynamics simulation study and molecular docking descriptors in structure-based QSAR on acetylcholinesterase (AChE) inhibitors. *SAR and QSAR in Environmental Research, 24*(9), 773–794. doi:10.1080/1062936X.2013.792877 PMID:23863115

Gozalbes, R., & Pineda-Lucena, A. (2010). QSAR-based solubility model for drug-like compounds. *Bioorganic & Medicinal Chemistry, 18*(19), 7078–7084. doi:10.1016/j.bmc.2010.08.003 PMID:20810286

Gregory, S., Sandeep Kumar, K., Jens, M., Edward, W., & Lowe Eric, L. B. (2014). Computational methods in drug discovery. *Pharmacological Reviews, 66*(1), 334–395. PMID:24381236

Hanyuan, D. (2011). On the Balaban Index of Trees. *Match (Mülheim an der Ruhr, Germany), 66*, 253–260.

Helen, W. (2015). Biological membranes. *Essays in Biochemistry, 59,* 43-69. doi:10.1042/bse0590043 PMID:26504250

Hirashima, A., Eiraku, T., Kuwano, E., & Eto, M. (2004). Comparative receptor surface analysis of agonists for tyramine receptor which inhibit sex-pheromone production in Plodiainterpunctella. *Combinatorial Chemistry & High Throughput Screening, 7*(2), 83–91. doi:10.2174/1386207043120775 PMID:15032656

Ishikawa, T., Hirano, H., Saito, H., Sano, K., Ikegami, Y., Yamaotsu, N., & Hirono, S. (2012). QSAR analysis to predict drug-drug interactions of ABC transporter ABCG2. *Mini-Reviews in Medicinal Chemistry, 12*(6), 505–514. doi:10.2174/138955712800493825 PMID:22587765

Jo-Lene, L., Rudi, B., Patrick, C. C., & Mei-Lin, G. (2007). Quantitative structure-activity relationship (QSAR) of indoloacetamides as inhibitors of human isoprenylcysteine carboxyl methyltransferase. *Bioorganic & Medicinal Chemistry Letters, 17*(4), 1025–1032. doi:10.1016/j.bmcl.2006.11.030 PMID:17157012

Khedkar, S. A., Malde, A. K., Coutinho, E. C., & Srivastava, S. (2007). Pharmacophore modeling in drug discovery and development: An overview. *Medicinal Chemistry (Shariqah, United Arab Emirates), 3*(2), 187–197. doi:10.2174/157340607780059521 PMID:17348856

Kortagere, S., Krasowski, M. D., & Ekins, S. (2009, March). The importance of discerning shape in molecular pharmacology. *Trends in Pharmacological Sciences, 30*(3), 138–147. doi:10.1016/j.tips.2008.12.001 PMID:19187977

Kunal, R. (2017). *Advances in QSAR modeling: applications in pharmaceutical, chemical, food agricultural and environmental sciences*. Springer.

Małgorzata, J., Katarzyna, S., & Anna, P. (2012). Quantification of Lipophilicity of 1, 2, 4-Triazoles Using Micellar Chromatography. *Chromatographia, 75*(9), 449–456. PMID:22593604

Marvin, C. (1978). Composition of the steric parameter as a function of alkyl branching. *The Journal of Organic Chemistry, 43*(21), 3995–4001. doi:10.1021/jo00415a002

Muhuo, L., & Bolian, L. (2010). Some properties of the first general Zagreb index. *Australasian Journal of Combinatorics, 47*, 285–294.

Pacák, P. (1989). Molar refractivity and interactions in solutions I. Molar refractivity of some monovalent ions in aqueous and dimethyl sulfoxide solutions. *Chemical Papers, 43*(4), 489–500.

Pengyu, R., Jaehun, C., Dennis, G. T., Michael, J. S., Marcelo, M., Jiajing, Z., & Nathan, A. B. (2012). Biomolecular electrostatics and solvation: A computational perspective. *Quarterly Reviews of Biophysics, 45*(4), 427–491. doi:10.1017/S003358351200011X PMID:23217364

Polamarasetty, A., Kakularam, K. R., & Pallu, R. (2012). Structure and ligand based drug design strategies in the development of novel 5-LOX inhibitors. *Current Medicinal Chemistry, 19*(22), 3763–3778. doi:10.2174/092986712801661112 PMID:22680930

Prija, P., Shikhar, G., Madhu, C., Rashmi, T., Anil, S. B., Garima, G., ... Hanumantharao, G. R. (2012). 2D-QSAR, docking studies, and in silico ADMET Prediction of polyphenolic acetates as substrates for protein acetyltransferasefunction of glutamine synthetase of Mycobacterium tuberculosis. *ISRN Structural Biology*.

Ravichandran, V., Harish, R., Abhishek, J., Shalini, S., Christapher, P. V., & Ram, K. A. (2011).. . *International Journal of Drug Design and Discovery, 2*(3), 511–519.

Roy, K., & Mitra, I. (2012). Electrotopological state atom (E-state) index in drug design, QSAR, property prediction and toxicity assessment. *Current Computer-aided Drug Design, 8*(2), 135–158. doi:10.2174/157340912800492366 PMID:22497469

Scott, A. W., & Gordon, M. C. (2002). Three-dimensional molecular descriptors and a novel QSAR method. *Journal of Molecular Graphics & Modelling, 21*(3), 161–170. doi:10.1016/S1093-3263(02)00147-X PMID:12463634

Sharma, P. C., Sharma, S. V., Archana, S., & Suresh, B. (2008). 3D-QSAR CoMFA study of some heteroarylpyrroles as possible anticandida agents. *Indian Journal of Pharmaceutical Sciences, 70*(2), 154–158. doi:10.4103/0250-474X.41447 PMID:20046704

Verma, J., Khedkar, V. M., & Coutinho, E. C. (2010). 3D-QSAR in drug design--a review. *Current Topics in Medicinal Chemistry, 10*(1), 95–115. doi:10.2174/156802610790232260 PMID:19929826

Vikramjeet, J., Rakesh, N., Deepika, S., Balasubramanian, N., & Pradeep, K. (2011). Hansch analysis for the prediction of antimycobacterial activity of ofloxacin derivatives. *Medicinal Chemistry Research, 20*(7), 826–837. doi:10.100700044-010-9400-8

Wenbo, Y., & Alexander, D. M. (2017). Computer-aided drug design methods. *Methods in Molecular Biology (Clifton, N.J.), 1520*, 85–106. doi:10.1007/978-1-4939-6634-9_5 PMID:27873247

Xin, L., Yu-Ze, Z., Zhi, J., Wen-Qing, J., Shu-Qing, W., Wei-Ren, X., & Xian-Chao, C. (2017). Molecular docking, 3D-QSAR and structural optimization of indolebiphenylcarboxylic acids as PPARγ antagonists. *Letters in Drug Design & Discovery, 14*(8).

Yap, C. W. (2011). PaDEL-descriptor: An open source software to calculate molecular descriptors and fingerprints. *Journal of Computational Chemistry, 32*(7), 1466–1474. doi:10.1002/jcc.21707 PMID:21425294

Yuan, H. Z., Michael, H. A., & Andreas, M. Z. (2003). Fast calculation of van der waals volume as a sum of atomic and bond contributions and its application to drug compounds. *The Journal of Organic Chemistry, 68*(19), 7368–7373. doi:10.1021/jo034808o PMID:12968888

Chapter 5
Virtual Screening and Its Applications in Drug Discovery Process

Gurusamy Mariappan
St. Mary's College of Pharmacy, India

Anju Kumari
St. Mary's College of Pharmacy, India

ABSTRACT

Virtual screening plays an important role in the modern drug discovery process. The pharma companies invest huge amounts of money and time in drug discovery and screening. However, at the final stage of clinical trials, several molecules fail, which results in a large financial loss. To overcome this, a virtual screening tool was developed with super predictive power. The virtual screening tool is not only restricted tool small molecules but also to macromolecules such as protein, enzyme, receptors, etc. This gives an insight into structure-based and Ligand-based drug design. VS gives reliable information to direct the process of drug discovery (e.g., when the 3D image of the receptor is known, structure-based drug design is recommended). The pharmacophore-based model is advisable when the information about the receptor or any macromolecule is unknown. In this ADME, parameters such as Log P, bioavailability, and QSAR can be used as filters. This chapter shows both models with various representative examples that facilitate the scientist to use computational screening tools in modern drug discovery processes.

INTRODUCTION

Lead discovery is the vital step in drug discovery programme. Advancements in genetics and computational biology boost up the modern drug discovery methods. The genetic scientists provide a lot of information about human genome along with gene requirement which codes for a particular protein that is prerequisite for the development of a particular organism. As a consequence, the targets for drugs and the mechanistic pathway can be traced with the support of genetic information. The drug targets may soon rise from 500 to 10,000 in future (Debouck C & Metcalf B, 2000).

DOI: 10.4018/978-1-5225-7326-5.ch005

Meanwhile, the advent of combinational chemistry also revolutionised the basic research to provide an infinite number of compounds in a short span of time. The high throughput screening (HTS) played a very vital role to automate the conventional assay methods (Hertzberg RP & Pope AJ, 2000). There are various combinatorial methods is available to create a wide range of chemical libraries like peptides, non-peptide oligomers, peptidomimetics, small molecules, and natural product-like organic molecules. Each combinatorial approach possesses unique high-throughput screening and encoding strategy. But still, it is in the infant stage due to its exorbitant economic implications. The virtual screening came to the practice as a complementary approach that can analyse the large databases.

The computational screening is otherwise known as *in silico* screening since the screening is done by silicon graphics interface (Walters WP 1998; Lyne PD 2002; Schneider G & Böhm HJ, 2002). Virtual screening is based on knowledge of either ligand or receptor. The virtual screening methods yield the information of the receptor based on the input information. For example, the three-dimensional image of the receptor is known, the virtual screening will direct as to receptor-based Drug Design . When the information about receptor is known, the virtual screening directs to pharmacophore drug discovery considering ADME parameters as a filter. In the following sections, application of virtual screening in drug discovery process are described with schematic representation.

VIRTUAL DRUG SCREENING

A pharmacophore is an abstract description of molecular features that are necessary for molecular recognition of a ligand by biological macromolecules. Gund proposed the pharmacophores could be used to search the database based on similarity in structure (Gund P, 1977). It paves the way to develop and apply 3D databases pharmacophore to discover novel leads (Kurogi Y & Guner OF, 2001; Langer T & Hoffmann RD, 2001). There are two steps in pharmacophore-based screening: one is identification of pharmacophore model and the second step is 3-D search based on the specific constraints. The most benefit of VS is that it can be applied to large databases.

Pharmacophore models are generally used when the active lead is identified, but the 3D image of the target is unknown. The active molecules are considered as training set and used for pharmacophore identification which is atoms/groups interact with the receptor.

The pharmacophore generation poses some problems due to conformational flexibility of the molecule Catalyst (Accelrys, (http://www.accelrys.com) Discotech and GASP (Tripos, (http://www.tripos.com; Jones G *et al.,* 1995) are commercially available programs for pharmacophore modeling. Conformational flexibility is the key feature to develop the algorithm which play pivotal role for the program development. These programs are based on the algorithms used for the alignment and the way in which conformational flexibility is handled. A pharmacophore model is obtained not only from active ligand but also from 3D receptor. Such a structure of receptor or receptor/ligand complex provides information on possible and essential points of interactions between receptor and drug. The active binding site in 3D receptor is analyzed and the same information which can be used in 3-D database screening. For instance, when a drug-receptor complex is available, the atoms of ligand which interacts with receptor can be defined as features in a pharmacophore modeling. The protein backbone atoms are also used in pharmacophore model. The information of protein backbone atoms are merged with the feature points into a single pharmacophore. When three-dimensional image is only protein, multiple queries are needed in order to correlate and explore various possible binding modes. The programmes such as UNITY (Tripos, http://

www.tripos.com) and CATALYST are available based on the structure of protein, since the preceptor structure is so complex it is important to trace the key feature to define the pharmacophore. The Drug Design module such as Cerius2 (Accelrys) is used for protein pharmacophore modeling and to design the ligand molecules (http://www.accelrys.com). The interaction map is generated from the active site of the receptor and analyzed for the parameters such as hydrophobicity, hydrogen donor and acceptor.

Virtual Screening Based Pharmacophore Model

Pharmacophore-based virtual screening is one of the advanced methods. Fox and Haaksma explained a computational process to identify ligands from the analysis of the 3-D structure of receptor (Fox T & Haaksma EEJ, 2000). These computational processes are explained into two stages. The first stage dealt with the specific interactions in the binding site with the program GRID (Goodford PJ, 1985). Some of the interactions types, typically including the hydrophobic, the alkyl hydroxyl group OH, organic halogen (Br, Cl), water, amides and amidine *etc.* The favourable interactions between receptor and ligand are translated into a database query. 2-D queries are specified by chemical substructures that have to be matched in the resulting GRID energies. The local minima of the interactions maps and the corresponding distances are measured to act as the mutual constraints between these features. In the second stage, the active compounds are identified from 3D database using UNITY. This approach was demonstrated with thrombin as the target. A pharmacophore model containing three-point interactions sites, one positively charged centre and two hydrophobic site hp1 and hp2 is given in Figure 1.

Fox *et al.* used benzamidine compounds as test databases, as the positive centre the amidine carbon atom of benzamidine (C_0) was used. The calculated 3-D flexible database search results shows the enriched hit lists with thrombin inhibitors compared to the total database. The Fox's approach lacunae are that it cannot be fully automated as the success will critically depend on the identification of an anchor fragment. An anchor fragment is a minimal recognition of the structure essential for specific binding. These fragments recognition are accomplished using the *de novo* design program LUDI.

Hindle *et al.* investigated the pharmacophore model with molecular docking (Hindle SA *et al.*, 2002). They proposed an advanced version of the flexible docking tool FlexX (Tripos, http://www.tripos.com), FlexX-PHARM, to study about the protein-ligand binding models into a docking calculation. This information is introduced as a simple set of constraints derived from receptor-based pharmacophore features. In FlexX-PHARM the active site is defined by two different types of constraint: namely interaction constraint and spatial constraints. In former, Flex X calculation surface in the active site that takes part

Figure 1. Pharmacophore model as derived from the GRID results and used in the UNITY database search; hp=hydrophobic center.

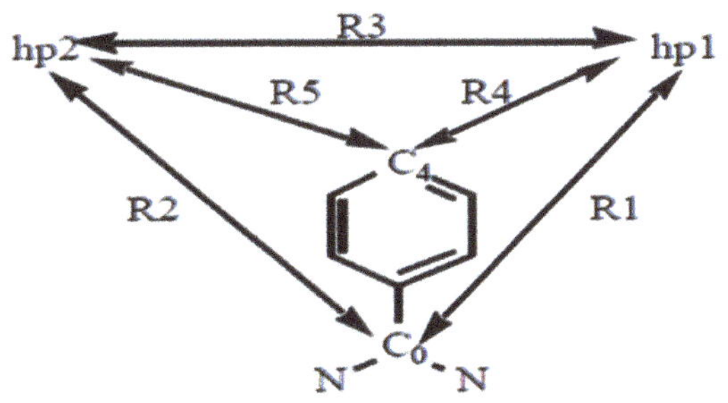

in interaction with ligand. The latter involves the inclusion volume. An interacting group and interaction type must be specified to define the interaction constraints. FlexX-PHARM ensures that interaction is ascertained between the specified interacting group in the active site and the ligand in a valid docking solution. The spatial constraint can be used to restrict ligand position in the active site and consists of a sphere plus an associated element type. The maximum potential is gained from FlexX-PHARM, and pro-docking checks were performed to eliminate these ligands devoid of pharmcophore constraints. Figure 2 shows four pharmacophore constraints in the active site of carbonic anhydrase. Examples are given where FlexX-PHARM significantly improved the results of docking in several PDB complexes

It was also tested as a tool on a small dataset of molecules for three target proteins including carbonic anhydrase, thermolysin, and dihydrofolate reductase. In two cases, FlexX-PHARM missed one or two of the active molecules due to the constraint selected. The challenge is that the constraints must first be obtained and then introduced into FlexX-PHARM.

Recently, VS based on pharmacophore model has been applied to discover novel ligands, and some examples are given in Table 1. Brenk *et al.* studied crystal structures of two ligands complexed with TGT by least squares method. UNITY was used to define the hydrogen donor and acceptor by picking the appropriate atoms of ligands. The directionality of the hydrogen bonds and the corresponding sites are related to the neighbouring atoms of the protein and the interstitial water molecules. The centroid of the benzoic ring of a ligand is characterised as hydrophobic moiety (Figure 3).

COMBINATORIAL DRUG DESIGN

Rational Drug Design is an optimization process to find the best combination of molecular fragments which can be constituted into a whole ligand and well placed in the active site of the receptor. In optimization process, the generated molecule should meet the given pharmacophoric features, which are

Figure 2. A set of four phamacophore constraints in the active site of carbonic anhydrase. Constraint 1: essential metal interaction at the zinc ion. Constraint 2: essential spatial constraint for a carbon atom. Constraint 3: optional hydrogen donor interaction at the backbone nitrogen of residue Thr199, and constraint 4: optional hydrogen acceptor interaction at the gamma oxygen of residue Thr199

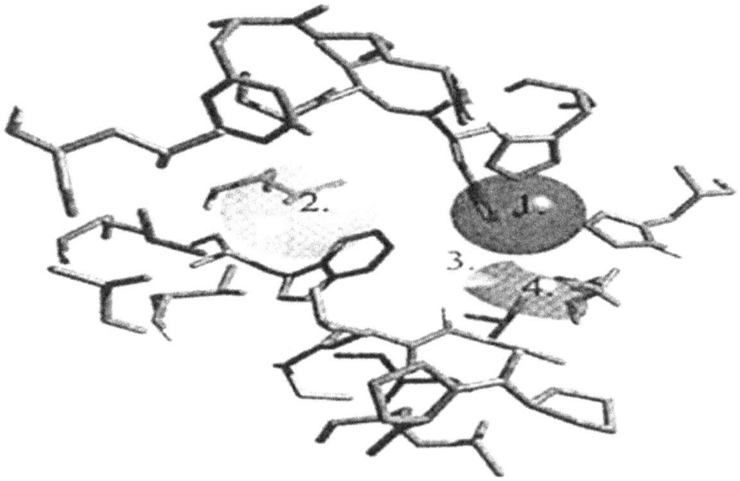

Figure 3. Structure-based pharmacophore hypothesis

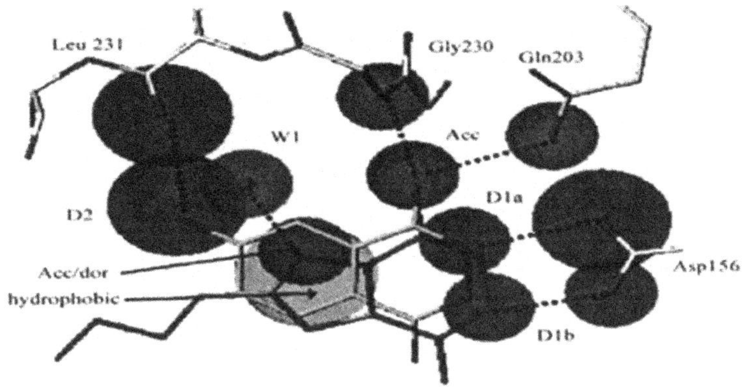

Table 1. Examples of bioactive molecules design using pharmacophore-based virtual screening

Molecular structure	Target	Method	Activity	Ref
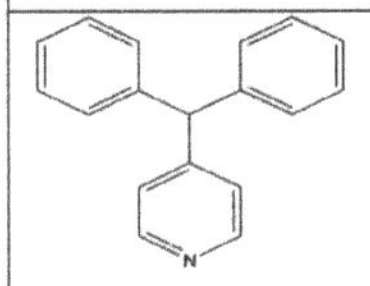	Dopamine transporter(DAT)	Quanta,Chem-X	0.255(Ki)	Enyedy IJ *et al.*, 2003
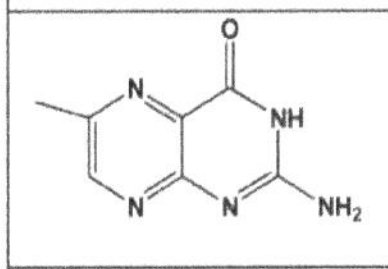	tRNA-guanine transglycosylase(TGT)	SuperStar, DrugScore, UNITY, FlexX	0.25(Ki)	Brenk R *et al.*, 2003
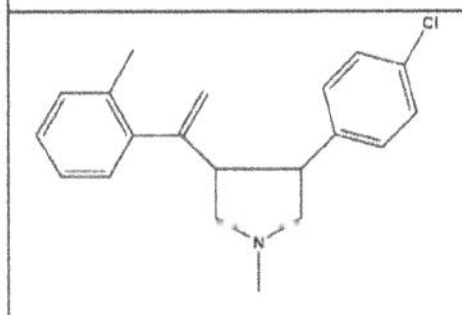	Dopamine transporter(DAT)	Quanta, Chem-X	0.084(IC50)	Enyedy IJ *et al.*, 2001

represented by the crucial receptor-ligand interaction points. These interaction points are usually generated by 3D-structure of receptor analysis (Koide Y,2003).

Some examples of *de novo* design methods applied in Drug Design is given Table **2**. The other approaches are developed before 2000 which have been reviewed in literature besides TOPAS and LEA (Murcko M,1997). The methods are divided into two categories: namely atom-based and fragment-based. The former techniques construct a molecule atom-by-atom, while later methods use sets of pre-defined molecular building blocks. Amongst them, fragment-based approaches are more advantageous appealing, because the virtual molecule can be constructed from combinatorial building blocks. In *rational Drug Design* methods shown in (Table **1**), LUDI (Accelrys, http://www.accelrys.com), Leapfrog (Tripos, http://www.tripos.com) and SPROUT (SimBioSys, http://www.simbiosys.ca) (Gillet VJ *et al.*, 1995 Mata P *et al.*, 1995) belong to fragment-based approaches. This approaches can be further divided into two subclasses: 1. sequential growth, 2. fragment-location and linking. The latter depends on a small

Table 2. Examples of denovo design methods

Method	Description	Ref.
CAVEAT	Fragment-based, fragment-based 3-D database search	Lauri G & Barlett PA, 1994.
CAVITY, FOUNDATION, DBMAKER, SPLICE	Fragment-based, generation of ligand by 3-D database search	Ho CMW & Marshall GR,1990; Ho CM. & Marshall GR,1993; Ho CM & Marshall GR,1995
CLIX	Fragment-based, fragment-based 3-D database search	Lawrence MC & Davis PC, 1992
CONCEPTS	Atom-based, stochastic search, MD optimization	Pearlman DA & Murcko MA.1993
CONCERTS	Fragment-based, stochastic search	Pearlman DA & Murcko MA 1996
DLD	Atom-based, structural sampling by Monte Carlo	Miranke A & Karplus M 1995
GenStar	Atom-based, sequential growth	Rotstein SH & Murcko MA 1993
GROW	Peptide design, sequential growth	Moon J & Howe W 1991
GrowMol	Fragment based, sequential growth	Bohacek RS & McMartin C 1994
HOOK	Fragment-based linker search	Eisen MB *et al.*, 1994
LEA	Fragment-based, genetic algorithm	Douguet D *et al.*, 2000
Leapfrog	Fragment-based, combinatorial search	LUDI (Accelrys, http://www.accelrys.com).
LEGEND	Atom-based, sequential growth	Nishibata Y & Itai A,1991
LUDI	Fragment-based, sequential growth, combinatorial search	Böhm HJ, 1992
MCDNLG	Atom-based, stochastic search	Gehlaar DK 1995
MCSS	Fragment-based, multiple-copy simultaneous sampling	Miranke A & Karplus M, 1991
NEWLEAD	Fragment-based, connecting pharmacophoric pieces	Tschinke V & Cohen NC, 1993
PRO_LIGAND	Fragment-based, sequential growth, combinatorial search	Clark DE *et al.*, 1995
SMOG	Fragment-based, sequential growth	DeWitt R & SMOG,1997
SPROUT	Fragment-based, sequential growth, combinatorial growth	Gillet VJ *et al.*, 1995

number of well-placed fragments, can provide a significant binding affinity. Both of these two classes of methods bear inherit advantages and disadvantages. These two LUDI and Leapfrog approaches are generally used.

The problem of most rational design methods may be synthetic inaccessibility which can be solved by using the program CLIX, SEEDS, CAVEAT to search the Available Chemicals Directory for scaffolds that contain designed ligands. To discover novel inhibitors of Factor Xa and DNA gyrase, the scaffold-based approach was used (Table **3**). The scaffold-based approach is almost similar to pharmacophore-based VS in much respect. These molecular fragments used as scaffolds can be considered as the pharmacophoric features in a pharmacophore model.

Applications of Combinatorial Drug Design

Genetic algorithm based Combinatorial Drug Design approaches are becoming important in this area. In (Table 2), both of TOPAS and LEA are based on genetic algorithm. In TOPAS (Schneider G *et al.*, 2000) a set of 24,563 molecular fragments serves as the building blocks, which were obtained by a straightforward fragmentation procedure from 36,000 known drugs. Several schemes were implemented for both fragmentation and building block assembly. This combination of drug assembly from building blocks and a restricted set of reaction schemes proved to be a key for the automation for novel structures. TOPAS is based on a simple evolutionary algorithm (EA), a (1, λ) evolution strategy. In optimization process, molecules were generated from a parent moiety by virtual synthesis and the best structure is selected as the parent for the subsequent TOPAS cycle. TOPAS was used to find the potential thrombin inhibitors. The first application of TOPAS was tried to develop molecules mimicking the NAPAP structure. The the fitness function was chosen asTanimoto index. After 12 optimization cycles the process converged at a high fitness level (0.86), and the best hit is similar to NAPAP (Figure 4). Moreover, it was used to the design of the peptide-analogues of the tripeptide D-Phe-Pro-Arg, an excellent natural thrombin substrate.

Compared with the other virtual screening approaches, the *rational* design methods do not show much progress in practical applications. However, it is used in lead generation methods. Recently, Ji *et al.* demonstrated several non-azole lead molecules by *de novo* design (http://www.molsoft.com.). All lead molecules exhibited potent inhibitory effects on CYP51 of *Candida albicans*. Table 3 shows the examples of bioactive molecules designed using *de novo* design.

VIRTUAL SCREENING BASED ON MOLECULAR DOCKING

Docking is defined as the fitting of ligands into exact position in receptor and applied as a very efficient way to study of protein-ligand interactions. The Structural information from ligand-receptor complex allowed us to trace the mechanism of molecular recognition, and to the predict binding affinities between receptor and ligands (Hou TJ *et al.*, 1999). It gives a detailed and exact computational model to identify a receptor-focused database. There are many docking programs available for use in virtual screening, differing in the sampling algorithm, scoring functions, the treatment of ligand flexibility with the receptor, and the docking time frame for a molecule to a given target. The commonly used docking programs are listed in (Table 4).

Figure 4. The structures afforded by (a) TOPAS (b) NAD NAPAP

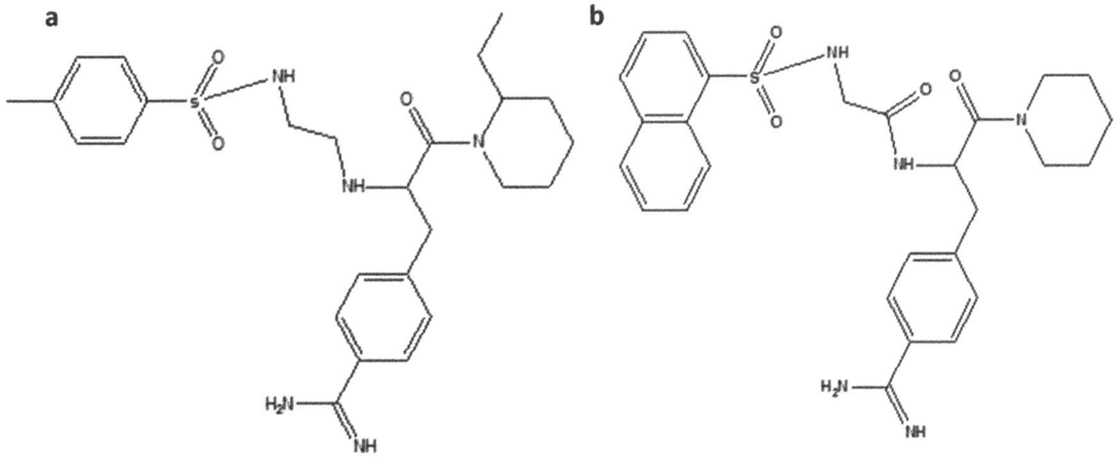

Table 3. Examples of bioactive molecules design using de novo design

MOLECULAR STRUCTURE	Target	Method	Activity	Ref.
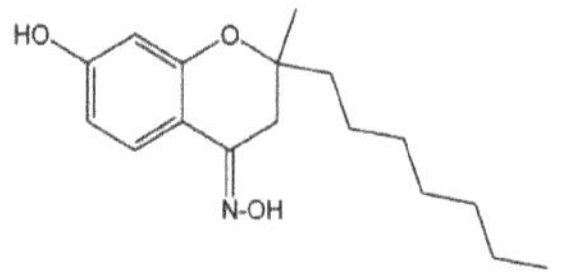	Lanosterol14α - demethylase(CYP51)	MCSS/LUDI	35.21(IC_{50})	Ji TT *et al.*, 2003
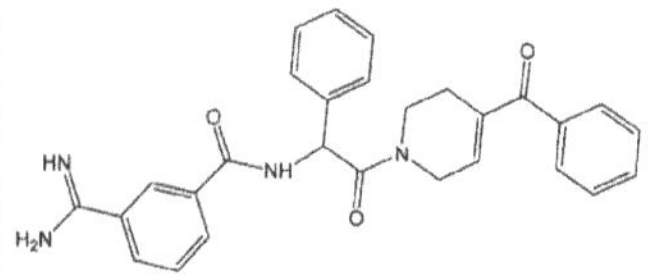	Factor X_a	PRO_SELECT	16nm(K_i)	Liebeschuetz JW *et al.*, 2002
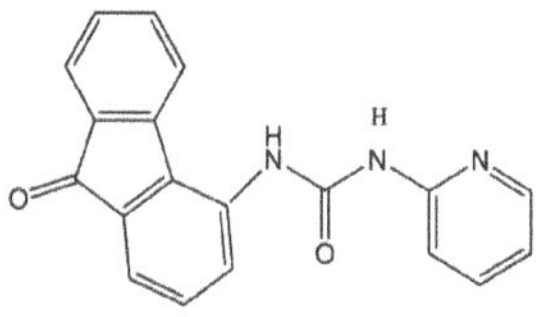	Cdk4	LEGEND/SEEDS	7.6(IC_{50})	Honma T *et al.*, 2001
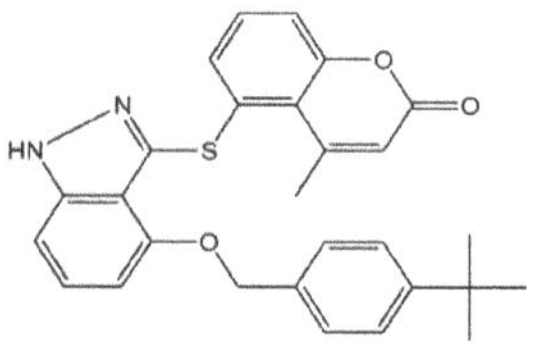	DNA gyrase	LUDI, CATALYST, MOLOC	0.03 (MNEC)	Boehm HJ *et al.*, 2000

Table 4. Commonly used docking programmes for virtual screening

Method	Sampling method	Scoring function	Speed	Ref.
DOCK	Incremental build	Force field, contact score, chemical complementary score	Fast	Ewing, TJ *et al.*, 2001
eHiTS	Exhaustive search	Empirical score	Fast	Zsoldos Z *et al.*, 2002
EUDOC	Exhaustive search	Force field	Fast	Pang YP *et al.*, 2001
FlexX	Incremental build	Empirical score	Fast	Rarey M *et al.*, 1996
LigandFit	Monte Carlo	Empirical score	Fast	Venkatachalam CM *et al.*, 2003
Fred	Conformational ensembles	Shape complementarity, Gaussian score	Fast	www.tripos.com
Slide	Conformational ensembles	Empirical score	Fast	Schnecke V & Kuln LA 2000
Glide	Exhaustive search	Empirical score	Slow	www.schrodinger.com
Gold	Genetic algorithm	Empirical score	Fast	Jones G *et al.*, 1997
QXP	Monte Carlo	Force field	Slow	McMartin C & Bohacek RS 1997

Molecular Docking and Successful Examples

In addition of traditional methods, such as DOCK, FlexX (Tripos, http://www.tripos.com), AutoDock, Gold (Cambridge Crystallographic Data Centre, http://www.ccdc.cam.ac.uk), ICM (MolSof, http://www.molsoft.com), some advanced docking programs have been released recently, including EUDOC, LigandFit (Accelrys, http://www.accelrys.com) and eHiTS (SimBioSys, http://www.simbiosys.ca). The EUDOC program has versatile in nature. Initially, the molecular flexibility of ligand and receptor is considered into account via either conformation selection theory or conformation substitution theory. Second, the program computes the intermolecular interaction energies of biologically important metal ions such as Zn^{2+}, Ca^{2+}, and Mg^{2+} that mediate the binding of a ligand to the receptor using a cationic dummy atom approach. Third, the program applies "spatial decomposition" to achieve maximum parallelism in computing. With the support of EUDOC program, the authors carried out a computational screening ACD (Available Chemicals Directory) database to identify prototypic inhibitors of FTase containing a zinc ion in the active site and found 21 compounds as potential inhibitor leads of FTase. Among these, 18 compounds have inhibitory activities against Ftase *in vitro* at 500 uM; and 4 compounds with *in vitro* IC_{50} values from 25 to 100 uM. The most active inhibitor also has inhibitory activity in human lung cancer cells. Furthermore, this lead molecule identified with the support of the EUDOC program, is more active than the recognized most strong inhibitor lead, kurasoin A.

Ligand Fit designed by Venkatachalam *et al.* belongs to a method used cavity tracing algorithm for detecting invaginations in the protein as candidate active site regions (Figure 5a). Monte Carlo conformational search with shape filter used for generating ligand poses consistently with the active site shape. The result is obtained after docking by alignment of the principal axes of the ligand to with receptor site (Figure 5b). Then the docking energy was used to as parameter to explore the best docking conformation of the drug. The docking energy is the sum of internal energy of the ligand and the interaction energy of ligand with the receptor. To minimize the errors from grid interpolation, a non-linear interpolation scheme was employed. The LigandFit was applied to 19 diverse protein-ligand complexes. The results are encouraging, reproducing the X-ray image ligand poses within an RMS of 2 Å in 14 out of 19 complexes. Moreover, HTP VS using LigandFit was applied to the thymidine kinase receptor. LigandFit yields outstanding results for a ligand pool seeded with known biological activities when combined with LigScore.

Figure 5. (a) Schematic diagram of the grid system enclosing the protein (black boundary), and (b) four orientations of the ligand matches the shape correlation between the ligand and the site

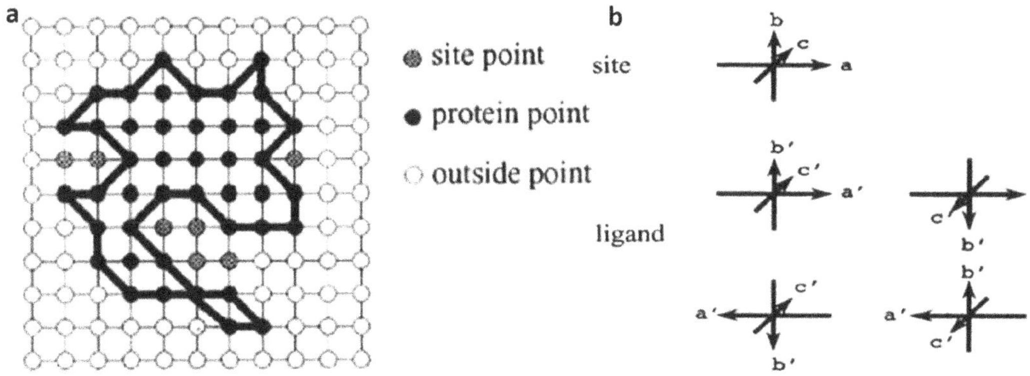

The eHiTs program was released by Sim Bio Sys, Inc. recently. In eHiTs, the algorithm applied is based on exhaustive graph matching that rapidly enumerates all possible mappings of interacting atoms between receptor and ligand. Then angles of rotatable bonds are computed as required by the positioning of the interacting groups. The optimal conformation can be found by using the algorithm. The scoring function is calculated by treatment of weak hydrogen bonds, aromatic -stacking and penalties for conflicting interactions. Alternatively, the target and its cavity details can be based on a pharmacophore model or a CoMFA study of overlaid lead compounds. A systematic and organized algorithm is used in eHiTs with no random, stochastic or evolutionary element and hence, it provides comprehensive search space coverage. eHiTs cut a ligand into rigid fragments which are docked in receptor and stores rigid fragment poses in Dock Table, a SQL database used to speed up the dockings by dynamically updating and retrieving molecular fragments.

All docking procedures suffer some methodological challenges: analysis of receptor-ligand conformations and evaluation of receptor-ligand matrix. In docking studies, the ligand is carefully treated with different computational techniques, such as incremental build and conformational search in DOCK and FlexX, the genetic algorithm in AutoDock and GOLD and pseudo-Brownian sampling in ICM etc. But the receptor flexibility remains a major challenge. The conformational changes and receptor flexibility induced by a ligand play very vital role in docking studies. The docking results may be questionable if the receptor flexibility is not given importance. Hou *et al.* verified the binding pattern of Quinazoline Type inhibitor complexed with EGF-R. DOCK calculations failed to give the proper orientation of inhibitor in EGF-R since it avoided the flexibility of the protein. (Hou TJ, 2003).

The receptor structures from NMR and molecular dynamics simulations are generally used to incorporate receptor flexibility. Recently, AutoDock was used to study several strategies for incorporating protein flexibility using receptor to generate Boltzmann-weighted grids which create the docking function (Osterberg F, 2002)

The reference crystal structures were super imposed, mapped and the structure of the possible receptor is generated. It is two-fold faster than explicit docking against all conformations when this assembly is used. (Claussen H *et al.*, 2001). The construction of receptor structures is computationally expensive because the docking process should be performed to each receptor structure, with an aim to identify all ligands that can bind to at least one conformational part of the receptor.

Now-a-days VS based molecular docking in rational Drug Design are very successful (Table 5),

Fcoring Functions

Docking of small molecules into their respective receptors is a novel tool in drug discovery process. The credibility of docking is based on precise scoring functions. These functions are used to trace the binding affinity of a novel molecule on active site of the receptor. Recently Scoring functions are a very active and becoming popular research area, in modern drug research. Here, a brief introduction of statistically-fit scoring functions, knowledge-based scoring functions, first-principle-based scoring functions and consensus scoring approach are given with suitable examples.

Statistically-fit scoring functions are widely used in molecular docking, and it assumes the total binding affinity of protein-ligand complexes to several empirical weighted-interaction terms, like metal-ligand interaction, hydrogen bonding, rotational entropy and hydrophobic interaction etc., (Gohlke H & Klebe G, 2002). The prime advantage of statistically-fit scoring functions are highly efficient and gives more

Table 5. Examples of drug molecules designed by Docking-Based Virtual Screening

Molecular Structure	Target	method	Activity	Ref.
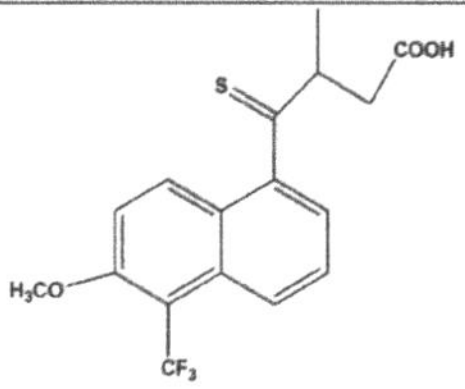	Aldol reductase(ALR2)	DOCK	0.10(IC_{50})	Rastelli *et al.*, 2002
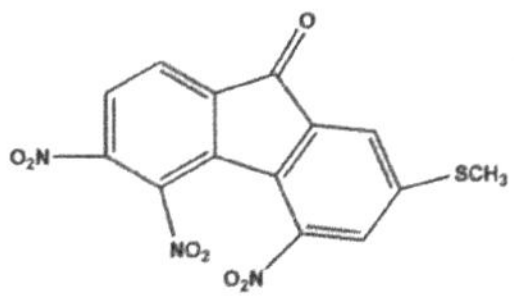	Adenovirus proteinase	EUDOC	3.09(k_i)	Pang YP *et al.*, 2001
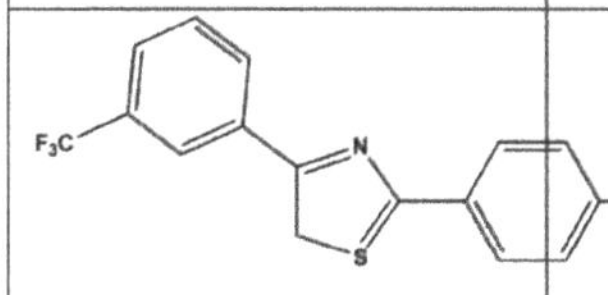	Retinoic acid receptor	ICM	2(ED_{50})	Schapira M *et al.*, 2000
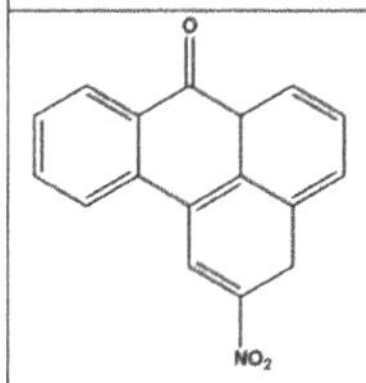	Protein tyrosine phosphate(PTPIB)	DOCK	21(Kis)	Sarmiento M *et al.*, 2000

intuitionistic knowledge of which specific force contributing to binding free energies. Unfortunately, it is limited to the training set.

In recent years, knowledge-based potentials are popular. It applies the statistical tool to extract rules on preferred binding geometries. The pseudo-potential based rules, which can be applied to predict the ligand binding conformations. These knowledge-based potentials implicitly incorporate physical effects such as (de) solvation and polarization. The knowledge-based potentials are derived from experimental crystal structures. Some examples are include SMoG (Grzybowski BA *et al.*, 2002; Ishchenko AV & Shakhnovich EI, 2002), PMF (Muegge I & Martin YC 1999), BLEEP (Mitchell JBO *et al.*, 1999), Drug Score (Gohlke H Hendlich M & Klebe G, 2000) and others (Verkhiver G *et al.*, 1995;Charifson PS,1999).

$$\Delta W_{ij}(r) \propto - \ln g_{ij}(r)/g_{ref}$$

where $g_{ij}(r)$ is the frequency or probability distribution of atom pairs of type i and j at a distance from each other, and g_{ref} corresponds to a reference distribution.

In these three knowledge-based potentials, Drug Score proposed by Gohlke *et al.* is the most practical one. The function used in Drug Score was developed by converting structural information for 1376 protein-ligand complexes, extracted from Relibase (Hendlich M,1998), into distance-dependent pair-potentials and solvent-accessible surface-dependent singlet-potentials using 17 different atoms. The sum was used to score protein-ligand interactions. For two test sets of 91 and 68 complexes, Drug Score reevaluated the multiple solutions proposed by FlexX, and gave the best solution. Moreover, Gohlke *et al.* compared the DrugScore and DOCK 4.0, and found that DrugScore is superior and predictive. DrugScore yields slightly superior results in flexible docking compared to the AutoDock Scoring function (Sotriffer CA *et al.*, 2002) and it is available in the SYBYL interface to FlexX.

Ishchenko reported SmolG2001 (Ischchenko AV *et al.*, 2002), an advanced knowledge-based scoring function of SMoG. In the advanced version, reference state defined in such a way that it ensured proper normalization of contact probabilities (sum of all values over atom types is equal to 1) and introduced to distance intervals ("bins") over which the contact statistics are computed. SMoG2001 reproduces the experimental binding constants with high accuracy and efficiency better than PMF and SCORE1 in LUDI, and comparable to DrugScore. Its predictive power will reduce when the affinities of ligands with metal ions and ligands that is large and flexible.

As compared to statistically-fit scoring functions, first-principle-based approaches calculate the total binding affinities to individual terms and computed from physico-chemical concept. first-principle-based approaches are theoretically rigorous as compared with scoring functions above, though they are relatively time-consuming and show more theoretical difficulties particularly entropy and de(solvation) effect. Kuntz groups have introduced PBSA (Possion-Boltzmann/surface area) and GBSA (Generalized Born/surface area) to evaluate de (solvation) contributions in molecular docking analysis (Zou X *et al.*, 1999). In First-principle-based approaches proposed by Kollman *et al., is* the 'MM-PBSA' approaches and play key role in this field (Kollman PA *et al.*, 2000). Here the binding free energy of a noncovalent associating for a protein-ligand system can be computed as:

$$\Delta G_{bind} = G_{complex} - G_{protein} - G_{ligand} = \Delta E_{MM} + \Delta G_{PB} + \Delta G_{NP} - T\Delta S \quad (2)$$

where G_{PB} is the polar solvation energy in continuum solvent, usually computed using a finite-difference Poisson-Boltzmann (PB) model, and G_{NP} is the nonpolar solvation energy, which is obtained from the solvent accessible surface area (SA). E_{MM} refers the sum of molecular mechanical (MM) energies of the molecules from internal, electrostatic and van der Waals energies. In equation 2 the final term denotes the solute entropy and estimated by a classical statistical formulas and normal mode analysis. The thermal energy terms in equation 2 are obtained from the MD sampling. The MM/PBSA technique was applied recently by Wang's *et al.*, to determine the binding mode between HIV-1 RT and efavirenz. The binding free energies between HIV-1 RT and efavirenz were calculated for the five possible binding modes, and recognized the exact one. Dupont Pharmaceuticals recently solved the crystal structure, and the RMSD of the ligand and its surroundings is 1.0 angstrom. Hou *et al.,* applied Molecular Dynamics simulations combined with MM-PBSA to determine the exact binding mode of the quinazoline inhibitor and EGF-R. The homology model of EGF-R was applied since the crystal structure of EGF-R is not available. When the crystal structure of quinazoline/EGF-R was reported, it is exciting to find that the best binding model predicted by MM-PBSA is very close to the structure (Hou TJ *et al.*, 2003). The crystal water molecules crucial to ligand binding were produced by the predicted model. In future research, MM/PBSA should be advanced to represent the entropic effects precisely and quickly.

In 1999, Charifson *et al.* used three scoring functions to classify the docked conformations (Charifson PS *et al.*, 1999). As Compared to a single scoring function, the hit rates can be effectively improved. Recently, Tripos introduced a module CScore (Consensus Score) (Tripos, http://www.tripos.com) to integrate a number of scoring functions for ranking the affinity of ligands bound to the active site of a target. The CScore module uses the consensus score and applies, five different scoring functions, namely G_score (Jones, G *et al.*, 1997), PMF_score(Muegge *et al.*, 1999), D_score(Kuntz *et al.*, 1982) and F_score, (Rarey *et al.*, 1996). In C Score, the range of scores are determined, above these range, the cutoff threshold are considered "good", and the consensus score is calculated by sum of the number of "good" results. The molecular docking can be improved by combining results from functions in CScore (Clark *et al.*, 2002), a consensus docking approach (ConsDock) proposed by Paul and Rogan that takes advantage of three widely used docking tools (Dock, FlexX and Gold) (Paul *et al.*, 2002). When applied to large data set it significantly does single docking with respect to the docking accuracy. Amongst all, ConsDock was able to predict the X-ray structure with 2 Å RMSD.

VIRTUAL SCREENING BASED ADME/TOX FILTERS

The failure of the Drug Design needs a predictive tool which eliminates the uncertainty factors. Almost the failures are resulting due to the complex uncertainty in pharmacokinetic properties. Hence computational screening should not be restricted only to binding affinity but also ADME/toxicity parameters.

In Silico Prediction of ADME Profiles

The "rule of 5" proposed by Lipinski *et al.* in 1997 played a vital role in tracking ADME profiles (Lipinski, CA 1997). Lipinski and coworkers analyzed a subset of 2245 drugs from the World Drug Index (WDI) and found that poor absorption and permeation are resulting in the conditions like a. the molecular weight is over 500, b. the octanol/water partition coefficient is over 5 (CLOGP) or 4.15 (MLOGP), c. The number of hydrogen-bond donors (OH and NH groups) is more than 5, and d. The number of hydrogen-bond acceptors (N and O atoms) is more than 10. The fast estimations of log*P* allow the "rule of 5" screening of library prior to enumeration. As per Lipinski, it is easier to optimize pharmacokinetic properties on early stage; therefore the receptor binding affinity can be optimized at a later stage (Lipinski CA, 2000).

ADME parameters are analyzed by many computational tools (Stenberg, P., *et al.* 2001; Chaturvedi PR *et al.*, 2001; Ekins S *et al.*, 2000). The properties like bioavailability, aqueous solubility, intestinal permeability, blood-brain barrier penetration, metabolism, drug-drug interactions, drug transport and toxicity are generally studied. The properties are predicted by two modeling methods: data modeling and molecular modeling. For molecular modeling, molecular mechanics, pharmacophore modeling, molecular docking, or quantum mechanics are used to explore the potential interactions between the small molecules and proteins in ADME processes. QSAR models ranging from simple multiple linear regression to modern multivariate analysis techniques or machine-leaning methods, such as partial least squares (PLS) (Cruciani G *et al.*, 2000), genetic algorithm (GA) (Hou TJ & Xu XJ, 2002), neural networks (NN) (Doniger S *et al.*, 2002), and support vector machines (SVM) are now being applied to analyze ADME data.

The predictions of aqueous solubility, blood-brain barrier penetration and intestinal permeability are usually based on the QSAR approaches. Most of the old predictive models for intestinal permeability or blood-brain barrier penetration are based on multiple linear regressions, and many used physicochemical properties, such as polar surface area, log*P*, volume, and hydrogen bonding capacity (Stenberg P *et al.*, 2001). Ghuloum *et al.* used a numerical molecular representation called molecular hashkey predict log*P* and intestinal absorption of a set of drugs (Ghuloum AM., 1999). In VolSurf, a 3D molecular field descriptor are transformed into a new set of descriptors, that was used as inputs for the construction of models for intestinal permeability, aqueous solubility, and blood-brain barrier penetration (van de *et al.*, 2003).

The relationships between oral bioavailability and molecular structures have been studied recently (Yoshica F & Toplss JG, 2000). The oral bioavailability prediction is difficult since it is based on absorption and liver first-pass metabolism. Yoshida and Topliss constructed QSAR model with a range of physiochemical parameters. The predictive power of the bioavailability model was evaluated using a separate test set of 40 compounds, of which 60% were correctly classified. Andrews *et al.* also proposed a QSAR model based on 591 compounds and 85 structural descriptors (Andrews CW *et al.*, 2000)

Moreover, compared with the Lipinski's rule of 5, the false negative predictions were reduced significantly. However, the predictability of these models is quite close to random, so it cannot be applied as a filter in virtual screening as the current form. Bans followed genetic programming to predict oral bioavailability (Bains W *et al.*, 2002). A slight improvement was observed than the Yoshida's results, although a direct comparison is difficult for four classes. Recently, Mandagere *et al.* proposed a graphical model for *in vitro* ADME data, such as Caco-2 permeability and metabolic stability in liver S9 or microsomes, to estimate %*F* into groups of low, medium, or high regions (Mandagere AK *et al.*, 2002). This graphical model provides a tool to estimate human oral bioavailability from *in vitro* ADME data to large databases. But the inputs to this model depend on other ADME-concerned properties, such as permeability and metabolic clearance, and thus cannot be used as high throughput fashion in virtual screening.

Theoretical studies of transporter proteins, especially P-Glycoprotein (p-gp) are active in recently because transport proteins are found in most organs involved in the uptake and removal of endogenous compounds and xenobiotics, including drugs (Ayrton A & Morgan P,2001). QSAR and pharmacophore modeling was applied to study the characteristic features of p-gp substrate, the interactions between substrate and P-gp (Wiese M & Pajeva IK, 2001; Pajeva IK. & Wiese M 2002). From the obtained results, we can give some explanations to the broad structural variety of the P-gp substrates and inhibitors and derive predicted models for discrimination between substrate and non-substrate, but at present, the accuracy of those models is too limited to be applied in computational screening.

The metabolism studies are also popular in recent years, due to the extent and rate of metabolism affect clearance, whereas the implications of enzymes might lead to issues related to the polymorphic nature of some of these enzymes and drug–drug interactions. Ekins *et al.* proposed pharmacophore modeling based on 3D/4D QSAR and to investigate the common structural features of cytochrome P450 (CYP) 2C9 inhibitors and interactions between competitive inhibitors and P4502C9 (Ekins S *et al.*, 2000; Ekins S, 2001). The obtained results from models of CYP inhibition will be useful for future prediction of drug-drug interactions. Cruciani *et al.* proposed MetaSite program to identify potential substrate of cytochrome P450s (Cruciani G, 2002), this model is based on pharmacophore model obtained from interaction fields for the protein structure and a fingerprint for the potential substrate. A linear PLS-based prediction system described by Zuegge for binary classification of drug-drug interaction liability is caused by cytochrome P450 A4 inhibition. It can be used as a valid filter in virtual screening because of its predictive power up to 95% of the training data, and 90% of a semi-independent validation dataset (Zuegge J *et al.*, 2002). Several approaches that use databases to predict metabolism are available or under development, including expert systems, such as MetabolExpert, META or Meteor and Metabolism (Langowski J & Long A, 2002; Ehrhardt PW,1999).

Overall, the number of ADME properties that can be predicted computationally is very limited. Due to the predictability of these approaches, properties including drug solubility, Caco-2 cell absorption, blood-brain barrier permeation, can be practically applied in rational screening. At present, the widely-used programs for ADME predictions include VolSurf (tripos, http://www.tripos.com) C2.ADME (accelrys, http://www.accelrys.com) and QikProp (schrödinger, http://www.schrödinger. com) .

VolSurf computes 3-D molecular interaction fields and uses image-processing methods to convert them into simple molecular descriptors that are easy to understand and interpret. These descriptors characterize the size, shape, polarity, and hydrophobicity of molecules, and the balance amongst them. Multivariate statistical methods within VolSurf also developed to relate its descriptors to biological properties. The ADME models included in VolSurf predict drug solubility, Caco-2 cell absorption, blood-brain barrier permeation, and drug distribution. These models have been developed from published experimental data from *in vitro* assays to correlate the in *vivo* behaviour of drugs. Recent studies have shown that models of membrane partitioning generated using VolSurf's descriptors are significantly more predictive than those generated from other descriptors. C2·ADME can give predictions for several ADME properties including passive intestinal absorption, blood-brain barrier (BBB) penetration, and a water solubility at 25°C. All three models are designed for analysis of combinatorial libraries, as well as individual molecules. The models were developed and validated using diverse compounds with data from the literature as well as data from Pharmacopeia Drug Discovery Services. C2·ADME overcome the necessity of 3-D structure generation which is laborious and time consuming.

Professor Bill Jorgensen has developed QikProp at Yale University; specifically, for drug discovery and results have been fitted to datasets of drug-like molecules, based on 2-D and 3-D descriptors reflecting Monte Carlo simulation studies as well as experiment. The calculated features of QikProp include Solubility, Blood/Brain barrier permeability, Caco-2 Cell Permeability Boehringer, Caco-2 Cell Permeability Affymax, MDCK Cell Permeability Affymax and Skin Permeability Coefficient.

In Silico Prediction of Toxicity

Toxicity is a key factor for many compounds failing to reach the market and for the withdrawal of a significant number of compounds from the market even after approved. The *in silico* prediction of toxicity can be divided into two basic categories: knowledge-based and statistically-based (Greene N, 2002; Durham SK & Pearl GM, 2001). Knowledge-based approaches adopt the rules based on relationships between structure and biological activity that are derived from human expert opinion and interpretation of toxicological data to predict the potential toxicity. But statistically-based approaches use the structural connectivity and statistical methods to acquire mathematical relationships for a training set of non-congeneric compounds in an unbiased manner. Currently, several commercial tools of *in silico* prediction of toxicity are available, which include; DEREK (LHASA Limited, http://www.chem.leeds.ac.uk), Hazard Expert, COMPACT, CASE and MCASE (MultiCASE, http://www.multicase.com), OncoLogic (LogiChem, http://www.logichem.com) and TOPKAT (accelrys, http://www.accelrys.com). The features, main strength and limitations of these programs have recently been reviewed . The primary emphasis of the current software packages is carcinogenicity and mutagenicity, teratogenicity, irritation, sensitization, immunotoxicology and neurotoxicity but the predictability of the commercial tools for toxicity prediction is quite limited. The National Toxicology Program has conducted several exercises to validate the predictability of the used programs. It analyzed 44 chemicals and the predictions made by Multi-CASE, TOPKAT, DEREK, and COMPACT were published in advance of the bioassays being performed. The predictions were then compared to the results from the experimental bioassays. The best prediction is given by DEREK, with a ratio of 59% and the predicted precision of the current programs should be promoted dramatically if necessary.

STRATEGIES FOR VIRTUAL SCREENING

If crystal structure of receptor and a prepared 3-D database are available, molecular docking can certainly be applied to obtain the best drug candidates. Usually, molecular docking is time-consuming, if the 3-D database, like ACDSC database, is very large, expensive. Figure 6 represents a typical strategy in virtual screening. First, one can use several ADME-concerned filters to minimize the size of the initial database. Common filtering protocols include "drug-like" property, Lipinski's rule or ADME properties. The rotatable bonds in molecules or polar surface areas can also be used as filters. Additional filters are

Figure 6. Structure based virtual screening

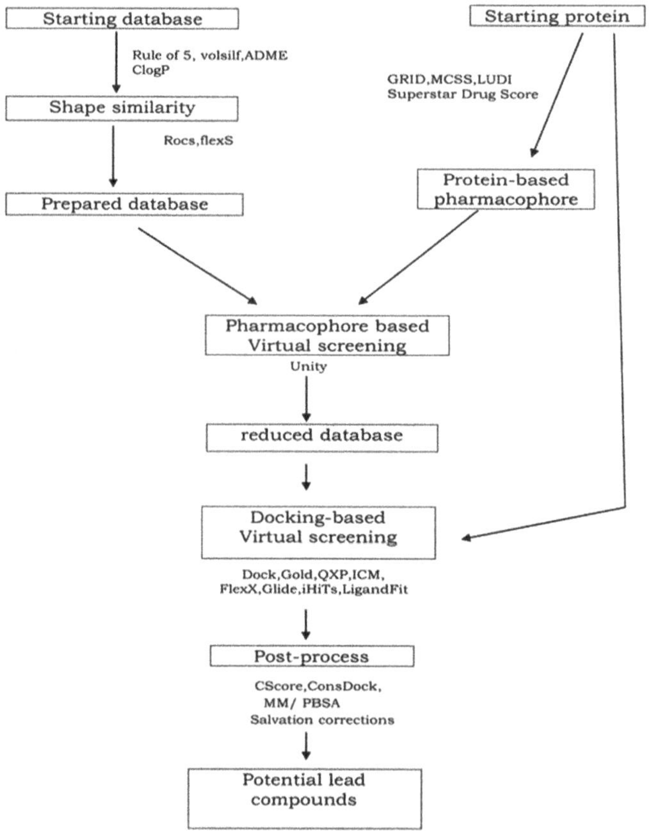

often applied to eliminate the compounds with poor chemical stability or toxicity. All of these filters can be applied to very large databases and are computationally inexpensive.

Second, if the inhibitors of a protein are available, then some computational tools can be used, such as FlexS (tripos, http://www.tripos.com) or ROCS (OpenEye, http://www.openeye.com), to reduce the database size by shape-similarity with known inhibitors. FlexS can rapidly overlay rigid ligands to the template molecule and screen large lists of ligands that make use of rapid rigid scoring, followed by flexible alignment of the best scoring ligands.

Then, the chemical characteristics of the binding site are analyzed to determine the functional group maps or hot spots for protein-ligand interactions, which can act as receptor-based pharmacophore model. This pharmacophore model combined with some steric constraints from receptor can be used as query of UNITY for 3-D database screening. After screening, only these compounds with appropriate chemical features complementary to the receptor-based pharmacophore model and suitable steric features survived. The receptor-based pharmacophore model is obtained from the analysis of the crystal complex structure or from computational programs such as GRID, MCSS, LUDI, Super Star. Virtual screening based on receptor-based pharmacophore model is slower than ligand-based screening, but much faster than molecular docking. After the above three stages of virtual screening, the size of the initial database was greatly reduced, and then processed through atom-based molecular docking screening.

The Maybridge (61,186 entries) and the Lead Quest (37, 841 entries) databases are used as a search engine. First, application of 5-rules reduced this initial set to 98,850 entries and then, UNITY search reduced to 5904 entries. In the next step, the favourable regions for protein-ligand interactions by using LUDI, GRID, Super Star and Drug Score are done. Flexible UNITY search were performed using the pharmacophore model based on the "hot spots" detected. Of the 5904 compounds, only 3314 entries satisfied the pharmacophore query. FlexS was used to superimpose all entries with two potent hCAII inhibitors and compute the similarity score concerning reference molecules. FlexS computed a superposition for 2237 compounds from selected 3314 compounds. In the final step, the 100 molecules from the FlexS filtering were docked into the binding pocket using FlexX. Visual inspection of binding modes of FlexX, together with the scoring values of FlexX, FlexS, and Drug Score, was used to select a small set of compounds for ordering and biological testing. Finally, 13 compounds were selected for biological assays, and 3 compounds have the inhibitory activities at the level of sub nanomolar, one is nanomolar, and rests are micromolar inhibitors.

Ultimately, virtual screening is knowledge-based, and we should apply a different strategy for a different problem in hand. It is recommended to use different combinations of virtual screening techniques and consider the subset of the database that satisfied the defined criteria. Certainly, the usage of whether this screening technique should be consistent with the available program and computational resources that can be used by researchers.

CONCLUSION

This chapter gives a summary of advanced technologies used in virtual screening, especially docking-based screening, scoring functions and ADME-based virtual screening. Furthermore, successful examples of VS are provided, demonstrating that VS has become a vital tool to find new lead compounds for the pharmaceutical industry. The quality of the scoring functions and ADME/Tox are still needs improvement. In molecular docking or *de novo* design approach, the scoring function is the central problem. all docking programs and scoring functions suffer from a significant number of false positives. Although, this problem has been partially solved by using several scoring functions, but still quality of the scoring functions should be needed to progress this technology further. Current models used to predict ADME/Tox are also very limited by low predictability. Further developments in virtual ADME/Tox are valuable for making this tool a reality and transforming more virtual molecules into real drugs. Hence it can be concluded that VS methods play a vital role in drug discovery programme and to intensify the research on various bio active molecules.

REFERENCES

Andrews, C. W., Bennett, L., & Yu, L. X. (2000). Predicting human oral bioavailability of a compound: Development of a novel quantitative structure-bioavailability relationship. *Pharmaceutical Research*, *17*(6), 639–644. doi:10.1023/A:1007556711109 PMID:10955834

Ayrton, A., & Morgan, P. (2001). The role of transport proteins in drug absorption, distribution and excretion. *Xenobiotica*, *31*(8-9), 469–497. doi:10.1080/00498250110060969 PMID:11569523

Bains, W., Gilbert, R., Sviridenko, L., Gascon, J. M., Scoffin, R., & Birchall, K. (2002). Evolutionary computational methods to predict oral bioavailability QSPRs. *Current Opinion in Drug Discovery & Development*, *5*, 44–51. PMID:11865672

Boehm, H. J., Boehringer, M., Bur, D., Gmuender, H., Huber, W., Klaus, W., ... Mueller, F. (2000). Novel inhibitors of DNA gyrase: 3-D structure based biased needle screening, hit validation by biophysical methods, and 3-D guided optimization A promising alternative to random screening. *Journal of Medicinal Chemistry*, *43*(14), 2664–2674. doi:10.1021/jm000017s PMID:10893304

Bohacek, R. S., & McMartin, C. (1994). Multiple highly diverse structures complementary to enzyme binding sites: Results of extensive application of a *de novo* design method incorporating combinatorial growth. *Journal of the American Chemical Society*, *116*(13), 5560–5571. doi:10.1021/ja00092a006

Brenk, R., Naerum, L., Grädler, U., Gerber, H. D., Garcia, G. A., Reuter, K., ... Klebe, G. (2003). Virtual screening for sub micromolar leads of tRNA-guanine transglycosylase based on new unexpected binding model detected by crystal structure analysis. *Journal of Medicinal Chemistry*, *46*(7), 1133–1143. doi:10.1021/jm0209937 PMID:12646024

Charifson, P. S., Corkerey, J. J., Murcko, M. A., & Walters, W. P. (1999). Consensus scoring: A method for obtaining improved hit rates from docking databases of three-dimensional structures into proteins. *Journal of Medicinal Chemistry*, *42*(25), 5100–5109. doi:10.1021/jm990352k PMID:10602695

Chaturvedi, P. R., Decker, C. J., & Odinecs, A. (2001). Prediction of pharmacokinetic properties using experimental approaches during early drug discovery. *Current Opinion in Chemical Biology*, *5*(4), 452–463. doi:10.1016/S1367-5931(00)00228-3 PMID:11470610

Chem-X version 96. (2001). Oxford Molecular Group, Inc.

Clark, D. E., Frenkel, D., Levy, S. A., Li, J., Murray, C. W., & Robson, B. (1995). PRO_LIGAND: An approach to *de novo* Drug Design. *Journal of Computer-Aided Molecular Design*, *9*, 13–32. doi:10.1007/BF00117275 PMID:7751867

Clark, R. D., Strizhev, A., Leonard, J. M., Blake, J. F., & Matthew, J. B. (2002). Consensus scoring for ligand/protein interactions. *Journal of Molecular Graphics & Modelling*, *20*(4), 281–295. doi:10.1016/S1093-3263(01)00125-5 PMID:11858637

Claussen, H., Buning, C., Rarey, M., & Lengauer, T. (2001). FlexE: Efficient molecular docking considering protein structure variations. *Journal of Molecular Biology*, *308*(2), 377–395. doi:10.1006/jmbi.2001.4551 PMID:11327774

Cruciani, G., Crivori, P., Carrupt, P. A., & Testa, B. (2000). Molecular fields in quantitative structure-permeation relationships: The VolSurf approach. *Theochem*, *53*(1-2), 17–30. doi:10.1016/S0166-1280(99)00360-7

Debouck, C., & Metcalf, B. (2000). The impact of genomics on drug discovery. *Annual Review of Pharmacology and Toxicology*, *40*(1), 193–207. doi:10.1146/annurev.pharmtox.40.1.193 PMID:10836133

DeWitt, R. & SMOG. (1997). *de novo* design method based on simple, fast, and accurate free energy estimates 2 case studies in molecular design. *J Am Chem Soc, 119*, 4608-17.

Doniger, S., Hofmann, T., & Yeh, J. (2002). Predicting CNS permeability of drug molecules: Comparison of neural network and support vector machine algorithms. *Journal of Computational Biology*, *9*(6), 849–864. doi:10.1089/10665270260518317 PMID:12614551

Douguet, D., Thoreau, E., & Grassy, G. A. (2000). Genetic algorithm for the automated generation of small organic molecules: Drug Design using an evolutionary algorithm. *Journal of Computer-Aided Molecular Design*, *14*(5), 449–466. doi:10.1023/A:1008108423895 PMID:10896317

Durham, S. K., & Pearl, G. M. (2001). Computational methods to predict drug safety liabilities. *Drug Disc Dev*, *4*, 110–115. PMID:11727316

Ehrhardt, P. W. (1999). *Drug Metabolism Databases and High–Throughput Testing During Drug Design and Development. Blackwell Science.*

Eisen, M. B., Wiley, D. C., Karplus, M., & Hubbard, R. E. (1994). HOOK: A program for finding novel molecular architectures that satisfy the chemical and steric requirements of a macromolecule binding site. *Proteins*, *19*(3), 199–221. doi:10.1002/prot.340190305 PMID:7937734

Ekins, S., Bravi, G., Binkley, S., Gillespie, J. S., Ring, B. J., & Wikel, J. H. (2000). Three- and four-dimensional quantitative structure-activity relationship (3D/4D-QSAR) analyses of CYP2C9 inhibitors. *Drug Metabolism and Disposition: the Biological Fate of Chemicals*, *28*, 994–1002. PMID:10901712

Ekins, S., De Groot, M., & Jones, J. P. (2001). Pharmacophore and three-dimensional quantitative structure-activity relationship methods for modeling cytochrome P450 active sites. *Drug Metabolism and Disposition: the Biological Fate of Chemicals*, *29*, 936–944. PMID:11408357

Ekins, S., Ring, B. J., Grace, J., McRobie-Belle, D. J., & Wrighton, S. A. (2000). Present and further *in vitro* approaches for drug metabolism. *Journal of Pharmacological and Toxicological Methods*, *44*(1), 313–324. doi:10.1016/S1056-8719(00)00110-6 PMID:11274898

Enyedy, I. J., Sakamuri, S., Zaman, W. A., Johnson, K. M., & Wang, S. M. (2003). Pharmacophore-based discovery of substituted pyridines as novel dopamine transporter inhibitors. *Bioorganic & Medicinal Chemistry Letters*, *11*, 1123–1135. PMID:12565962

Enyedy, I. J., Zaman, W. A., Sakamuri, S., Kozikowski, A. P., Johnson, K. M., & Wang, S. M. (2001). Pharmacophore-based discovery of 3, 4-disubstituted pyrrolidines as a novel class of monoamine transporter inhibitors. *Bioorganic & Medicinal Chemistry Letters*, *11*(9), 1113–1118. doi:10.1016/S0960-894X(01)00132-9 PMID:11354356

Ewing, T. J., Makino, S., Skillman, A. G., & Kuntz, I. D. (2001). DOCK 40: Search strategies for automated molecular docking of flexible molecule database. *Journal of Computer-Aided Molecular Design*, *15*(5), 411–428. doi:10.1023/A:1011115820450 PMID:11394736

Fox, T., & Haaksma, E. E. J. (2000). Computer based screening of compound database: 1 preselection of benzamidine-based thrombin inhibitor. *Journal of Computer-Aided Molecular Design*, *14*(5), 411–425. doi:10.1023/A:1008167012101 PMID:10896314

Gehlaar, D. K. (1995). *De novo* design of enzyme inhibitors by Monte Carlo ligand generation. *Journal of Medicinal Chemistry*, *38*(3), 466–472. doi:10.1021/jm00003a010 PMID:7853340

Ghuloum, A. M., Sage, C. R., & Jain, A. N. (1999). Molecular hash keys: A novel method for molecular characterization and its application for predicting important pharmaceutical properties of molecules. *Journal of Medicinal Chemistry*, *42*(10), 1739–1748. doi:10.1021/jm980527a PMID:10346926

Gillet, V. J., Myatt, G., Zsoldos, Z., & Johnson, A. P. (1995). SPROUT, HIPPO AND CAESA: Tools for *de novo* structure generation and estimation of synthetic accessibility. *Perspectives in Drug Discovery and Design*, *3*(1), 34–50. doi:10.1007/BF02174466

Glide. (n.d.). Retrieved from www.schrodinger.com

Gohlke, H., Hendlich, M., & Klebe, G. (2000). Knowledge-based scoring function to predict protein-ligand interactions. *Journal of Molecular Biology*, *20*(2), 337–356. doi:10.1006/jmbi.1999.3371 PMID:10623530

Gohlke, H., & Klebe, G. (2002). Approaches to the description and prediction of the binding affinity of small-molecule ligands to macromolecular receptors. *Angewandte Chemie International Edition*, *41*(15), 2644–2676. doi:10.1002/1521-3773(20020802)41:15<2644::AID-ANIE2644>3.0.CO;2-O PMID:12203463

Goodford, P. J. (1985). A computational procedure for determining energetically favorable binding sites on biologically important macromolecules. *Journal of Medicinal Chemistry*, *28*(7), 849–857. doi:10.1021/jm00145a002 PMID:3892003

Greene, N. (2002). Computer systems for the prediction of toxicity: An update. *Advanced Drug Delivery Reviews*, *54*(3), 417–431. doi:10.1016/S0169-409X(02)00012-1 PMID:11922956

Grzybowski, B. A., Ishchenko, A. V., Shimada, J., Whitesides, G. M., & Shakhnovich, E. I. (2002). From knowledge-based potentials to combinatorial lead design *in silico*. *Accounts of Chemical Research*, *5*(5), 261–269. doi:10.1021/ar970146b PMID:12020163

Gund, P. (1977). Three-dimensional Pharmacophore Pattern Searching. *Progress in Molecular and Subcellular Biology*, *5*, 117–143. doi:10.1007/978-3-642-66626-1_4

Hendlich, M. (1998). Databases for protein-ligand complexes. *Acta Crystallographica. Section D, Biological Crystallography*, *54*(6), 1178–1182. doi:10.1107/S0907444998007124 PMID:10089494

Hertzberg, R. P., & Pope, A. J. (2000). High-throughput screening: New technology for the 21st century. *Current Opinion in Chemical Biology*, *4*(4), 445–451. doi:10.1016/S1367-5931(00)00110-1 PMID:10959774

Hindle, S. A., Rarey, M., Buning, C., & Lengauer, T. (2002). Flexible docking under pharmacophore type constraints. *Journal of Computer-Aided Molecular Design*, *16*(2), 129–149. doi:10.1023/A:1016399411208 PMID:12188022

Ho, C. M., & Marshall, G. R. (1993). FOUNDATION: A program to retrieve all possible structures containing a user-defined minimum number of matching query elements from three-dimensional databases. *Journal of Computer-Aided Molecular Design*, *7*, 623–647. doi:10.1007/BF00125322 PMID:8473917

Ho, C. M., & Marshall, G. R. (1995). DBMAKER: A set of programs designed to generate three-dimensional databases based upon user-specific criteria. *Journal of Computer-Aided Molecular Design*, *9*(1), 65–86. doi:10.1007/BF00117279 PMID:7751871

Ho, C. M. W., & Marshall, G. R. (1990). Cavity search: An algorithm for the isolation and display of cavity-like binding regions. *Journal of Computer-Aided Molecular Design*, *4*(4), 337–354. doi:10.1007/BF00117400 PMID:2092080

Honma, T., Hayashi, K., Aoyama, T., Hashimoto, N., Machida, T., Fukasawa, K., ... Morishima, H. (2001). Structure-based generation of a new class of potent Cdk4 inhibitors: New *de novo* design strategy and library design. *Journal of Medicinal Chemistry*, *44*(26), 4615–4627. doi:10.1021/jm0103256 PMID:11741479

Hou, T. J., Wang, J. M., Chen, L. R., & Xu, X. J. (1999). Automatic docking of peptides and proteins using a hybrid method combined with genetic algorithm and tabu search. *Protein Engineering*, *12*, 639–647. doi:10.1093/protein/12.8.639 PMID:10469824

Hou, T. J., & Xu, X. J. (2002). ADME Evaluation in Drug Discovery: Applications of genetic algorithms on the prediction of blood-brain partitioning of a large set drug. *Journal of Molecular Modeling*, *8*(12), 337–349. doi:10.100700894-002-0101-1 PMID:12541001

Hou, T. J., Zhu, L. L., Chen, L. R., & Xu, X. J. (2003). Mapping the binding site of a large set of quinazoline type EGF-R inhibitors using molecular field analyses and molecular docking studies. *Journal of Chemical Information and Computer Sciences*, *43*(1), 273–287. doi:10.1021/ci025552a PMID:12546563

Ischchenko, A. V., & Shakhnovich, E. I. (2002). Small molecular growth 2001 (SMoG2001): An improved knowledge-based scoring function for protein-ligand interactions. *Journal of Medicinal Chemistry*, *45*(13), 2770–2780. doi:10.1021/jm0105833 PMID:12061879

Ji, T. T., Zhang, W. N., Zhang, M., Kudo, M., Aoyama, Y., Yoshida, Y., ... Zhu, J. (2003). Structure-based *de novo* design, synthesis, and biological evaluation of non-azole inhibitors specific for lanosterol 14α-demethylase of fungi. *Journal of Medicinal Chemistry*, *46*(4), 474–485. doi:10.1021/jm020362c PMID:12570370

Jones, G., Willett, P., Glen, R., Leach, A. R., & Taylor, R. (1997). Development and validation of a genetic algorithm for flexible docking. *Journal of Molecular Biology*, *267*(3), 727–748. doi:10.1006/jmbi.1996.0897 PMID:9126849

Koide, Y., Tatsui, A., Hasegawa, T., Nurakami, A., Satoh, S., & Yamada, H. (2003). Identification of a stable chymase inhibitor using a pharmacophore-based database search. *Bioorganic & Medicinal Chemistry Letters*, *13*(1), 25–29. doi:10.1016/S0960-894X(02)00853-3 PMID:12467610

Kollman, P. A., Massova, I., Reyes, C., Kuhn, B., Huo, S. H., Chong, L., ... Cheatham, T. E. (2000). Calculating structures and free energies of complex molecules: Combining molecular mechanics and continuum models. *Accounts of Chemical Research*, *33*(12), 889–897. doi:10.1021/ar000033j PMID:11123888

Kuntz, I. D., Blaney, J. M., Oatley, S. J., Langridge, R., & Ferrin, T. E. (1982). A geometric approach to macromolecule-ligand interactions. *Journal of Molecular Biology*, *161*(2), 269–288. doi:10.1016/0022-2836(82)90153-X PMID:7154081

Kurogi, Y., & Guner, O. F. (2001). Pharmacophore modeling and three-dimensional database searching for Drug Design using catalyst. *Current Medicinal Chemistry*, *8*(9), 1035–1055. doi:10.2174/0929867013372481 PMID:11472240

Langer, T., & Hoffmann, R. D. (2001). Virtual screening: An effective tool for lead structure discovery? *Current Pharmaceutical Design*, *7*(7), 509–527. doi:10.2174/1381612013397861 PMID:11375766

Langowski, J., & Long, A. (2002). Computer systems for the prediction of xenobiotic metabolism. *Advanced Drug Delivery Reviews*, *54*(3), 407–415. doi:10.1016/S0169-409X(02)00011-X PMID:11922955

Lauri, G., & Barlett, P. A. (1994). CAVEAT: A program to facilitate the design of organic molecules. *Journal of Computer-Aided Molecular Design*, *8*(1), 51–66. doi:10.1007/BF00124349 PMID:8035213

Lawrence, M. C., & Davis, P. C. (1992). CLIX: A search algorithm for finding novel ligands capable of binding proteins of known three-dimensional structure. *Proteins*, *12*(1), 31–41. doi:10.1002/prot.340120105 PMID:1313175

Liebeschuetz, J. W., Jones, S. D., Morgan, P. J., Murray, C. W., Rimmer, A. D., Roscoe, J. M. E., ... Wilkinson, K. (2002). PRO_SELECT: Combining structure-based Drug Design and array-based chemistry for rapid lead discovery 2 the development of a series of highly potent and selective factor Xa inhibitors. *Journal of Medicinal Chemistry*, *45*(6), 1221–1232. doi:10.1021/jm010944e PMID:11881991

Lipinski, C. A. (2000). Druglike properties and the causes of poor solubility and poor permeability. *Journal of Pharmacological and Toxicological Methods*, *44*(1), 235–249. doi:10.1016/S1056-8719(00)00107-6 PMID:11274893

Lipinski, C. A., Lombardo, F., Dominy, B. W., & Feeney, P. J. (1997). Experimental and computational approaches to estimate solubility and permeability in drug discovery and development settings. *Advanced Drug Delivery Reviews*, *23*(1-3), 3–25. doi:10.1016/S0169-409X(96)00423-1 PMID:11259830

Lyne, P. D. (2002). Structure-based virtual screening: An overview. *Drug Discovery Today*, *7*(20), 1602178. doi:10.1016/S1359-6446(02)02483-2 PMID:12546894

Mandagere, A. K., Thompson, T. N., & Hwang, K. K. (2002). A graphical model for estimating oral bioavailability of drugs in humans and other species from their Caco-2 permeability and *in vitro* liver enzyme metabolic stability rates. *Journal of Medicinal Chemistry*, *45*(2), 304–311. doi:10.1021/jm010152k PMID:11784135

Mata, P., Gillet, V. J., Johnson, A. P., Lampreia, J., Myatt, G. J., Sike, S., & Stebbings, A. L. (1995). SPROUT-3D structure generation using templates. *Journal of Chemical Information and Computer Sciences*, *35*(3), 479–493. doi:10.1021/ci00025a016

McMartin, C., & Bohacek, R. S. (1997). QXP: Powerful, rapid computer algorithms for structure-based Drug Design. *Journal of Computer-Aided Molecular Design*, *11*(4), 333–344. doi:10.1023/A:1007907728892 PMID:9334900

Miranker, A., & Karplus, M. (1991). Functionality maps of binding sites: A multiple copy simultaneous search method. *Proteins*, *11*(1), 29–34. doi:10.1002/prot.340110104 PMID:1961699

Miranker, A., & Karplus, M. (1995). An automated-method for dynamic ligand design. *Proteins*, *23*(4), 472–490. doi:10.1002/prot.340230403 PMID:8749844

Mitchell, J. B. O., Laskowski, R. A., Alex, A., & Thornton, J. M. (1999). BLEEP-potential of mean force describing protein-ligand interactions: I generating potential. *Journal of Computational Chemistry*, *20*(11), 1165–1176. doi:10.1002/(SICI)1096-987X(199908)20:11<1165::AID-JCC7>3.0.CO;2-A

Moon, J., & Howe, W. (1991). Computer design of bioactive molecules: A method for receptor-based *de novo* ligand design. *Proteins*, *11*(4), 314–328. doi:10.1002/prot.340110409 PMID:1758885

Muegge, I., & Martin, Y. C. (1999). A general and fast scoring function for protein-ligand interactions: A simplified potential approach. *Journal of Medicinal Chemistry*, *42*(5), 791–804. doi:10.1021/jm980536j PMID:10072678

Murcko, M. (1997). Recent advances in ligand design methods. *Reviews in Computational Chemistry*, *11*, 1–66.

Nishibata, Y., & Itai, A. (1991). Automatic creation of drug candidate structures based on receptor structure-starting point for artificial lead generation. *Tetrahedron*, *47*(43), 8985–8990. doi:10.1016/S0040-4020(01)86503-0

Osterberg, F., Morris, G. M., Sanner, M. F., Olson, A. J., & Goodsell, D. S. (2002). Automated docking to multiple target structures: Incorporation of protein mobility and structural water heterogeneity in Auto Dock. *Proteins*, *46*(1), 34–40. doi:10.1002/prot.10028 PMID:11746701

Pajeva, I. K., & Wiese, M. (2002). Pharmacophore model of drugs involved in P-glycoprotein multidrug resistance: Explanation of structural variety (hypothesis). *Journal of Medicinal Chemistry*, *45*(26), 5671–5686. doi:10.1021/jm020941h PMID:12477351

Pang, Y. P., Perola, E., Xu, K., & Prendergast, F. G. (2001). Predergast FG. EDUDOC: A computer program for identification of drug interaction sites in macromolecules and drug leads from chemical databases. *Journal of Computational Chemistry*, *22*(15), 1750–1771. doi:10.1002/jcc.1129 PMID:12116409

Pang, Y. P., Xu, K., Kollmeyer, T. M., Perola, E., McGrath, W. J., Green, D. T., & Mangel, W. F. (2001). Discovery of a new inhibitor lead of adenovirus proteinase: Steps towards selective, irreversible inhibitors of cysteine proteinases. *FEBS Letters*, *502*(3), 93–97. doi:10.1016/S0014-5793(01)02672-2 PMID:11583118

Paul, N., & Rognan, D. (2002). ConsDock: A new program for the consensus analysis of protein-ligand interactions. *Proteins*, *47*(4), 521–533. doi:10.1002/prot.10119 PMID:12001231

Pearlman, D. A., & Murcko, M. A. (1993). CONCEPTS: New dynamics algorithm for *de novo* drug suggestions. *Journal of Computer-Aided Molecular Design*, *14*, 1184.

Pearlman, D. A., & Murcko, M. A. (1996). CONCERTS: Dynamics connection of fragments as an approach to *De novo* ligand design. *Journal of Computer-Aided Molecular Design*, *39*, 1651–1663. PMID:8648605

QikProp. (n.d.). Retrieved from http://www.schrodinger.com

Rarey, M., Kramer, B., Lengauer, T., & Klebe, G. A. (1996). Fast Flexible Docking Method using an Incremental Construction Algorithm. *Journal of Molecular Biology*, *261*(3), 470–489. doi:10.1006/jmbi.1996.0477 PMID:8780787

Rastelli, G., Ferrari, A. M., Costantino, L., & Gamberini, M. C. (2002). Discovery of new inhibitors of aldose reductase from molecular modeling and database searching. *Bioorganic & Medicinal Chemistry*, *10*(5), 1437–1450. doi:10.1016/S0968-0896(01)00410-2 PMID:11886806

Rotstein, S. H., & Murcko, M. A. (1993). GenStar: A method for *de novo* Drug Design. *Journal of Computer-Aided Molecular Design*, *7*(1), 23–43. doi:10.1007/BF00141573 PMID:8473916

Rotstein, S. H., & Murcko, M. A. (1993). Group Build: A fragment-based method for *de novo* Drug Design. *Journal of Medicinal Chemistry*, *36*(12), 1700–1710. doi:10.1021/jm00064a003 PMID:8510098

Sarmiento, M., Wu, L., Keng, Y. F., Song, L., Luo, Z. W., Huang, Z. W., ... Zhang, Z.-Y. (2000). Structure-based discovery of small inhibitors targeted to protein tyrosine phosphatase 1B. *Journal of Medicinal Chemistry*, *3*(2), 146–155. doi:10.1021/jm990329z PMID:10649970

Schapira, M., Raaka, B. M., Samuels, H. H., & Abagyan, R. (2000). Rational discovery of novel nuclear hormone receptor antagonists. *Proceedings of the National Academy of Sciences of the United States of America*, *97*(3), 1008–1013. doi:10.1073/pnas.97.3.1008 PMID:10655475

Schnecke, V., & Kuln, L. A. (2000). Virtual screening with solvation and ligand-induced complementarity. *Perspect Drug Des Discov*, *20*(1), 171–190. doi:10.1023/A:1008737207775

Schneider, G., & Böhm, H. J. (2002). Virtual screening and fast automated docking methods. *Drug Discovery Today*, *7*, 63–70. doi:10.1016/S1359-6446(02)00004-1 PMID:11790605

Schneider, G., Lee, M. L., Stahl, M., & Schneider, P. (2000). *De novo* design of molecular architectures by evolutionary assembly of drug-derived building blocks. *Journal of Computer-Aided Molecular Design*, *14*(5), 487–494. doi:10.1023/A:1008184403558 PMID:10896320

Sotriffer, C. A., Gohlke, H., & Klebe, G. (2002). Docking into knowledge-based potential fields: A comparative evaluation of DrugScore. *Journal of Medicinal Chemistry*, *45*(10), 1967–1970. doi:10.1021/jm025507u PMID:11985464

Stenberg, P., Norinder, U., Luthman, K., & Artursson, P. (2001). Experimental and computational screening models for the prediction of intestinal drug absorption. *Journal of Medicinal Chemistry*, *44*(12), 1927–1937. doi:10.1021/jm001101a PMID:11384238

Tschinke, V., & Cohen, N. C. (1993). The NEWLEAD program: A new method for the design for the design of candidate structures from pharmacophoric hypotheses. *Journal of Medicinal Chemistry*, *36*(24), 3863–3870. doi:10.1021/jm00076a016 PMID:8254618

van de Waterbeemd, H., & Gifford, E. (2003). ADMET *in silico* modeling: Towards prediction paradise? *Nature Reviews. Drug Discovery*, *2*, 192–204. PMID:12612645

Venkatachalam, C. M., Jiang, X., Oldfield, T., & Waldman, M. (2003). LigandFit: A novel method for the shape-directed rapid docking of ligands to protein active sites. *J Mol Graphics Mol Mod*, *21*(4), 289–307. doi:10.1016/S1093-3263(02)00164-X PMID:12479928

Verkhiver, G., Appelt, K., Freer, S. T., & Villafrancda, J. E. (1995). Empirical free energy calculations of protein-ligand crystallographic complexes I knowledge-based ligand-protein interaction potentials applied to the prediction of human immunodeficiency virus 1 protease binding affinity. *Protein Engineering*, *8*(7), 677–691. doi:10.1093/protein/8.7.677 PMID:8577696

Walters, W. P., Stahl, M. T., & Murcko, M. A. (1998). Virtual screening-an overview. *Drug Discovery Today*, *3*(4), 160–178. doi:10.1016/S1359-6446(97)01163-X

Wiese, M., & Pajeva, I. K. (2001). Structure-activity relationships of multidrug resistance reversers. *Current Medicinal Chemistry*, *8*(6), 685–713. doi:10.2174/0929867013373138 PMID:11281849

Yoshica, F., & Toplss, J. G. (2000). QSAR model for drug human oral bioavailability. *Journal of Medicinal Chemistry*, *43*(13), 2575–2585. doi:10.1021/jm0000564 PMID:10891117

Yoshida, K., & Niwa, T. (2006). Quantitative Structure–Activity Relationship Studies on Inhibition of HERG Potassium Channels. *Journal of Chemical Information and Modeling*, *46*(3), 1371–1378. doi:10.1021/ci050450g PMID:16711756

Zou, X., Sun, Y., & Kuntz, I. D. (1999). Inclusion of solvation in ligand binding free energy calculations using the generalized-Born model. *Journal of the American Chemical Society*, *121*(35), 8033–8043. doi:10.1021/ja984102p

Zsoldos, Z., Johnson, A. P., Simon, A., & Szabo, I. (2002). *eHiTS: Novel algorithm for fast, exhaustive flexible ligand docking and scoring*. Presentation at the *224th ACS National Meeting*, Boston, MA.

Zuegge, J., Fechner, U., Roche, O., Parratt, N. J., Engkvist, O., & Schneider, G. (2002). A fastvirtual screening filter for cytochrom450 3A4 inhibition liability of compound libraries. *QSAR*, *21*, 249–256.

Chapter 6
Computational Investigation of Versatile Activity of Piperine

Thenmozhi Marudhadurai
Selvam College of Technology, India

Navabshan Irfan
Anna University, India

ABSTRACT

Piperine is known for its versatile therapeutic activity. It has been used for various disease conditions (e.g., cold, cough, etc.). Piperine is an alkaloid found in black pepper. It possesses various pharmacological actions like anti-inflammatory, anti-oxidant, anti-cholinergic, and anti-cancerous. The above-mentioned properties will be studied by selecting target proteins COX-2 protein, angiotensin converting enzyme, acetylcholineesterases, and survivin using computational docking study. This chapter explains the inhibition property of piperine against selected target protein from the results of docking studies. Based on the docking scores and protein-ligand interactions, piperine was found to bind well in the active site of the selected target proteins. It ensures the binding efficacy of piperine against selected target proteins. Docking scores and protein-ligand interactions plays an important role in its therapeutic activity.

INTRODUCTION TO PIPERINE

Piperine is an alkaloid widely present in the fruit of black pepper. Pepper is obtained from the medicinal plant, *Piper nigerum* and belongs to *piperacea* family (Figure 1) (Zoheir and Aftab, 2014). Piperine (Figure2) has wide therapeutic activity like anti-inflammatory, anti-oxidant property, antimicrobial activity, etc. (Vijaya kumar *et al*., 2014, Nisar ahmad *et al*., 2012). Many experimental studies revealed that it enhances oral bioavailability of certain drugs, nutrients and vaccines by inhibiting certain enzymes (Majeed and Prakash, 2000, Keith singletssry, 2010).

DOI: 10.4018/978-1-5225-7326-5.ch006

Figure 1. Black pepper

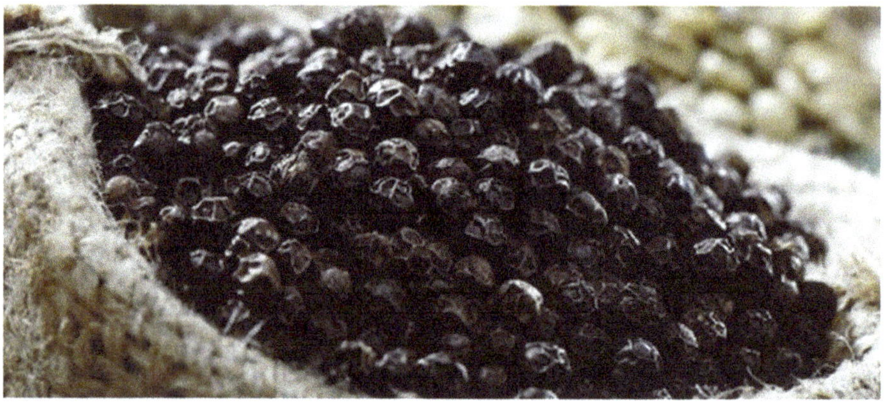

Figure 2. Piperine extracted from black pepper

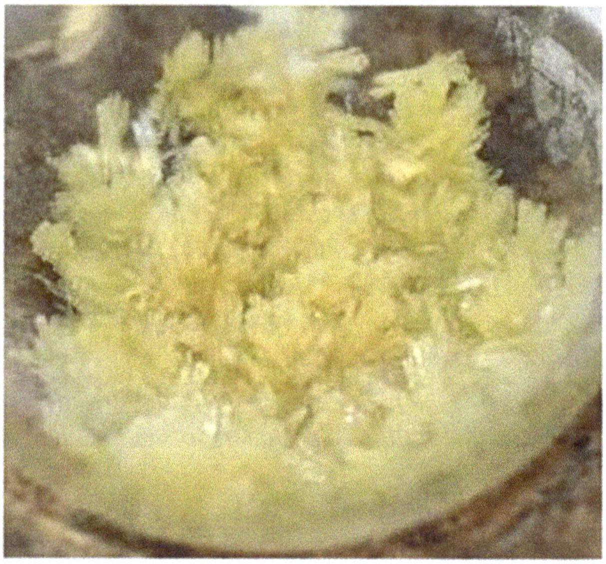

STRUCTURE OF PIPERINE

The structure of piperine (Figure 3) consists of methylenedioxyphenyl ring, basic piperidine moiety attached through a carbonyl amide linkage and side chain with conjugated double bond.

THERAPEUTIC ACTIVITY OF PIPERINE

Anti-inflammatory, Anti-oxidant, Anti-cholinergic, Anti-cancerous activity of piperine will be studied using selected protein targets which are as follows cyclooxygenase-2 enzyme(COX-2), Angiotensin converting enzyme, Acetylcholinesterase, Survivin.

Figure 3. Piperine structure

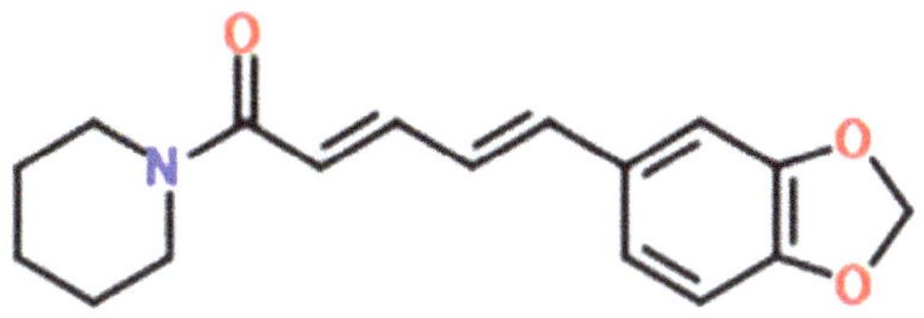

TARGET PROTEINS

Anti-Inflammatory

Experimental studies shows that the piperine controls the prostaglandin synthesis thereby control the cause of fever and severe pain. COX-2enzyme stimulates the release of prostaglandin. COX enzyme was selected to study the anti-inflammatory action of piperine. COX enzymes convert archidonic acid into prostaglandins. By blocking or inhibiting this enzyme, the synthesis of prostaglandins is blocked, which in turn relieves some of the effects of pain and fever (Subbaramaiah *et al.,* 2000, Dubois *etal.,*1998).

Cyclooxygenase Enzyme-2 (COX-2)

COX-2 is absent from most normal tissues and in some specific regions in the uterus, kidney and brain. Inflammatory cytokines such as Tumor Necrosis Factor (TNF) and interleukins (IL) induced the COX-2 expression. Mutation in c-src, Ras, APC, p53 and STK11/Lkb1, also encourage COX-2 transcription (Christopher *et al.*, 1999, Tsuji *et al.*, 2001). Furthermore, COX-2 has been shown to be induced in response to chemotherapy and radiotherapy (Steinauer *et al.*, 2000, Subbaramaiah, *et al.,* 2000). Increased synthesis of prostaglandins in found in neoplasic and inflamed tissues due to COX-2 expression (Dubois *et al.,* 1998, Subbaramaiah & Dannenberg, 2003). In most human cancers, COX-2 expression has been documented (Koki *et al.*, 2002). Tumor cells, activated stromal fibroblasts, tumor infiltrating inflammatory cells and angiogenic endothelial cells can also express COX-2 (Masferrer *et al.*, 2000)(Figure 4).

The α-helix represents in red color, yellow color represents β-sheets, and green color represents loops.

Antioxidant Activity

Angiotensin II receptor type-1(AT_1) mediate the production of oxygen free radical through angiotensin-II (Sohn *etal.,*2000). Angiotensin II receptor type-2 subtype functionally antagonizes AT_1 receptor induced production of oxygen free radical using tyrosine phosphatase pathway (Sohn *etal.,* 2000). Production of nitric oxide and oxygen ions in response to angiotensin II simulation, has been recently demonstrated *in vitro* (Pueyo *et al.*, 1998) as well as in humans (Dijkhorst-oei *et al.*, 1999). It has been studied that the angiotensin II stimulate the formation of $ONOO^-$, in cultured endothelial cells, indicated by the increase in luminal-dependent chemiluminescence and by the inhibitory effects of superoxide dismutase and nitric oxide synthase III inhibitors on chemiluminescence signals (Pueyo *et al.,* 1998). Likewise, angiotensin II-induced vasoconstriction was greatly dilated in response to consequent treatment with vitamin C. (Dijkhorst-Oei *et al.,* 1999; Chopra *etal.,*1992).

Figure 4. X-ray crystallographic structure of COX-2 with 1.9 Å resolution (PDB ID: 5f19)

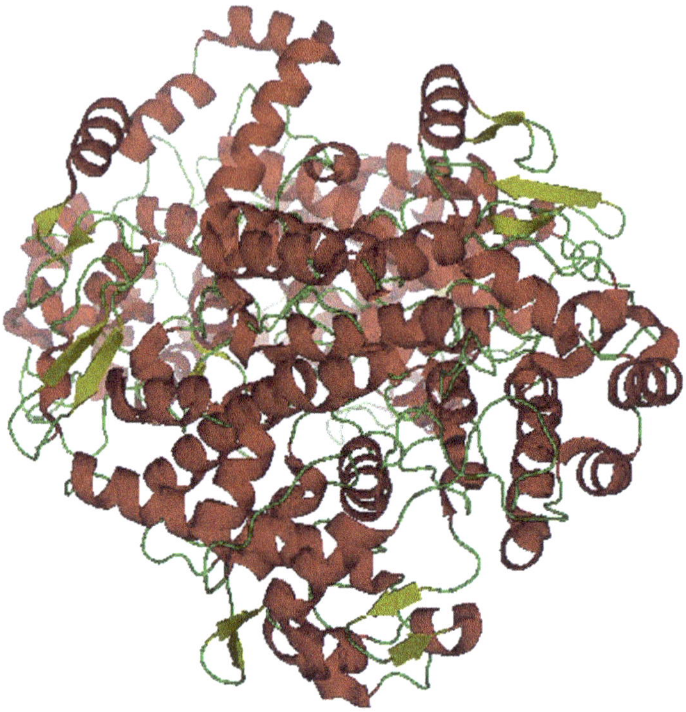

NAD(P)H oxidase activity is simulated by several growth factors and hormones including platelet-derived growth factor, tumour necrosis factor-α and angiotensin-II. Angiotensin-II increases NAD(P)H-related superoxide production in muscle cells and glomerular mesangial cells. Inhibition of Angiotensin converting enzyme controls the conversion of Angiotensin-II. There by, it controls free radical production through NAD(P)H oxidase enzyme (William, 2008).

Angiotensin Converting Enzyme (ACE)

Angiotensin-1 converting enzyme (ACE) is a metallopeptidase which consists of two catalytic domains namely N and C. Both domains have different substrate specificities. C-domain consists of somatic ACE which has no specific amyloid beta binding specificities. N terminal has selectivity for the amyloid peptide conferred through THR358 residue. Disorder of the hinge region in the crystal structure suggests that the N-domain can accommodate larger substrates through movement of the N-terminal helices. (Larmuth *et al.,* 2016) (Figure 5).

Anticholinergic Activity

Cholinergic is the term referred to acetylcholine. Neurologically, acetylcholine exclusively used to send messages is said to have cholinergic activity. During neurotransmission, acetylcholine is released from the presynaptic neuron into the synaptic cleft and binds to Acetylcholine receptors on the post synaptic membrane which rely on the signal from the nerve.

Figure 5. X-ray crystallographic structure of Angiotensin converting enzyme with 1.9 Å resolution (PDB ID: 5am8). The α-helix represents in red color, yellow color represents β-sheets, and green color represents loops

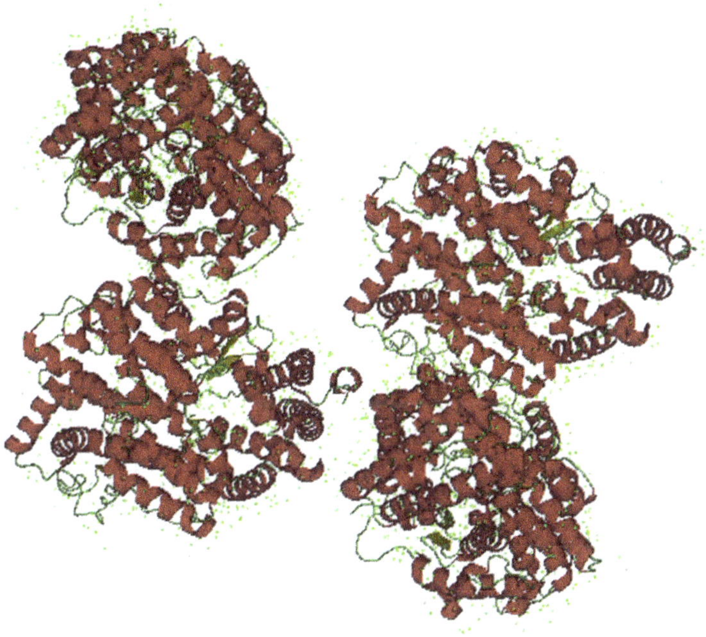

Acetylcholinesterase is an enzyme which prevents acetylcholine binding to its receptor by hydrolyzing acetylcholine into acetate and choline (Figure 3). It terminates neurotransmission by breakdown the acetylcholine and other cholinesterase which serves as neurotransmitter. By inhibition, acetylcholinesterase helps to restore the cholinergic activity which improves neurotransmission.

Acetyl Cholinesterase Enzyme

Human acetylcholinesterase enzyme with the length of 543 amino acids with a single chain A, it belongs to the carboxylesterase family (Figure 7). Carboxylesterase family classified into three types A,B and C on the different basis of inhibition pattern by organophosphatase. Serine, a glutamate or aspartate and a histidine are the catalytic triad for esterases in the case of lipases and serine proteases (Nachon *et al.,* 2005,Myres *et al.,* 1988,Sussman *et al.,* 1993,Chatonnet, *etal.,*1991).

Anticancer Activity

Survivin is a protein which is a member of Inhibitor Protein family. Inhibitor protein family inhibits caspase and blocks cell death. In the condition of abnormal cell proliferation, apoptosis is the process which helps to control cell proliferation. Survivin existence increases the chances of caspase dependent cell death. Caspase dependent cell death (Apoptosis) will proceed by inhibiting survivin protein (Figure 8) (Olivier *et al.,* 2003, Praveen Kumar *et al.*, 2015, Xun chen *et al.,* 2016).

Figure 6. After signaling, acetylcholine is released from receptors and broken down by acetyl-cholinesterase to be recycled in a continuous process(McGleenon et al., 1999)

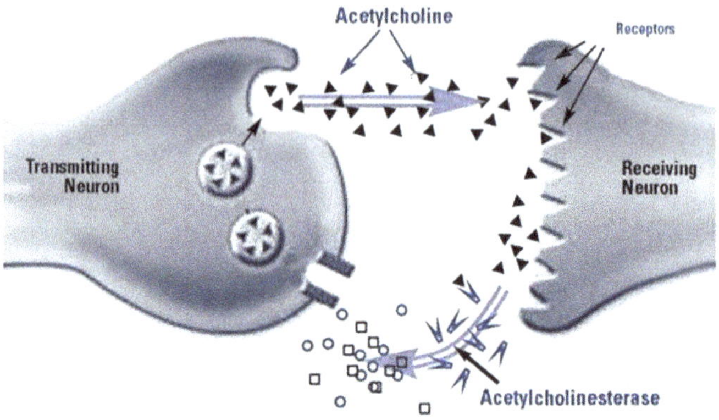

Figure 7. X-ray crystallographic structure of human acetylcholinesterase enzyme with 2.9Å resolution(PDB ID: 4PQE). The α-helix represents in red color, yellow color represents β-sheets, and green color represents loops

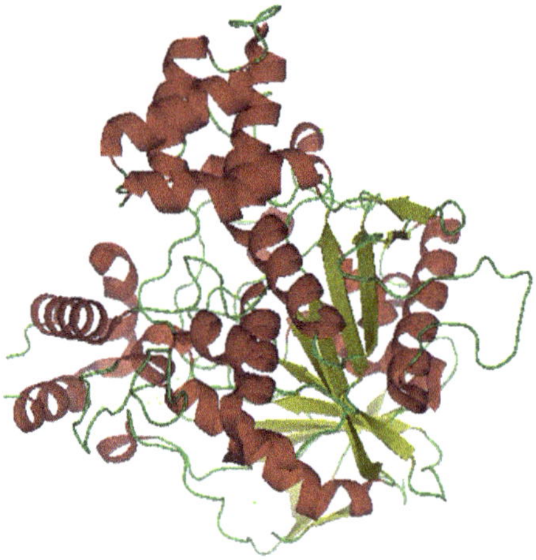

Figure 8. Survivin blocks the apoptosis process. Inhibition of survivin helps to enhance apoptosis (Xun Chen, 2016)

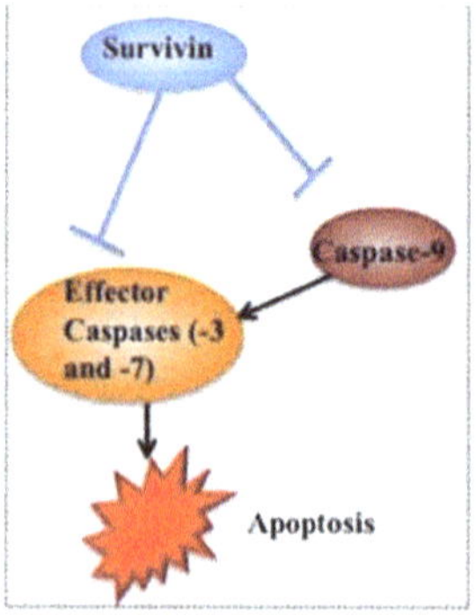

SURVIVIN

Survivin is a 16.5kDa protein which expressed during G2/M phase of the cell cycle and it inhibits a default apoptosis. Survivin consist of two domains, one is N terminal Zn^{2+} binding BIR domain linked to a 65 amino acids possess both hydrophilic and hydrophobic parts in C terminal alpha helix.. This crystal structure helps to understand that a basic amino acids acting as a sulfate phosphate-binding module, an acidic cluster projecting off the BIR domain and a solvent accessible hydrophobic surface residing on the C-terminal amphipathic helix, are suggestive of functional protein-protein interaction surfaces (Verdecia *et al.,* 2000)(Figure 9).

COMPUTATIONAL DOCKING STUDY

AutoDock tool is employed to study the piperine inhibition activity against selected target protein.

AutoDock is a semi-empirical force that includes intramolecular terms, a full desolvation model, and also it considers directionality in hydrogen bonds. The sum of torsional degrees of freedom calculates the conformational entropy. Water molecules are not modeled explicitly though, but pair-wise atomic terms are used to estimate the water contribution (dispersion/repulsion, hydrogen bonding, electrostatics, and desolvation), where weights are added for calibration (based on experimental data). For evaluation, the energy of ligand and protein in the unbound state is calculated and the energy of the protein-ligand complex is also calculated, then the difference between these two energies results in the net result of docking.

$$\Delta G = (V_{bound}^{L-L} - V_{unbound}^{L-L}) + (V_{bound}^{P-P} - V_{unbound}^{P-P}) + (V_{bound}^{P-L} - V_{unbound}^{P-P} + \Delta S_{conf})$$

Where *P* refers to the protein, *L* refers to the ligand, *V* are the pair-wise evaluations mentioned above, and ΔS~conf~ denotes the loss of conformational entropy upon binding (Huey et al., 2006).

Figure 9. X-ray crystallographic structure of human anti-apoptotic protein surviving with 2.58Å resolution(PDB ID: 1F3H). The α-helix represents in red color, yellow color represents β-sheets, and green color represents loops

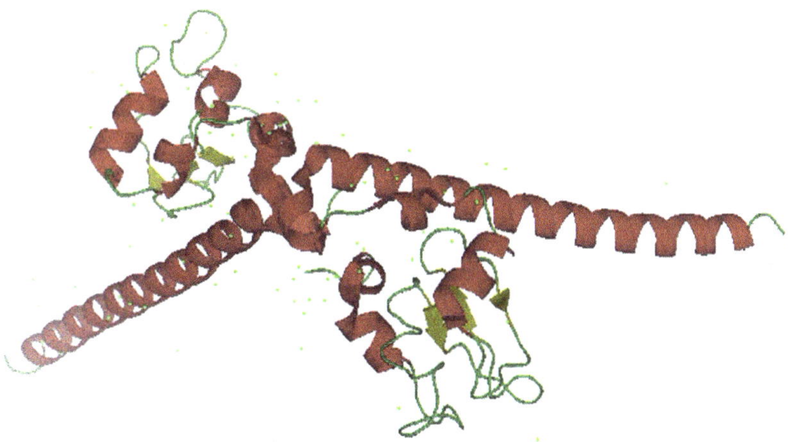

Protein Preparation

Protein structures were downloaded and prepared using autodock software, where kollman charges and polar hydrogen's were added and converted the structure format to .pdbqt file format(Gasteiger and Marsili, 1980).

Ligand Preparation

Downloaded ligand was prepared by detecting the rotatable bonds, and set the aromatic criterian, and ligand structure format converted to .pdbqt format (Jakalian *etal.,* 2002).

Grid Generation

Grid parameter file was prepared for docking study. Grid wasgenerated by selecting grid size before performing docking study. Grid size helps the ligand to identify its binding pocket.

Docking Parameter File Preparation

Docking parameter file was prepared for docking calculations by choosing macromolecule, as well as ligand file and finally, docking parameter file written using lamrickan algorithm.

Molecular Docking Studies

Cygwin terminal used to perform docking calculations, using the following command autodock4.exe –p a.dpf –l a.dlg&. Finally the .dlg file written inside the specified folder.

PROTEIN-LIGAND INTERACTIONS

Protein-ligand stability was studied based on protein-ligand interactions. Docked ligand piperine made hydrogen bond interactions with the amino acids which were present in the active site of the target proteins. Active site residues have the ability to inhibit/activate the corresponding protein. In this study, piperine wasselected to inhibit the target proteins to exhibit the following property which are as follows Anti-inflammation, Anti-oxidant, Anticholinergic, Anticancerous.

Cyclooxygenase-2 (COX-2): Piperine bound well in the active site of COX-2 enzyme based on the hydrogen bond interactions with the amino acids of active site. Piperine binds in the heme peroxidase domainof COX-2 enzyme. Hence, it has the ability to inhibit the COX-2 enzyme to reduce the pain and fever during inflammatory action(Tamatam *etal*., 2010)(Figure 10a).

Angiotensin Converting Enzyme (ACE): Piperine interactedtheamino acids,GLN582, GLN 586 found in catalytic center of ACE. Piperine interactionswith GLN 582, GLN586, LEU592 helps to inhibit the ACE there by control the conversion of Angiotensin I to AngiotensinII enzyme(Vukic *etal.,*2016)(Figure10b).

Acetylcholinesterase (AChE): According to AChE,VAL294 is a common residueinteracting with piperine. Piperine made hydrogen bond with carboxylesterase domain of acetylcholinesterase enzyme. It ensures piperine alsohasthe ability to inhibit the acetylcholinesterase enzyme and exhibit anticholinergic activity(Jiansongfang *etal.,*2014) (Figure 10c).

Survivin:In Survivin, the C-terminaldomainfound to be a catalytic domain whichhelpsto inhibit the protein. Piperine made a hydrogen bond with TRP10 which is one among the C-terminal amino acid. It indicated that the survivin protein action will be inhibited due to the binding of piperine(Verdecia*etal.,*2000) (Figure 10d). Table2explains the interacting residues of target proteins with piperine.

Table 1. Amino acids binding sites of piperine in target proteins

Drugs	PDBID 5F19	PDBID5AM8	PDBID4PQE	PDBID1F3H
	Cyclooxygenase-2	Angiotensin Converting Enzyme	Acetylcholinesterase	Survivin
Piperine	ASN375, ARG120, LEU145	ASN224, GLN582, GLN586, LEU592	PHE295, VAL294, ARG296	TRP10

Figure 10. Hydrogen bond interactions of piperine against its target protein

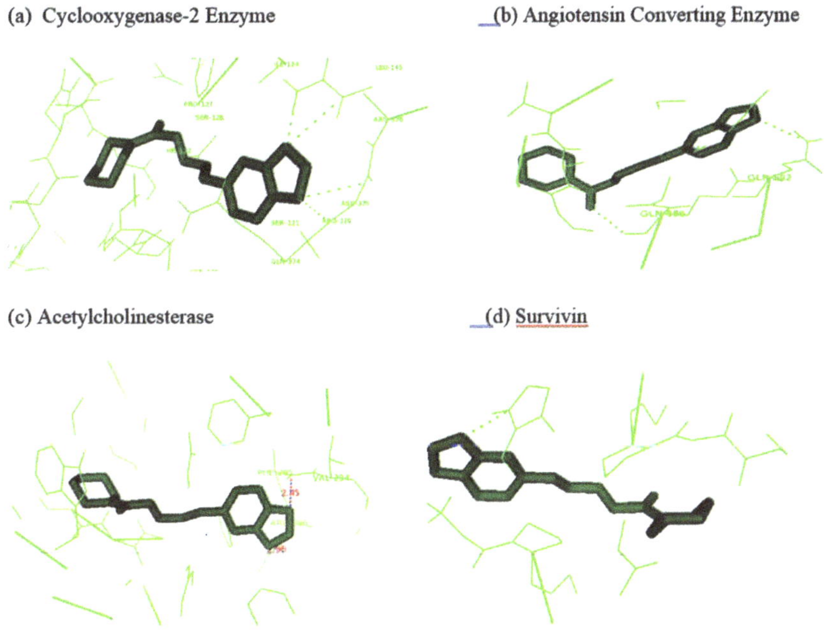

Table 2. Molecular docking score of selected target proteins and its selected ligand

S.No	Protein Name	Ligand Name	Binding Energy kcal/mol
1	Cyclooxygenase-2(COX2)	Piperine	-7.67
2	Angiotensin converting enzyme		-5.68
3	Acetycholinesterase		-4.07
4	Survivin		-6.39

SCORING FUNCTIONS

According to docking score more negative score reflects more binding affinity towards its target protein. In this present investigation following docking scores were observed -7.67 kcal/mol, -5.68 kcal/mol, -4.07 kcal/mol, -6.39 kcal/mol for piperine against its target proteins respectively cyclooxygenase-2 enzyme, angiotensin converting enzyme, acetylcholinesterase, survivin protein(Table 2). Table 2 discussed about the docking score of target proteins and its selected ligand piperine.

Based on the scores piperine has better binding affinity towards its target proteins.

CONCLUSION

Computational study is an attempt to strengthen and bring scientific evidence to prove its activity authentically. *Insilico* tools are the best one to study their actions and mechanism of the chemical constituents present in herb. It also helps to identify putative new leads of drugs, and summarise and/or visualize the complex patterns embedded within the output generated through associated with genomics and proteomics studies. *Insilico* studies is an economic way exploring the problem landscape and they can thus aid in the formulation of appropriate hypotheses for subsequent testing (*invivo* and *invitro*) laboratory studies.

The use of computational methods for drug discovery in natural products has increased during the previous decade. It would give great insight about therapeutic activity of plant preparations. Nevertheless, scientists should consider the quality of the data and computational models used.

In this chapter, the author has discussed the effect of piperine ondofferent targets and its ability to inhibit the selected target proteins were studies using AUTODOCK software. More negative score favors more ligands binding affinity towards its target protein. Piperine made sufficient hydrogen bond made in the catalytic center of all the target proteins.

Therefore it is expected piperine might down regulating the levels of proteins such as COX-2, Angiotensin converting enzyme, Acetylcholinesterase and Survivin to exhibit anti-inflammatory, antioxidant, anticholinergic and anticancerous property respectively.

REFERENCES

Ahmad, Fazal, & Abbasi. (2012). Biological role of piper nigrum L. (Black pepper): A review. *Asian Pacific Journal Tropical Biomedicine,* 1945-1953.

Araz, Jac., & Bayly. (2002). Fast, Efficient Generation of High-Quality Atomic Charges. AM1-BCC Model: II. Parameterization and Validation. *Journal of Computational Chemistry, 23*(16), 1623–41.

Chandramohan Reddy, T., Aparoy, P., Kishore Babu, N., Anil Kumar, K., Kumar Kalangi, S., & Reddanna, P. (2010). Kinetics and docking studies of a COX-2 inhibitor isolated form terminalia bellerica fruits. *Protein and Peptide Letters, 17*(10), 1251–1257. doi:10.2174/092986610792231537 PMID:20441561

Chatonnet, A., Krejci, E., Duval, N., Vincens, P., & Massoulie, J. (1991). Cholinesterase-like domains in enzymes and structural proteins: Functional and evolutionary relationships and identification of a catalytically essential aspartic acid. *Proceedings of the National Academy of Sciences of the United States of America*, *88*(15), 6647–6651. doi:10.1073/pnas.88.15.6647 PMID:1862088

Chen, Duan, Zhang, & Zhang. (2016). Survivin and tumorigenesis: molecular mechanism and therapeutic strategies. *Journal of Cancer, 7*(3), 314-323.

Chopra, M., Beswick, H., Clapperton, M., Dargie, H. J., Smith, W. E., & McMurray, J. (1992). Antioxidant effects of angiotensin-converting enzyme (ACE) inhibitors: Free radical and oxidant scavenging are sulfhydrl dependent, but lipid peroxidation is inhibited by both sulfhydryl-and non sulfhydryl-containing ACE inhibitors. *Journal of Cardiovascular Pharmacology*, *19*(3), 330–340. doi:10.1097/00005344-199203000-00005 PMID:1378110

Christopher, S. (1999). The role of cyclooxygenases in inflammation, cancer, and development. *Oncogene*, *18*(55), 7908–7916. doi:10.1038j.onc.1203286 PMID:10630643

Damanhouri & Ahmad. (2014). A review on therapeutic potential of *Piper nigrum* L. (Black Pepper): The king of spices. *Medicinal & Aromatic Plants*, *3*(3), 1–6.

Dijkhorst-Oei, L. T., Stroes, E. S., Koomans, H. A., & Rabenlink, T. J. (1999). Acute simultaneous stimulation of nitric oxide and oxygen radicals by angiotensin II in humans invivo. *Journal of Cardiovascular Pharmacology*, *33*(3), 420–424. doi:10.1097/00005344-199903000-00012 PMID:10069678

Dubois, R. N., & Abramson, S. B. (1998). Cyclooxygenase in biology and disease. *The FASEB Journal*, *12*(12), 1063–1073. doi:10.1096/fasebj.12.12.1063 PMID:9737710

Fang, Wu, Yang, Gao, Li, Wang, … Du. (2014). Inhibition of acetylcholinesterase by two geinstein derivatives: Kinetic analysis, molecular docking and molecular dynamics simulation. *Acta Pharmaceutica (Zagreb, Croatia)*, *4*(6), 430–437.

Gasteiger & Marsili. (1980). Iterative Partial Equalization of Orbital Electronegativity—a Rapid Access to Atomic Charges. *Tetrahedron*, *36*(2), 3219–3228.

Koki, A. T., Khan, N. K., Woerner, B. M., Seibert, K., Harmon, J. L., Dannenberg, A. J., ... Masferrer, J. L. (2002). Characterization of cyclooxygenase-2 (COX-2) during tumorigenesis in human epithelial cancers: Evidence for potential clinical utility of COX-2 inhibitors in epithelial cancers. *Prostaglandins, Leukotrienes, and Essential Fatty Acids*, *66*(1), 13–18. doi:10.1054/plef.2001.0335 PMID:12051953

Kumar, P. (2015). Survivin:Amolecular biomarker in cancer. *The Indian Journal of Medical Research*, *141*(4), 389–397. doi:10.4103/0971-5916.159250 PMID:26112839

Larmuth, K. M., Masuyer, G., Douglas, R. G., Schwager, S. L., Acharya, K. R., & Sturrock, E. D. (2016). Kinetic and structural characterization of amyloid-β peptide hydrolysis by human angiotensin-1-converting enzyme. *The FEBS Journal*, *283*(6), 1060–1076. doi:10.1111/febs.13647 PMID:26748546

Majeed & Prakash. (2000). The medicinal uses of pepper. *The International Pepper News*, *1*, 23-31.

Masferrer, J. L., & Leahy, K. M. (2000). Antiangiogenic and Antitumor Activities of Cyclooxygenase-2 Inhibitors. *Cancer Research*, *60*(5), 1306–1311. PMID:10728691

McGleenon, B. M., Dynan, K. B., & Passmore, A. P. (1999). Acetylcholinesterase inhibitors in Alzheimer's disease. *British Journal of Clinical Pharmacology*, *48*(4), 471–480. doi:10.1046/j.1365-2125.1999.00026.x PMID:10583015

Myers, M., Richmond, R. C., & Oakeshott, J. G. (1988). On the origins of esterases. *Molecular Biology and Evolution*, *5*(2), 113–119. PMID:3163407

Olivier, R., Daniel, I., & Elizabeth, D. (2003). Constitutive nuclear localization and initial cytoplasmic apoptotic activation of endogenous caspase-3 evidenced by confocal microscopy. *International Journal of Experimental Pathology*, *84*(2), 75–81. doi:10.1046/j.1365-2613.2003.00339.x PMID:12801281

Pueyo, M. E., Arnal, J. F., Rami, J., & Michel, J. B. (1998). Angiotensin II stimulates the production of NO and peroxynitrite in endothelial cells. *The American Journal of Physiology*, *274*(1), C214–C220. doi:10.1152/ajpcell.1998.274.1.C214 PMID:9458730

Ruth, Morris, Olson, & Goodsell. (2007). A Semiempirical Free Energy Force Field with Charge-Based Desolvation. *Journal of Computational Chemistry, 28*(6), 1145–52.

Singh, Singh, Mishra, Patel, Kamalesh, & Yadav. (2014). Piperine: Delightful surprise to the biological world, made by plant pepper and a great bioavailability enhancer for our drugs and supplements. *World Journal of Pharmaceutical Research*, *3*(6), 2084-2098.

Singletary, K. (2010). Black Pepper and health. *Nutrition Today*, *45*(1), 43–47. doi:10.1097/NT.0b013e3181cb4539

Sohn, H. Y., Raff, U., Hoffmann, A., Gloe, T., Heermeier, K., Galle, J., & Pohl, U. (2000). Differential role of angiotensin II receptor subtypes on endothelial superoxide formation. *British Journal of Pharmacology*, *131*(4), 667–672. doi:10.1038j.bjp.0703566 PMID:11030714

Steinauer, K. K., Gibbs, I., Ning, S., French, J. N., Armstrong, J., & Knox, S. J. (2000). Radiation induces upregulation of cyclooxygenase-2 (COX-2) protein in PC-3 cells. *International Journal of Radiation Oncology, Biology, Physics*, *48*(2), 325–328. doi:10.1016/S0360-3016(00)00671-4 PMID:10974444

Subbaramaiah, K., & Dannenberg, A. J. (2003). Cyclooxygenase 2: A molecular target for cancer prevention and treatment. *Trends in Pharmacological Sciences*, *24*(2), 96–102. doi:10.1016/S0165-6147(02)00043-3 PMID:12559775

23. Subbaramaiah, K., Hart, J. C., Norton, L., & Dannenberg, A. J. (2000). Microtubule-interfering Agents Stimulate the Transcription of Cyclooxygenase-2. *The Journal of Biological Chemistry*, *275*(20), 14838–14845. doi:10.1074/jbc.275.20.14838 PMID:10809726

Sussman, J. L., Cygler, M., Harel, M., Silman, I., Schrag, J. D., Doctor, B. P., & Gentry, M. K. (1993). Relationship between sequence conservation and three-dimensional structure in a large family of esterases, lipases, and related proteins. *Protein Science*, *2*(3), 366–382. PMID:8453375

Tsuji, S., Tsuji, M., Kawano, S., & Hori, M. (2001). Cyclooxygenase-2 Upregulation as a Perigenetic Change in Carcinogenesis. *Journal of Experimental and Clinical Cancer Research*, *20*(1),117-130.

Verdica, M. A., Huang, H., Dutil, E., Kaiser, D. A., Hunter, T., & Noel, J. P. (2000). Structure of the human anti-apoptotic protein surviving reveals a dimeric arrangement. *Nature Structural & Molecular Biology*, *7*(7), 602–608. doi:10.1038/76838

Vukić, V., Vukić, D., Milanović, S., Iličić, M., Kanurić, K. (2016). Molecular docking and stimulation through the angiotensin converting enzyme by inhibition by milk peptides. *Food Technology Quality and Safety*, *10*, 42-45.

Welch. (2008). Angiotensin II dependent superoxide effects on hypertension and vascular dysfunction. *Hypertension*, *52*, 51-56.

Chapter 7
Target Identification of HDAC8 Isoform for the Treatment of Cancer

A. Umamaheswari
Anna University, India

A. Puratchikody
Anna University, India

Sakthivel Balasubramaniyan
Anna University, India

ABSTRACT

Target identification has been considered as a chief parameter in drug discovery as it fully characterizes on-target and off-target effects of drug binding. Cell signaling receptors, structural proteins, and post-translational modifications of histones by histone deacetylases are the most widespread targets that are progressively being explored. The FDA approved histone deacetylases inhibitors and the majority of HDACi in and out of clinical trials based on the activities of 11 isoforms of the enzyme in non-selective influence approach. Unfortunately, reported HDACi does not possess a high degree of structural specificity and ultimately lessens the therapeutic index with many dose limiting toxicities. This chapter illustrates how different approaches are incorporated into the novel inhibitors discovery that are truly isoform-selective and which are specifically involved in targeting only a particular isozyme. Further, it highlights the aspects relating to provide a wider therapeutic index with an improved toxicity profile of lead like epigenetic modulators.

INTRODUCTION TO CANCER

Cancer is a heterogeneous disease with a wide range of clinical profile and diverse underlying mechanism. Cancer with ~14 million new cases and 8.2 million cancer-related deaths in 2012 is considered as the leading cause of morbidity and mortality worldwide. In the next two decades, the expected number of new cases of cancer is ~ 70% (Stewart & Wild, 2014).

DOI: 10.4018/978-1-5225-7326-5.ch007

There has been a prolonged targeting approach for the development of new cancer therapies, distinctive and appropriate for each individual. Surgery, intravenous cytotoxic chemotherapy and radiation are the major hallmark of treatment for cancer (David, 2008). These drugs target rapidly dividing cells in addition to certain normal tissues. Consequently, many patients get susceptible to therapy-related immediate and long-term toxicities like gastrointestinal symptoms, alopecia and myelosuppression that are often dose limiting.

Anti cancer drugs fail in the clinic for two main reasons; the first is that they do not act and the second is that they are not safe. Hence, innovative medications are in demand for the management of severe therapeutic conditions including cancer, autoimmune, infectious and metabolic diseases. Now, patients diagnosed with cancer very frequently shift to newer and more personalized treatment strategies. A noteworthy progress in the treatment of cancer in the past decades is the recent concept of targeted therapies which have been very much supportive in channelizing the path “from the bench to the bed” (Yoh *et al.,* 2012).

A drug candidate is not a one size-fits-all-diseases stratagem instead its pathway has to be identified and validated appropriately. Hence, a target-based strategy for the development of new drug through drug discovery is essential. For the last two decades, researchers of biotech and pharmaceutical organisations and universities work in the area of target-based drug discovery (Terstappen *et al*., 2007).

There is a need for drug discovery to move from the slow and too expensive trial and error approach. Over the last two to three decades, the shift in focusing towards target based discovery has been a foremost landmark in drug discovery research. Computational modelling and drug design forms significant constituents of new-age biology for the reason that they are crucial to understand the large-scale data produced by high-throughput screening experiments and to create hypotheses, which are in general recapitulated with experimental validation.

Target Therapies

A target is a broad terminology applied to a series of biological entities that includes proteins, genes, RNA, monoclonal antibodies, antibody fragments, recombinant fusion proteins and peptides. A good target desires to be efficacious, safe, satisfies clinical and commercial needs and, above all, it should be ‘druggable’. A ‘druggable’ target upon binding to either a small drug molecule or larger biological, produce a desired biological response that can be quantified both *in vitro* and *in vivo* techniques. The first stage in drug discovery process is to acquire the knowledge about the disease mechanism, utilize cellular and genetic approaches and finally identify potential drug targets either for a particular disease or phenotypes (e.g. HIV replication within T-cells). Subsequently, genomics and proteomics helps in providing gene sequence and gene expression data for disease tissues compared to normal tissues.

Generally, in a diseased condition genes as well as their protein products are highly expressed when compared to low expression in normal tissues and hence become apparent potential targets for therapy. The selected disease targets are modulated and behavioural changes of diseased cells are validated by *in vitro* research, usually cell-based and animal models proving themselves to prioritize for future research. Identification of good target and validation enables increased confidence in the relationship between disease and target and explore whether modulation in the target will direct to mechanism-based side effects (DiMasi *et al.,* 2003). Targeted therapies pave a way to develop specific treatments for severe medical conditions however, concurrently ensuing little to no off-target toxicity. The goal in tumor therapies are aimed to stop the multiplication of the cancer cells by focussing at a particular tumor target and, confidently, leading to desired treatment strategies with fewer side effects. The purpose of this chapter is to help the researchers to understand targeted therapies and what it really mean for. In cancer treatment, targeted therapies work in similar ways but some of the drugs produce more effect in certain subtypes of cancer.

Small molecules penetrate more easily through cell membrane and interact with targets available inside a cell. Generally, they are designed to block the target proteins enzymatic activity. Some examples of small molecules (Al-Hussaini, 2014) are imatinib (tyrosine kinase inhibitor), seliciclib (cyclin-dependent kinase inhibitor) and bortezomib (proteasome inhibitor). Many therapeutic proteins are significant in alleviating disease with high potential. Of the new anticancer drugs approved by the U.S. Food and Drug Administration (FDA) since 2000, 15 have been targeted therapies, compared with only five traditional chemotherapeutic agents (Centerwatch, 2007).

Target Identification Tools

Bio and Cheminformatics tools, plays a vital role in identifying target molecule which could be a potential drug (Sreenivasa Reddy *et al.,* 2011). Not all small molecules can be drugs, and not all proteins can be drug targets. A protein to which the small molecule binds must have a binding site that must be complementary to the druggable properties of the small molecule to fit in the pharmacophoric region of the protein. Chemoinformatic tools have become a remarkable potential tool to advance drug design and discovery through *in silico* techniques and to provide integration of information in different levels to improve the conformity of data outcomes. The success of the drug response depends on the competing ability for protein binding site with endogenous small molecule. The recent prevailing hypothesis in drug discovery seeks to identify a particular small molecule inhibitor to bind to a specific receptor, a macromolecular target by *in silico* research. However, discovery of the novel biological targets depends on the ability of efficient methods to manipulate organic small molecules. Several approaches and databases are applied for the discovery of existing and new drug targets.

One of the most important application of databases in the discovery of target is to deduce relative gene expression levels in a given cell or tissue. Gene expression levels are important because the phenotype is determined by the small portion of genes that are expressed at any given time in a cell or tissue type and gene expression changes can be associated with disease.

Thus, novel drug targets can be identified by *in silico* methods by comparing gene expression levels in normal and disease states. Proteins associated with metabolic pathways and specific to micro-organism are of particular interest. A drug interacting with such target is less likely to interact with a human homologue. A drug-discovery program typically starts with the suitable drug targets identification and ends with the production of new drug candidate and finally ends up with selling of the drug candidate in the market after successful get through in clinical trials.

Target identification can also be studied through network-based drug discovery, a field integrating different levels of information in drug-protein and protein-disease networks. This approach involves a highly mutual interaction between databases and its correlations across different factors like genomics, proteomics, metabolomics, transcriptomics, microbiome and pharmacogenomics. Target identification highly depends on the recent developments of pertinent computational and systems biology tools for the interpretation of data (Barabasi *et al.,* 2011). Such approaches, for instance relating pharmacological and genomic spaces are used to develop computational frameworks for drug target identification (Zhao & Li, 2010). Another recent network-based application is the integration of large-scale structural genomics and disease association studies, to generate three-dimensional human interactome, which results in the identification of candidate genes for unknown disease-to-gene associations with proposed molecular mechanisms (Wang *et al.,* 2012). To facilitate gaining in-depth knowledge of disease mechanisms and/or phenotypes, information technologies are greatly needed today more than ever (Buchan *et al.,* 2011). In order to study the disease mechanisms and/or related phenotypes instead of investigating a particular gene or protein study, entire set of biomolecules is analyzed (Gentles & Gallahan, 2011).

Computer-Aided Drug Design

Computer modeling has played a significant role in understanding the enzyme-drug interactions, identifying potent inhibitors and obtaining quantitative structure activity relationships of potential lead molecules.

Traditionally, high-throughput screening (HTS) of libraries of compounds identified potential inhibitors from about tens to hundreds of thousands of small molecules tested against a given assay in order to discover various novel drugs. However, this approach can be very expensive and resource intensive. Though high throughput screening identifies hit compounds, its success rate are often very low due to their failure rates during the testing of physicochemical parameters. Once effective target is identified, a panel of *in silico* tools can be used to initiate drug design process based on the nature of the target and available information on the system. In the past decade, computer aided drug design (CADD) has offered valuable tools in the identification of compounds, minimizing the risk of later rejection of lead compounds. CADD plays a vital role in high success rates of hit compound identification (Doman *et al.,* 2002), as well as the precedence of HTS active compounds. One such example predicting the importance of CADD compared to HTS was the identification of transforming growth factor-β 1 receptor kinase inhibitors.

A variety of computational techniques can help to reduce the size of chemical library by focusing on those compounds that are predicted to be most likely active by *in silico* modeling. The design of improved lead molecule for the drug target can be made using computational methods that are expected to play a crucial role in understanding the precise molecular recognition events of the target macromolecule with candidate hits (Shaikh *et al.,* 2007). Generally, there are two diverse methods for computational drug design viz. structure based and ligand based (Figure 1). These two methods are solely dependent on the information available on the identified target. The information on the 3-D structure and active sites of the target protein can be retrieved from X-ray crystallography, nuclear magnetic resonance, or 3-D structure databases. The 3-D structure and active sites are then incorporated into a computer model and new compounds are designed and binding conformations are assessed for their proper fit to the target (Cavasotto & Phatak, 2009). This approach is known as "structure-based drug design (SBDD)". Some of the techniques more often used in this approach are docking and molecular dynamics simulation (Ivanov *et al.,* 2009). Docking software is used to screen potent ligands from molecule database (Chen, *et al.,* 2009). Two decades ago, Captopril was the first drug where X ray structural information was used as a guide for small molecule design. Although the template used for discovery of captopril was a homology model derived from the X-ray structure of bovine carboxypeptidase A, the credit of this homology model was a milestone (Hardy *et al.,* 2003). On the other hand, molecular dynamics simulations are used to determine the interaction of a molecule with target protein and other properties such as membrane permeability of the molecule (Wang *et al.,* 2010; Bemporad *et al.,* 2005). Alternatively, where appropriate data of the 3-D structure of a target protein are not available, drug can be designed using the known ligands of a target protein. This approach is known as "ligand-based drug design (LBDD)". Molecular

Figure 1. Types of drug design and steps for identification of lead molecules

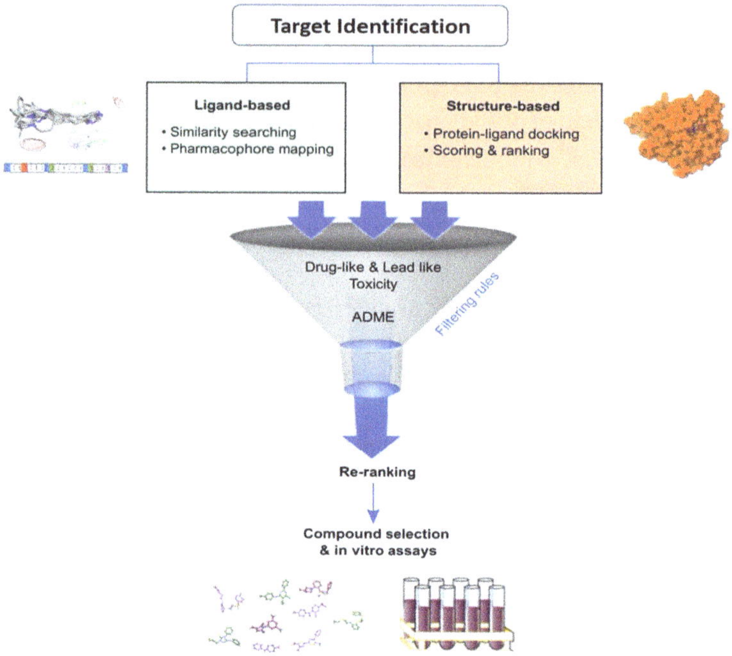

similarity approaches, quantitative structure-activity relationships (QSAR) and pharmacophore models are frequently used methods in the ligand-based drug design process (Tintori *et al.,* 2010).

Generally, the most commonly used methods in hit compound identification rely on virtual screening techniques on the targets' binding site. These methods depend on docking large libraries of small molecules such as ZINC (Irwin *et al.,* 2012), or chemical information on known compounds such as Pubchem (Kim *et al.,* 2015) using docking or pharmacophore modeling tools.

Ultimately, virtual screening of chemical libraries provides an alternative approach to finding active chemical entities and structural scaffolds for the development of novel cancer therapeutic agents. For the structural modification, computer-aided scaffold replacement method can be used wherein a portion of the molecule could be replaced, or a particular group might be added to accomplish a specific polar or steric interaction that might improve and enhance the binding affinity. The inexpensive virtual screening method employs either a target based or a ligand based approach.

DRUG TARGETS

The completion of the Human Genome Project had led to the identification of new targets for drug therapy (Figure 2) (Hopkins & Groom, 2002). It is now evident that only a segment of 30,000 proteins encoded for by the human genome are probable to the intervened by small drug molecule. The size of the human "druggable genome" (human genes encoding proteins are supposed to contain efficiently crucial binding pockets with appropriate structures for interactions with drug-like molecules) is more than 3000 target proteins (i.e., about 10% of the genome), of which, the most significant portion is the presence of enzymes (Hopkins & Groom, 2002).

Figure 2. Distribution of marketed drugs by biochemical target class

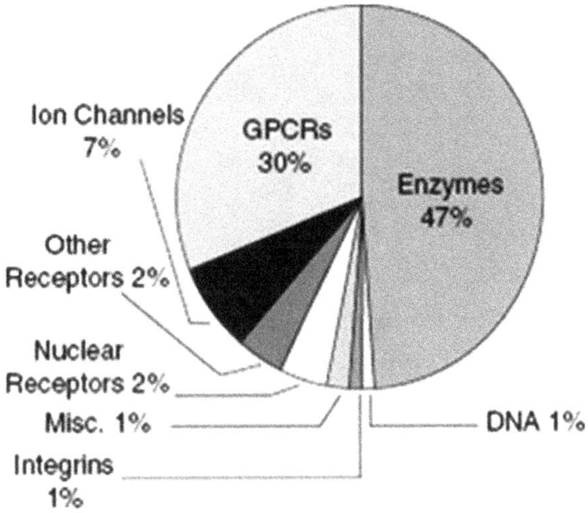

The drug molecules undergo various conformations to electrostatic, stereochemical, hydrophobic, and other physiochemical properties so that the drug targets create binding pockets for these drug molecules that demonstrate structural and electronic complementarity. Accordingly a "druggable target" contains a "druggable binding pocket" as part of its 3-D structure, and the druggable binding pocket conforms to specific structural and chemical requirements (Andrew & Colin, 2002).

Drug binding pockets are referred to cavities or clefts along the protein surface, with small molecular volumes relative to that of the entire protein of around 1000 Å^3 (Liang *et al.*, 1998). On contrary to the drug molecules, ligand binding pockets often consists of specific loci for hydrogen bonding, salt bridge formation, and other noncovalent, electrostatic interactions between the binding partners. A considerable surface complexity in drug binding pockets occurs due to the combination of electrostatic determinants of binding, the general hydrophobicity of the pockets, and surface roughness (Hajduk *et al.*, 2005).

Ligand binding pockets are composed of hydrophobic amino acids and usually designed excluding bulk solvent. Nevertheless, the pockets that contain highly ordered water molecules, incorporated as water molecules destruct the specific architectural pattern participating in ligand interactions. Ultimately, this exclusion favors the formation of stronger hydrogen bonds and other electrostatic interactions between the protein and the ligand. Druggable binding pockets on protein surfaces have largely evolved to bind physiologically relevant small molecular weight ligands, such as nucleotide analogs (e.g., ATP, GTP, NADH), amino acids, steroid hormones, metabolites, peptides, cofactors (e.g., flavins, hemes). The interactions of these natural ligands with the protein binding site typically effect a change in the biological activity of the target protein often leading to post-translational modification of cytosolic domains of the receptor protein. These post-translational modifications lead to recruitment and/or activation of various proteins, thus initiating cellular signal transduction cascades that are critical for a number of cellular activities, such as cell proliferation, mobility, and programmed cell death (Copeland, 2013).

The most common drug targets of currently marketed drugs include:

- Membranes
- Nucleic acid

- RNA
- Enzymes
- G protein coupled receptors
- Ion channels
- Species-specific genes
- Proteins

Membranes as Drug Targets

Cell membrane proteins act as a barrier segregating everything that goes into and out of a cell via proteins and maintain the integrity of the cell. It tightly controls most of the nutrients, ions, waste products, and even DNA and proteins. Membrane proteins act as bestowed arena for an entire collection of cellular functions such as cell proliferation, adhesion, migration, and intracellular trafficking. Since, drugs normally target membrane proteins, they are considered for molecular recognition. Hence, an understanding of the structural and dynamic functions of the membranes (e.g., plasma membranes and intercellular membranes) may perhaps put in more information for a more rational design of drug molecules with superior permeation characteristics and specific membrane effects to cure diseases. Many general anesthetics, different classes of antibiotics, antifungals and toxins are believed to work on planar lipid bilayers causing transmembrane pores (Singh *et al.,* 2006).

Nucleic Acid as Drug Targets

Nucleic acids are considered to be warehouse of genetic information. DNA itself has been shown to be the presumed target for many drugs clinically used in cancer and other diseases. Thus, they are used in chemotherapies as drug targets (Drews, 2000).

DNA binds with drugs, expresses/represses genes and creates protein and are thus considered a key target for the delivery of drugs. In fact, there are very few ways by which drugs bind to DNA. One key way is by controlling the transcription factors via special enzymes where the drugs target proteins that bind to the DNA. Sometimes, molecules bind to the double helix parts of DNA and interfere with the interactions between DNA and proteins. Telomerase inhibitors are one such type of target that is related to cancer treatment. Telomeres are present at chromosome ends and they protect the ends from damage and help to make sure DNA replication occurs as intended. Telomerase inhibitors inhibit the action of reverse transcriptase telomerase that helps tumour cells keep the telomere ends stable, and hence starts apoptosis by inhibiting its action.

DNA replication stands as an essential mechanism for the proliferation and survival of all living forms ranging from simple virus to more complex organisms including humans. The significance of DNA replication is frequently emphasized by various pathological states such as ataxia telangiectasia (Kulkarni & Wilson, 2008). The foremost objective in biomedical science is to develop therapeutic agents to combat these pathological states of hyperproliferative diseases such as cancer, autoimmune conditions, and viral/bacterial infections. There are several approaches currently used to inhibit DNA replication. DNA damaging agents, chemotherapeutic agents such as temozolomide and cisplatin mutate the entire composition and structure of DNA and inhibit DNA synthesis thus preventing cellular proliferation (Havelka *et al.,* 2007). The second strategy is to alter the activity of individual enzymes involved in

DNA replication. Agents such as etoposide inhibit the activity of topoisomerase causing apoptosis by the breaking single and double-stranded DNA through disruption of DNA synthesis (Baldwin & Osheroff, 2005). The third approach includes reducing the availability of dNTPs that are the building blocks for DNA synthesis. By inhibition of certain enzymes involved in nucleotide metabolism, anti-metabolites such as methotrexate decrease the number of nucleotide groups and somehow hamper DNA synthesis (Mc Guire, 2003). However, the use of nucleoside analogs that target the enzymatic reactions of DNA polymerase is the most appropriate method of direct targeting (Anderson & Perry, 2007).

DNA polymerase catalyses the addition of mononucleotides to a large polymer by taking the template of either DNA or RNA as a basis for each addition. Various mechanisms such as chemical modification, cross linking of DNA (cisplatin) or cleavage of the DNA (bleomycin) are involved for this enzymatic reaction. In addition, researchers have reported intercalation of a polyaromatic ring system into the double stranded helix (actinomycin D, ethidium) and binding to the major and minor grooves of DNA (e.g., netropsin) (Haq, 2002). DNA has been shown to be the target for chemotherapy with efforts to design sequence-specific reagents for gene therapy.

RNA as Drug Target

RNAs serve as the messenger between DNA and Proteins. They are considered to be potential targets for drugs that bind directly to RNA or RNA- protein complexes (Drews, 2000). RNA was thought to be an exclusively elastic molecule without noteworthy structural complexity.

Innovative technologies for the determination of the complex structure and function of RNA have created new opportunities extensively for the pharmaceutical industries to target RNA with small molecules. Perhaps more importantly, certain drugs bind to RNA in such a manner that they produce extraordinary effects that cannot be accomplished by the drugs that bind to proteins (Ecker & Griffey, 1999). There are many proven records that reveal different classes of natural products binding to RNA or RNA-protein complexes. The binding sites on RNA are hydrophilic and relatively open as compared to proteins. The potential for small molecule recognition based on shape is enhanced by the deformability of RNA. The molecules bind to specific RNA targets can be verified by global conformation, charge distribution, aromaticity and hydrogen bonding groups. The major groove of RNA provides many sites for specific hydrogen bonding with a ligand. The rich structural and sequence diversity of RNA proves that ligands can be designed with high affinity and specificity for their target. Despite the role of RNA in the replication of bacteria, the rising problem of antibiotic resistance makes the search for novel RNA binders of crucial importance. Certain small molecules can bind and block essential functions of RNA.

Aminoglycoside antibiotics and drugs such as erythromycin bind to bacterial rRNA and releases peptidyl-tRNA and mRNA. These drugs produce their antibacterial effects by targeting specific sites in the bacterial ribosome.

On the other hand, structurally related antibiotics for example neamine, ribostamycin, neomycin B, and paromomycin, the binding site has been confined to the A-site of the prokaryotic 16S ribosomal decoding region RNA (Moazed & Noller, 1987). Binding of aminoglycosides to this RNA target hampers the conformation of mRNA translation and ends up in miscoding and truncation, consequently leading to the death of bacterial cell (Alper *et al.,* 1998).

Enzymes as Drug Target

Enzymes are the best targets as small molecules can be easily fitted in their pocket (Singh *et al.,* 2006). Enzymes are a classic target for therapeutic intervention and numerous well-studied examples exist. The macromolecule accountable for the catalysis of biochemical reactions are an apparent target when a disease state is associated with production of a biologically active species.

Despite enzymes are very much essential for life, deregulated enzymatic activity pave way for causing diseased condition. A survey in the year 2000 reported that approximately 30% of all drugs in clinical use extend their therapeutic efficacy through enzymatic reactions (Drews, 2000). Later, Hopkins and Groom (2002) updated this survey by incorporating newly launched drugs and found that nearly half (47%) of all marketed drugs inhibit enzymes as their molecular target. The sale of small molecule drugs such as enzyme inhibitors crossed over 65 billion dollars in 2001 worldwide and this market was expected to grow to more than 200 billion dollars by 2020. Some contraction of the worldwide market has occurred due to withdrawal of several products since 2005.

Mutations in genes encoding enzymes can lead to abnormally high concentrations of the enzyme within a cell due to overexpression. Alternatively, point mutations can lead to an enhancement of the catalytic efficiency of the specific enzyme because of structural changes in the catalytically critical amino acid residues. These two mechanisms are responsible for irregular levels of the reaction product's formation thus resulting in specific pathologies. Hence, human enzymes are also commonly targeted for pharmacological intervention in many diseases. Traditional medicinal chemistry enzyme targets include hydrolases, kinases, phosphodiesterases, proteases and phosphotases. In view of the fact that the target should be unique, no other pathway should be able to associate the function of the target and prevails the presence of the inhibitor through exploitation of the structural and biochemical differences between the normal and pathogenic forms. Undeniably, the target should be competent enough to inhibit small molecule binding.

G Protein Coupled Receptors (GPCRs)

G-protein-coupled receptors (GPCRs) are the signaling proteins responsible for various biological processes like cell proliferation, inflammation, neurotransmission etc. It is obvious that they represent the most important target proteins in modern pharmacology and 50% of the drugs available on the market target them. GPCRs have been commonly targeted by antihypertensive and antiallergy drugs (Rask-Andersen *et al.,* 2011).

This may be due to their functional and stereochemical properties they mediate especially within brain and peripheral nervous system. Besides managing a great number of physiological processes, such as signal transduction (Davies *et al.,* 2007; Lagerstrom & Schioth, 2008) ligand diversity and unique tissue expression (Ma & Zemmel, 2002), GPCRs exist in majority and encompass the property of ''ligand binding specificity'' (Lagerstrom and Schioth, 2008). About 80% of hormones and neurotransmitters exert their pharmacological effects by interacting with GPCRs (Birnbaumer *et al.*, 1990). Consequently, these properties make GPCRs as ideal therapeutic targets for various diseases.

Many pharmaceutical companies have identified agents that target GPCRs (Lagerstrom and Schioth, 2008; Overington *et al.*, 2006) and involved in exploring the factors that influence GPCRs' activity (Ghanemi *et al.*, 2013) during drug development. So far, quite a few drugs with an activity based on the interaction with GPCR-related system includes opiates, antihistamines, α- and β-blockers, β agonists, dopamine receptor blockers, angiotensin receptor blockers, angiotensin – converting enzyme inhibitors and selective serotonin reuptake inhibitors have been investigated (Whalen *et al.*, 2011).

Ion Channels

Ion channels are protein molecules that cross the cell membrane and switches to open and close states. They guard the entry or exit of specific ions across the cell membrane in their open state. Ion channels are gated and have particular triggers that allow for highly selective opening for the ions. There are two forms of gating – ligand gated ion channels, which are an intergral part of a receptor and are opened either by G-proteins directly, or downstream effector molecules such as cAMP. The second is the voltage gated ion channels which opens up in counter to differences in voltage across cell membrane. These channels open when the membrane becomes depolarized and is generally short lasting. Drugs bind directly within the ion channel and prevent the flow of ions. Sometimes, they bind to another place on the molecule and increase or decrease the probability of the channel opening in response to a change in voltage. Class I antiarrhythmic drugs (Vaughan-Williams, 1984) target the fast acting cardiac Na^+ channels during phase 0.

These drugs act as Na^+ channel blockers and inhibit the permeability of the membrane to Na^+, in that way decrease rate/velocity/magnitude of the depolarization that arises in phase 0 of the cardiac action potential (Milne *et al.,* 1984).

Species-Specific Genes as Drug Targets

Specific genes conserved in different genomes are very much essential as they are attractive targets for new therapeutics. Through genomic analysis, it is revealed that the most promising candidates for drug targets are the conserved genes. Species specific protein coding genes laid a strong platform for the design of drugs against a particular or narrow group of pathogens (Galperin & Koonin, 1999). Complete genome sequences available in the databases offer the first insights into drug discovery and development approaches in near future (Galperin & Koonin, 1999).

A remarkable advancement in the prediction of potential drug targets referred to as differential genome display has been proposed by Huynen and co-workers (Huynen *et al.*, 1997).

This approach depends on the fact that genome of parasitic bacterium are normally much smaller and code for fewer proteins than the genomes of free-living organisms. The genes that are present in the genome of a parasitic microorganisms but missing in a closely related genome of free pathogenicity can be deemed to be potential drug targets. For an instance, an extensive assessment of *H.influenzae* and *E.coli* gene products resulted in the identification of 40 *H. influenzae* genes that have been exclusively found in pathogens and accordingly represent potential drug targets.

Proteins as Drug Targets

Proteins are continuously believed to have noteworthy consideration as important source of potential drug targets. Proteins afford a crucial link between genes and disease and are considered to be the key to understand the disease pathology, diagnosis, and treatment. In the year 2006, about 324 drug targets were recommended for all classes of approved therapeutic drugs (Overington, 2006). About 668 proteins in the non-target set of 3573 small molecular weight chemical compound (SMOL) were identified to have target-like properties. Hence, these SMOL had the prospective of considering innovative targets (Bakheet and Doig 2009). Moreover, proteins are currently highly concentrated as major targets by the drug discovery and in the near future, nucleic acids might achieve foremost importance as drug targets (Peter *et al.,* 2006; Davidson, 2011).

Currently, addressed target classes and the mode of action for therapeutics are summarized in Table 1.

Rask-Andersen *et al.* (2011) have identified 435 effect-mediating drug targets in the human genome after modulation of 989 unique drugs through 2242 drug–target interactions. Receptors constitute the largest group of drug targets with 193 proteins which constitutes for about for 44% of human drug targets (Rask-Andersen, 2011). The Drug target database (Table 2) is considered one of the most important sources of information for drugs and drug targets (Knox *et al.,* 2011).

A lot of key target proteins are available in ample quantity to make them acquiescent not only to biological assays, NMR studies in solution and to crystallization for X-ray analysis. The number of protein structures solved using X ray or NMR has begun to rise sharply and more than 60,230 protein three dimensional structures have been deposited in the Protein Data Bank till date (Feb, 2018) (www.rcsb.org/pdb/).

The target should be essential in such a way that in spite of its crucial role in cell cycle its elimination should lead to the pathogen's death. Proteins (specifically histones) controlling epigenetic events are therefore of increasing interest in drug discovery and development aspects. Selective destruction of malignant tumour cells without damaging normal cells is a key goal for safer and more effective cancer chemotherapy (Glenn *et al.*, 2004).

Table 1. Target classes addressed by SMOLs, BIOLs and nucleic acids and their modes of action

Drug	Covered target classes	Mode of action
Small molecular weight chemical compound (SMOL)	Enzymes	Inhibitors, activators [a]
	Receptors	Agonists, antagonists, modulators, allosteric activators, sensitizers
	Transcription factors	Inhibitors, activators
	Ion Channels	Inhibitors, openers
	Transport proteins	Inhibitors
	Protein-Protein interface	Inhibitors of protein- protein interaction [a]
	Nucleic acids	Alkylation, Complexation, intercalation
Biologics (BIOL)	(Extracellular) Proteins	Antibodies
	Transmembrane receptors, extracellular proteins	Recombinant proteins
	Cell surface receptors	Antibody-drug conjugates (ADCs)
	Substrates and metabolites	Enzyme cleavage
Nucleic acids	RNA	RNA interference

[a]Novel approaches

Table 2. Drug target databases Websites (Yan-Fen & Xing-Ming, 2015)

Drug target databases	Websites
DrugBank	http://www.drugbank.ca/
STITCH	http://stitch.embl.de/
ChEMBL	https://www.ebi.ac.uk/chembldb/
Superdrug	http://bioinformatics.charite.de/superdrug2/
DGIdb	http://dgidb.genome.wustl.edu/
Binding DB	http://www.bindingdb.org/bind/index.jsp
CLiBE	http://xin.cz3.nus.edu.sg/group/clibe/clibe.asp
The TDR Targets database	http://tdrtargets.org/
Comparative Toxicogenomics Database	http://ctdbase.org/
IUPHAR-DB	http://www.iuphar-db.org/index.jsp
PROMISCUOUS	http://bioinformatics.charite.de/promiscuous/
KEGG BRITE	http://www.genome.jp/kegg/brite.html
Potential Drug Target Database	http://www.dddc.ac.cn/pdtd/
Therapeutic Target Database	http://bidd.nus.edu.sg/group/ttd/ttd.asp

Histone Deacetylases /Classification of HDAC Enzymes and Their Localization

A promising strategy to meet the objective of safer therapy is the use of differentiating agents such as Histone deacetylases inhibitors (HDACi) derived from amino acids which can differentiate cancer cells from normal cells (Kahnberg *et al.*, 2006). Histone deacetylases (HDACs) are a new class of potential therapeutic agents, have attracted a great deal of interest for both research and clinical applications. So far, 18 genes were found to encode HDAC family, which are grouped according to class I to IV (Witt *et al.*, 2009). Aberrant regulation of classic HDACs (class I, II, and IV) has been reported in various cancer types suggesting significance of HDAC in carcinogenesis. Increasing efforts have been focused on the discovery of HDAC inhibitors and some HDAC inhibitors have been approved as a new target for anti-cancer drug development for use in cancer therapy.

HDAC8 as Target for Cancer

Among them, HDAC8 belongs to the class I group. HDAC8 is differentially expressed and associated with various cancers. It was reported that HDAC8 is relevant in neuroblastoma (Oehme *et al.*, 2009); its inhibition induces apoptosis in T-cell cancers such as leukemia (Gryder *et al.*, 2012; Balasubramanian *et al.*, 2008). The significant concentrations of HDAC8 found in colorectal, cervical, and gastric cancers cells (Song *et al.*, 2005, Zhu *et al.*, 2004) indicate that HDAC8 inhibitors may be chemotherapeutic agents for colon, cervical, and gastric cancers.

The HDAC8 enzyme contains 377 long amino acids and this isoform is ubiquitously found in the nucleus. This enzyme is with stand-alone deacetylase activity and a key participant in a growing number of biological processes and tumor cell lines (Buggy *et al.*, 2000). The other functional HDACs are found as multimeric complexes of higher molecular weight whereas HDAC8 appears as single peptides. It was observed that most of the purified HDAC enzymes are functionally inactive (Vannini *et al.*, 2007; Bolden *et al.*, 2006). This enzyme is one of the regulatory components that enables the tight epigenetic control over the chromatin and has shown to regulate p53 levels (Yan *et al.*, 2012). HDAC8 is involved in tumorigensis in some tissues as it regulates telomerase activity.

Moreover, an RNA interference study exhibited that HDAC8 is the only deacetylase found overexpressed than other HDACs (Waltregny *et al.*, 2005). This protein binds with the leukemic inv (16) protein, an abnormal fusion protein formed during acute myeloid leukemia (Durst *et al.*, 2003). By considering the drug discovery perspective, HDAC8 is deemed to be the preeminent target among other mammalian HDACs. HDACi are elating anticancer agents that stimulate tumour cell death, differentiation and/or cell-cycle arrest. In addition to their inherent special effects on tumour cells, HDACi acts by regulating host immune responses and tumour vasculature damage to control the survival of neoplastic tissues. A major advantage of HDACi is its resistance to normal cells (Burgess *et al.*, 2004; Insinga *et al.*, 2005; Ungerstedt *et al.*, 2005) when compared to tumor cells. They are more sensitive and undergo growth arrest, inhibited differentiation and cell death. However, pan-HDAC inhibitors lack isotype selectivity, simultaneously inhibiting multiple HDAC isotypes.

Many clinical trials have assessed the efficacy of HDACi against individual isoforms from different classes. Disappointingly, very few inhibitors in clinical trials have shown a broadband inhibition profile, moderately selective for one HDAC class but not for a particular isotype. The prevalence of drug-induced side effects was also observed to be very high: constitutive (gastrointestinal (anorexia 81% and diarrhea 56%), fatigue 62%, and hematologic (thrombocytopenia 50%) (Duvic *et al.,* 2007).

Another limitation of current HDAC inhibitors is their tissue and drug specific action and relatively narrow therapeutic window for off- target effects. Many on target effects are dependent on still poorly understood host factors, and the mutual redundancy of individual HDACs needs further study. Many HDACi effects on biological targets require sustained dosing, as effects are reversible upon drug removal. In addition, the mechanisms of resistance to HDAC inhibitors need to be further explored in order to maximize clinical efficacy of the drugs in the market. (Zheng *et al.,* 2017).

Despite the limited understanding of the mechanisms underpinning HDACi action, there is mounting clinical evidence demonstrating an acceptable toxicity profile for the most HDACi.

This leaves open a narrow window of speculation that the decreased therapeutic efficacy and observed side effects may be most likely due to non specific HDAC isoform inhibition. Further insight into the molecular mechanisms that govern the inhibition of HDACs could help to design more specific and potent drugs. Thus, the development of selective HDAC8 inhibitors is of high interest in the etiology and treatment of various cancers.

The proposed chapter is focused on the understanding of the molecular function of HDAC8 in cancer to find rationally targeted treatment combinations for clinical application of HDAC8-selective inhibitors. This chapter also will also demonstrate superiority of selective HDAC isozyme targeting versus pan-HDAC inhibition in terms of reduced toxicity and with greater efficacy in a tumor that is dependent on HDAC8. By executing this approach, inhibition of the activity of HDAC8 specifically will pertain to yield full therapeutic potential restricting/ limiting side effects. Finally, HDAC8-selective targeting can be effective in cancer exhibiting HDAC8 isozyme-dependent tumor growth *in vitro.*

Targets for HDAC8 on Adult T Cell Leukemia/Lymphoma

Even though HDAC8 was the first human HDAC to be crystallized with bound inhibitors, (Somoza *et al.*, 2004; Vannini *et al.*, 2007; Dowling *et al.*, 2008). A few years later, startlingly very little information was recognized on the role of HDAC8 in physiology or pathophysiology. HDAC8 remains one of the least understood HDACs with no identified direct transcriptional target or corepressor partner (Delcuve *et al.*, 2013; Mihaylova & Shaw, 2013). Other class I HDACs (1, 2 and 3) is predicted to associate with gene promoters in repressor complexes, but promoter interactions with HDAC8 have neither reported nor regulatory gene targets of HDAC8 clearly revealed (Delcuve *et al.*, 2013). An activated fusion protein, PML-RAR by drafting in nuclear corepressor complexes has been shown to inhibit cellular differentiation. Such complexes play vital role to maintain HDAC in various hematologic lineage specific gene promoters. This HDAC-dependent transcriptional repression emerges out as common pathway for the development of leukemia and embodies a crucial target for new therapeutic agents (Martinez-Mancilla *et al.*, 2006).

Many inventors spot out their efforts for developing isoform specific and selective HDAC8i pretending to the verity that the enzyme HDAC8 is expressed at high levels in Jurkat, K562 and HuT78 cell lines (Ononye *et al.*, 2012). Importantly, an HDAC8-specific inhibitor, PCI-34051 was reported to induce caspase-dependent apoptosis through activation of phospholipase 1 in T-cell lines derived from Adult T-cell leukemia/lymphoma (ATL) or CTCLs but not in other hematopoietic or solid tumor cell lines (Balasubramanian *et al.*, 2008). The reason for such selective activity is not clear but may be related to the dominant expression of phospholipase C1 in T cells. Although PCI- 34051 have not been tested for ATL but, the results strongly suggested that PCI-34051 would be highly effective on ATL. In fact, a pan-HDAC inhibitor, **4** was shown to have a potent antiproliferative effect on ATL (Hasegawa *et al.*, 2011).

Undeniably by considering the above facts, it is concluded that there is quest for the HDAC8 targets by which isoform selectivity and the mechanism responsible for its specificity could be targeted so as to design much more HDAC8 specific inhibitors, as it is ubiquitously expressed.

COMPUTATIONAL MAKE OF HDAC 8 INHIBITORS AND ITS VALIDATION BY *IN VITRO* STUDIES: A CASE STUDY

HDACi characteristically follow a structural motif comprised of a surface recognition cap moiety (a) that can tolerate extraordinary variability, a linker group (b) that traverses tunnel of the active site and a zinc binding group (ZBG (c) that chelates active site zinc ion (Gryder *et al.,* 2012). By modifying these different pieces of pharmacophore, the structural basis for HDACi potency, isoform selectivity and efficacy against cancer can be explored. Modification of the linker group, with different chain length, saturated or unsaturated hydrocarbons, including cyclic hydrocarbons have also displaced variations in the inhibitory activity. It is a tough task to identify novel compounds that belong to these structural classes or to entirely new structural classes that can act as a therapeutic agent for cancer specifically by inhibiting the responsible HDAC8 activity. A slight modification of the zinc binding group (ZBG), linker and hydrophobic cap group has individually contributed to the selective inhibitory nature of the compounds. Eventually, such modifications have led to the class-selective rather than isoform-selective inhibitors (Krennhrubec *et al.*, 2007; Estiu *et al.*, 2010). The active site in HDAC8 has a long narrow tunnel that leads to the cavity of catalytic machinery. During the deacetylation reaction, the tunnel is presumably dwelled by the four methylene groups of the acetylated lysine. The rim of the tunnel is formed by three conserved hydrophobic, Phe152, Phe208, and Met274 (Krennhrubec *et al.*, 2007). These residues are conserved across the class I HDACs, whereas in other family members in lieu of Met274, Leu is placed (Somaza *et al.*, 2004). In HDAC8, the Zn (II) that facilitates amide hydrolysis is found at the bottom of the tunnel.

The active site region of the isoenzymes of HDAC is significantly conserved among the family members. This makes the design of isoform-selective inhibitors very complicated. Literatures have reported that the exposed surface of the active site entrance is less conserved among HDAC isoforms and this region can be exploited for the design of isoform selective inhibitors (Estiu *et al.*, 2010). The hydrophobic cap zone is predominantly accountable for selectivity. It is capable of binding to the HDAC besides other complex components available near the active site (Salisbury & Cravatt, 2007).

The three dimensional X-ray crystal structure of human HDAC8 was the first to be deposited in PDB. Presently, there are 14 human HDAC8 structures co-crystallized with different inhibitors with PDB codes 1T64, 1T67, 1T69, 1VKG, 2W22, 2V5W, 2V5X, 3EW8, 3EWF, 3EZF, 3EZT, 3F06, 3F07 and 3FOR.

Depending on the type of inhibitor bound with HDAC8, the active site has revealed greater topological differences. In addition, conformational flexibility mediated by the L1 and L2 active site loops have helped in sorting out unique features of HDAC8 for catalysis. These changes instigate from the existence of two profound pockets, one leading to the active site and the other adjacent to the active site lined by Tyr306 and Phe152 (Figure 3) (Source: Somaza *et al.*, 2004, Structure, vol.12, no.7, pp. 1325-1334).

The second deep pocket is open in the structure 1T64 whereas it remains closed and well defined in the bulk of the protein in the SAHA-co-crystallized structure of 1T69 (Estiu *et al.*, 2010). The opening of the second pocket is intervened by a movement of loop L1 (Somoza *et al.*, 2004). This pocket is created by movement of amino acid residue Phe152 away from its normal position packed against amino

Figure 3. Complexes of HDAC8 with TSA, MS-344, SAHA and CRA-A
[Source: Somaza et al., 2004, Structure, vol.12, no.7, pp. 1325-1334]

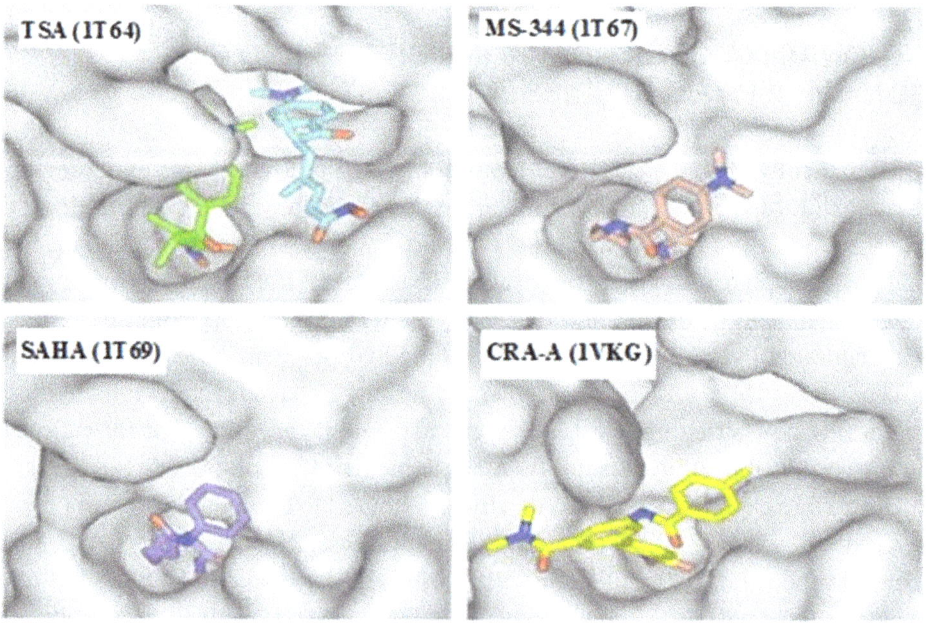

acid residue, Met274 of HDAC8 and forms the lip of the active site tunnel. Beeler *et al.* (2014) reasoned that this sub-pocket could be targeted by a new HDAC8i scaffold. If this pocket is accessible only to HDAC8, inhibitors that bind to it should be selective for HDAC8.

Further, it was proposed that the compounds which possess a ZBG linked to a moiety or group of moieties that are positioned to a hydrophilic subpocket between HDAC8 residues Met274 and Phe152 near the active site Zn (II) may be selective for HDAC8.

Reported HDAC8 Inhibitors

Very few HDAC8 selective inhibitors have been designed adhoc and reported (Hu *et al.*, 2003 & Tang *et al.*, 2011). Previous reports of selective HDAC8i included short (**1-3**) (Suzuki *et al.* 2014) and linkerless hydroxamates (**4-6**) (Krennhrubec *et al.*, 2007).

The highthroughput screening efforts by many researchers have produced libraries of small molecule HDACi with hydrazide aryl hydroxamic acids as a new linker motif (**7** and **8**) that exhibits selectivity for HDAC8 on contrary to the general pharmacophoric features (Tang *et al.*, 2011).

Researchers from Novartis also reported two lead HDACi that have an (R)-α- amino-ketone moiety (**9** and **10**) as a unique ZBG. These compounds have recorded themselves as selective HDAC8i by an interaction with the acetate exit tunnel of HDAC8 (Whitehead *et al.*, 2011).

Drugs in the clinical trial and their specificity under class I HDAC category are shown in table 3.

Estiu *et al.*, (2010) stated that the exposed surface of active site entrance is less conserved among HDAC isoforms and this region can be exploited for the design of isoform selective inhibitors. The hydrophobic cap zone is predominantly accountable for selectivity. Salisbury & Cravatt (2007) reported that the cap group (**a**) is capable of binding to the HDAC besides other complex components available near the active site. Partial changes in the linker (**b**) distinguish HDAC8 from other classes that endow direct specificity by exact fit into the widened catalytic pocket of HDAC8 (Falkenberg & Johnstone

Figure 4. Structures of HDAC8 inhibitors

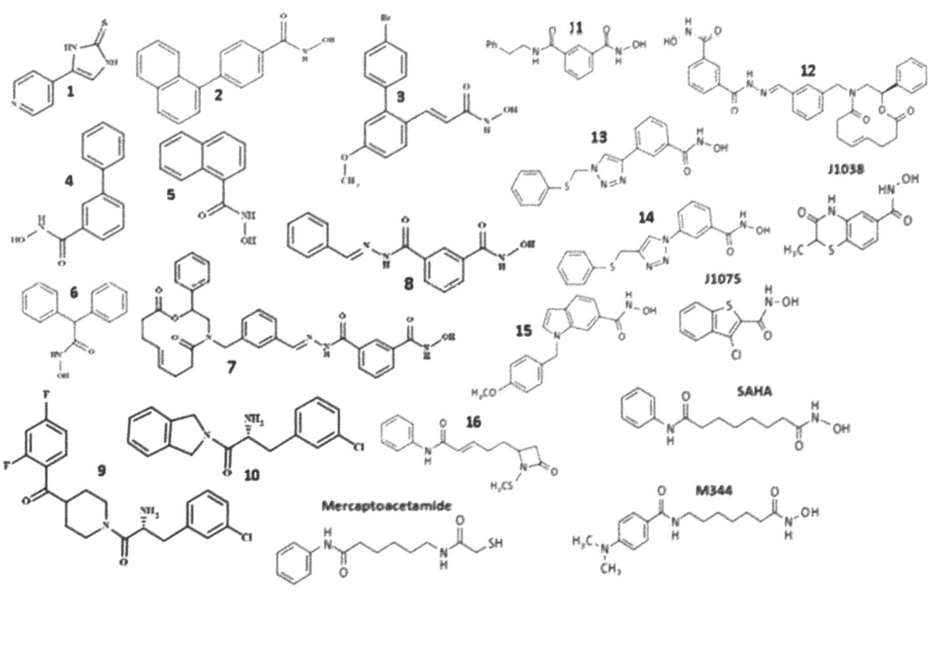

Table 3. Specificity of Class I HDAC for drugs in clinical trials

Compound	Class I HDACs				Reference
	HDAC 1	HDAC2	HDAC3	HDAC8	
1	ni[a]	-	ni[a]	0.5 μM	(Hu *et al.*, (2003)
2	>100 μM	-	-	0.3 μM	(Krennhrubec *et al.*, (2007)
3	4.5 μM	>20 μM	4.8 μM	5.7nM	(Huang *et al.*, (2012)
9	>30 μM	>30 μM	-	200nM	(Whitehead *et al.*, (2011)
11	12 μM	9 μM	23 μM	0.12 μM	(Olson *et al.* (2013)
12	-	3.6 μM	15 μM	0.023 μM	(Tang *et al.*, (2011)
13	38 μM	>100 μM	68 μM	0.070 μM	(Suzuki *et al.*, (2014)
14	>100 μM	>100 μM	>100 μM	0.053 μM	(Suzuki *et al.*, (2014)
15	4 μM	>50 μM	>50 μM	0.01 μM	(Balasubramanian *et al.*, (2008)
16	>1000 μM	> 1000 μM	>1000 μM	4.53 μM	(Galletti *et al.*, (2009)
J1038	23.6 μM	-	12.3 μM	0.97 μM	(Martin *et al.*, (2013)
J1075	19.4 μM	-	1.9 μM	3.1 μM	(Martin *et al.*, (2013)
Mercapto-acetamide	-	-	-	200 μM	(Stolfa *et al.*, (2014)
SAHA	117 nM	-	123.8nM	0.4 μM	(Martin *et al.*, (2013) Stolfa *et al.*, (2014)
M344	43.1nM	-	17.62nM	2.9 μM	(Martin *et al.*, (2013) Stolfa *et al.*, (2014)

[a]Abbreviations: ni, no inhibition ;- values not reported.

2014; Tessier *et al.*, 2009). The literature on pharmacophoric features revealed that minor changes near the ZBG moiety (**c**) produces interruption in the existing catalysis due to high sequence similarity (Bieliauskas & Pflum, 2008).

Fortunately, HDAC8 exhibits a number of unique characteristics allowing the development of selective inhibitors. One interesting feature in this regard is the formation of the foot pocket (also called acetate release channel). This subpocket is observed in class I HDACs (HDAC1, 2, 3 and 8), but not in class II isotypes (HDAC4 and 7) x-ray structures. Another very special characteristic structural feature of HDAC8 is the presence of the side pocket. Human HDAC8 demonstrate opening of this subpocket, while in other class I HDACs (1–3), it is not observed (Melesina *et al.*, 2015). This pocket is created by movement of amino acid residue Phe152 away from its normal position packed against amino acid residue, Met274 of HDAC8 and forms the lip of the active site tunnel. Beeler *et al.*, (2014) reasoned that inhibitors which bind to this pocket are exclusively selective for HDAC8 isoform alone. Further, the findings reported by Smil *et al.*, (2009) suggest that HDAC isoform selectivity can be achieved by chiral specific molecules. The above findings were validated by Umamaheswari *et al.*, (2015) using *in silico* approaches, and found that opening of adjacent pocket facilitated the HDA8 specificity while interacting with chiral molecules. Hence, this method can be used to achieve catalysis of designed inhibitors for isoform specific HDAC8 inhibitors for our proposed study.

Pharmacophore Modeling

Structural elements responsible for selective binding of the therapeutically relevant HDAC8 isoforms are traced out by pharmacophore modeling. A three dimensional (3D) chemical feature based pharmacophore model make available an efficient way to confer the isoform selective HDAC8i. It is the chemical features generated by the pharmacophoric modeling which might be responsible for the selectivity of HDAC8i in comparison with the classical pan-HDAC pharmacophore model. On the other hand, molecular docking is highlighted by the chemical interactions features of the ligand with the receptor. The best binding poses evaluated assists the identification of ligand properties and the amino acid residues in HDAC8 accountable for activity and selectivity (Ortore *et al.*, 2009). The results of pharmacophore modeling and docking altogether contribute to the understanding of the chemical features and binding orientation underlying the selectivity of HDACi respectively. It also suggested a possible target region to design novel selective HDAC specific inhibitors (Zhu *et al.*, 2010).

ADMET

ADMET descriptors make use of pre-built validated models for a broad range of critical pharmacological end points. These models provide an early assessment of compounds being investigated by calculating the predicted absorption, distribution, metabolism, excretion and toxicity (ADMET) properties for collections of molecules such as synthesised candidates, vendor libraries, and screening collections. It predicts aqueous solubility, Blood-Brain Barrier penetration, human intestinal absorption, hepatotoxicity, plasma protein binding and CYP2D6 binding for the molecules being investigated. The results obtained from these predictions helps to eliminate compounds with adverse ADMET characteristics. As a consequence, helps to propose structural refinements in drug design with improved ADMET properties prior to synthesis (http://accelrys.com/).

TOPKAT

TOPKAT (TOxicity Prediction by Komputer Assisted Technology) is an established *in-silico* method for assessing toxicity prediction of organic compounds. TOPKAT can help to assess environmental fate, ecotoxicity, toxicity, mutagenicity, and reproductive/developmental toxicity of chemicals. It utilizes strong and cross-validated Quantitative Structure Toxicity Relationship (QSTR) models for evaluating a different range of measures of toxicity and utilizing the patented Optimal Predictive Space validation method to support in construing the results. The toxicological endpoints available are Ames mutagenicity - rodent carcinogenicity, weight of evidence carcinogenicity, carcinogenic potency TD_{50}, developmental toxicity potential, rat oral LD_{50}, rat maximum tolerated dose, rat inhalation toxicity LC_{50}, rat chronic LOAEL, skin irritancy and sensitization, eye irritancy, aerobic biodegradability, fathead minnow LC_{50}, daphnia magna EC_{50} and log P (http://accelrys.com/).

There is an assumption that analogues with multi-substituents in the diverse hydrophobic cap moiety would display more potent inhibition compared to single cap moiety in SAHA. Choi *et al.*, (2011 & 2012) illustrated that SAHA analogues with substituents adjacent to the capping group were potent nM inhibitors and more tolerant to HDAC proteins whereas, those close to the hydroxamic acid proved μM IC_{50} values. These facts suggested that any substitutions along the linker might tolerate well but the potency diminishes when positioned near the metal binding moiety. It was also noted that HDAC isoform selectivity can be achieved by using chiral specific molecules (Smil *et al.*, 2009).

The US FDA guidelines necessitate that absolute stereochemistry be established early in drug development (Brooks *et al.*, 2011). Recent studies with various single enantiomers proved to be many fold therapeutically active with low doses and fewer adverse effects than its racemates (Sumithira & Sujatha 2013; Slovakova & Hutt, 1999).

Ligand Preparation

There are now several drugs on the market that originated from this structure-based design approach; (Larry & Antony, 2003) list >40 compounds that have been discovered with the aid of structure-guided methods and that have entered clinical trials. The structure-based design methods used to optimize these leads into drugs are now often applied much earlier in the drug discovery process. Previous reports has shown the active site of HDAC8 with a stretched, tapered and hydrophobic tunnel produced by Gly151, Phe152, His180, Phe208, Met274 and Tyr306 (Vijayakumar *et al.*, 2011). Based on the pharmacophore of HDAC8, a series of 52 chiral hydroxamic acid derivatives were designed by structure-based design approach (SBDD approach) and represented in Figure 5. Molecular interaction studies were carried out for the designed ligands. All the ligands designed were typed with CharmM force field (Brooks *et al.*, 1983) and subjected to energy minimization using smart minimizer. The unwanted forces present in the molecules were removed and the energy level of the molecules was lowered. The designed ligands were saved in .mol format.

Figure 5. Structures of Chiral hydroxamic acid derivatives designed by structure-based design approach

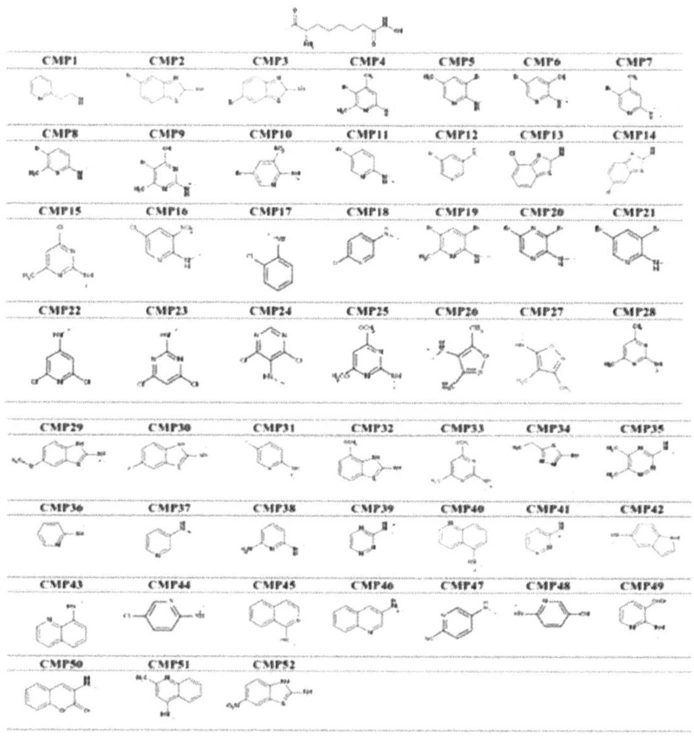

Protein Preparation

To determine the binding of HDAC8 with the designed set of ligands, the X-ray crystal structure of human HDAC8 complexed with SAHA was recovered from Protein Data Bank (PDB: 1T69). This structure was saved as standard PDB file. The protocol sets the protein by incorporating the missing atoms, assigning correct bond orders and fixing of the charges. Redundant substances like water and ligand molecules are eliminated prior to minimization. After applying CharmM force field, macromolecule 1T69 was assigned as receptor.

Molecular Docking

Molecular docking studies were performed with C DOCKER method. The target protein was loaded into the software and the active site was observed. A sphere of 8.3633Å radius around the bound inhibitor was selected as the active site sphere. And then, the designed ligands saved as.mol format were examined so as to generate the best pose by analyzing the binding interactions. The docking scores, hydrogen bond interactions, ligand atoms coordinating Zn (II) in the catalytic pocket were determined and their poses were saved for further studies. The top 12 scoring conformations of the ligands were considered for evaluating the hits. The final hits were selected based on the binding mode and molecular interactions observed at the active site.

Ligand receptor interactions reveal the binding mode of enzyme inhibitors and enzyme (Yuhong *et al.*, 2012). In addition to the best pharmacophore model generated, molecular docking was used to envisage the binding orientations of the designed ligands and their interactions with the active site amino acid residues. The designed ligands along with SAHA were docked at the active site of the target and the pictorial representation of the docked ligand is shown in Figure 6.

Figure 6. Docked complex of the ligand with HDAC8

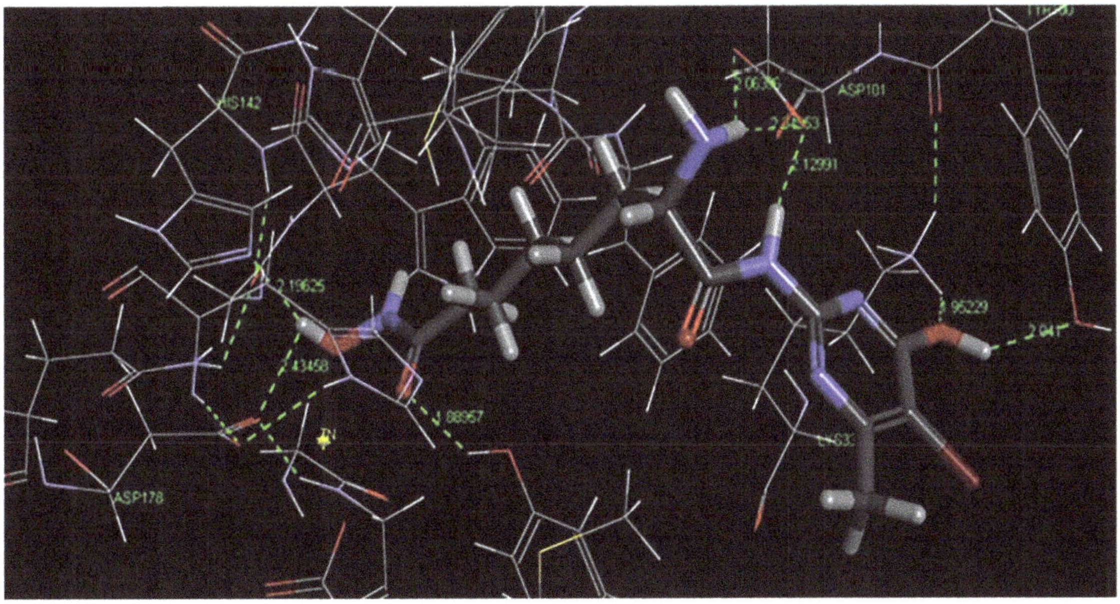

The docking energy of the bound conformation was considered to be responsible for best binding orientation of the ligands at the active site. When compared to SAHA, all the ligands maintained six hydrogen bond interactions with the active site residues, namely, Lys 33 (HZ2), Tyr 306 (HH), Asp 101 (OD1), His 142 (NE2), Asp178 (OD1) and Asp 101 (OD2). These ligands have shown hydrogen bonding with Asp 101 which confirmed that the ligands were well fitted to the substrate and is responsible for HDAC8 specificity. Earlier reports revealed that the crystal structures of HDAC8 have shown an extremely conserved binding configuration with the amino acid residues, Tyr100 and Asp101, in that way allowing for interaction with different amino acid residues in the distal part of the L2 loop (Dowling *et al.*, 2008).

On the other hand, the L1 loop located at the entrance to the catalytic site and directly above an internal cavity was supposed to play an active role in the catalytic mechanism (Haider *et al.*, 2011). It was deemed to function as an exit tunnel for the acetate product after catalysis. The C position of Lys33 in this loop demonstrated the flexibility and ability to undergo more binding. Hence it was proved that, the L1 and L2 loops equally, were essential for catalytic function of HDAC8 (Kunze *et al.*, 2013). Further, Vannini and his research group have shown that Asp101 had formed hydrogen bonds with the backbone of HDAC8 substrate by which, the substrate make itself positioned and stabilized for the deacetylation reaction (Vannini *et al.*, 2007). The presence of chiral $-NH_2$ in the designed inhibitor have shown hydrogen bonding with Asp101 side chain oxygen of the backbone amides which was considered important for inhibiting the deacetylation of HDAC8 (Dowling *et al.*, 2008).

In our findings, the most promising scaffold seemed to be associated with chiral linker, which can fit into the open-groove conformation unique to HDAC8 enzyme. The huge miscellany in the heteroaromatic cap moiety connected by a chiral amine linker assisted in the opening of second pocket by displacement of Phe152 away from its normal position. Among the shortlisted compounds, **CMP 9** has formed hydrogen bonding with Asp101, Tyr100 as well as Lys33 exhibiting a structurally highly conserved binding configuration and stabilizing the substrate for the acetylation reaction.

The hydroxamates ionize to form unique stable 5-membered ring chelates with Zn (II) (Holmes & Matthews, 1981). It has established hydrogen bonds with His142, His143 and Tyr306, and coordinated Zn (II) in a bidentate fashion, with one of the oxygen atoms replacing the active-site water molecule. The aliphatic linker present in different inhibitors complexed with the HDAC8 has shown several interactions within the active site tunnel (Somaza *et al.*, 2004; Vannini *et al.*, 2004). The aliphatic linker present in the designed ligands occupies within the hydrophobic channel and makes apolar interactions with Met274, Cys153, Phe152 and Phe208. The binding of designed ligands at the active site is shown in Figure 7 and it is presumed that all other hydroxamic acid based inhibitors bind in the similar manner as well. This suggested that a strong chelating interaction and stabilization of the compounds in the active site in addition to the hydrophobic and H-bond binding resulting in enhanced interaction of the molecule with the protein.

The docking analysis suggested that Asp101, His142, Tyr306, Asp178, Tyr100 and Lys33 are very important for HDAC8 inhibition. The significance of interaction of the inhibitor-bound structures described above shows the startling performance of the conserved Asp101 residue not only for HDAC8 substrate recognition, but a boon for the design of new HDAC8i as well. The results obtained from the docking report in Figure 6 prove that the above said distinctive features are deemed to justify the high affinity consequently resulting in antitumor effects of HDAC8i.

Figure 7. CMP 9 with Asp101 and Tyr100 exhibiting a structurally highly conserved binding configuration in the HDAC8 substrate

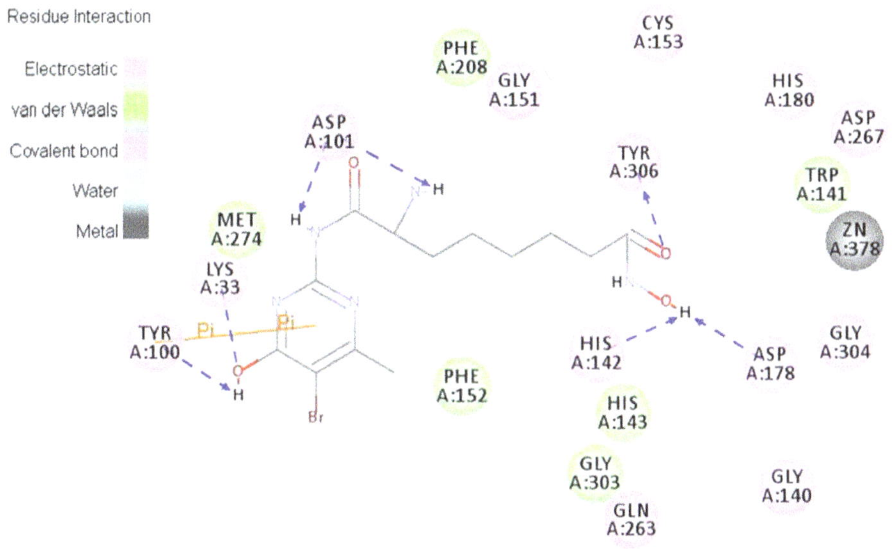

HDAC8 Enzyme Inhibition

The influence of substitutions at the heteroaromatic ring of the synthesized compounds **CMP 1e-5e** on HDAC8 inhibition activity was examined. The results of the enzyme assays are shown in Table 4.

The results showed that **CMP 1e** and **5e** inhibited HDAC8 much more significantly at 0.1 M concentration when compared to the standard drug SAHA. The percentage of inhibition for all the compounds tested was found to be in the range of 56.3 -78.5%. Even though, greater steric tolerance existed at the HDAC8 active site near the entrance of the capping group than the metal binding moiety region, the pyridimine (**CMP 1e, 2e & 4e**) and pyridine analogues (**CMP 5e**) displayed the greatest inhibitory activity at IC_{50} 0.1 μM. The polarity of the nitrogen atom and the inductive effect of the substituents might interact favorably in the binding area of the HDAC8 active site. Not surprisingly, similar trends are observed across the pyrimidines and pyridine nucleus.

Introduction of bromine at the m-poistion of the pyrimidine ring in **CMP 1e** enhanced its activity to 78.5% at 0.1 μM. This result was similar to the one reported in Dai *et al*., (2003) for the phenyl ring. Improved potency was observed when a $-OCH_3$ group introduced to *o*- and *p*- position due to positive inductive effect (68.80% in **CMP 2e**). The position of substitution seems to have little impact on activity. This is exemplified by **CMP 2e** and **4e**. Introduction of two $-CH_3$ groups in **CMP 3e** exhibited potency equal to SAHA. However, replacement of the isoxazole nucleus (**CMP 3e**) with a pyrimidine nucleus led to a greater increase in potency. As a result, the selectivity was attained not only by the diversity of subsituents but also the polarity of the pyridylamino group (**CMP 5e**) of equal size to that of the pyrimidinyl group (**CMP 1e, 2e & 4e**) at IC_{50} 0.1 μM.

These data suggested that the addition of diverse substituents at the cap position likely promotes interaction between the entrance area of HDAC8 active site and the inhibitor. The influence of the chiral amino group with bulky or polar groups near the capping group had allowed assessing the struc-

Figure 8. Structures of the synthesized compounds

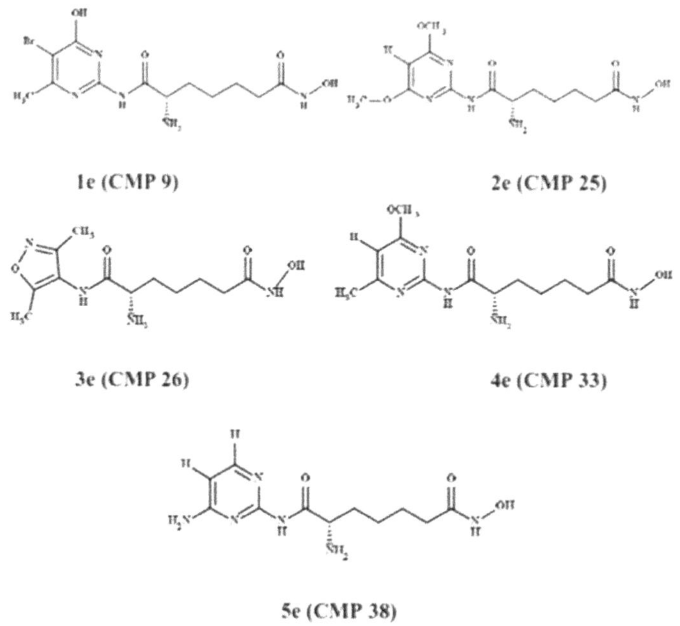

Table 4. Percentage of inhibition observed for CMP 1e - 5e by HDAC8 enzyme assay

Compound	0.025 µM	0.05 µM	0.1 µM
SAHA	34.07 ± 0.1764	43.20 ± 0.5196	56.47 ± 0.1764
CMP 1e	77.13 ± 0.1202	77.50 ± 0.1732	78.50 ± 0.3464
CMP 2e	60.07 ± 0.6386*	62.00 ± 0.5196*	65.13 ± 0.2603*
CMP 3e	56.37 ± 0.4410	57.20 ± 0.4619	58.00 ± 0.1732
CMP 4e	65.37 ± 0.2963	67.50 ± 0.2309	68.80 ± 0.5196
CMP 5e	75.03 ± 0.1764*	76.00 ± 0.05773*	78.20 ± 0.2082*

Blank - 1356.5, Total Activity – 4608

Values are expressed as mean ± SEM. Significant at *P value ≤ 0.05 as compared to the standard using Graphpad prism version 5.0.

tural requirements of the inhibitors in detail. These data suggests that small geometric differences in heteroaryl rings and linker have an effect on HDAC8 inhibitory activity and its selectivity. Among the five compounds tested for selective inhibition, **CMP 9 (CMP 1e)** is considered predominant. Hence, the obtained results are on par with *in silico* and all the *in vitro* studies.

Based on our interesting results, it is concluded that the yield of compounds **CMP 1e-5e** obtained ranges between 63-76% by the assistance of MW. This MW approach is more eco-friendly compared to previous methods used. Further, it has been proved that the modifications carried out by varying the substitutions in the heteroaromatic cap region along with a decrease in linker length retained the selectivity towards HDAC8 with increased potency.

A combination of computational modeling and MW synthesis served as a solution for drug design problem. This effort also provided some interesting insights of how small structural changes contribute to isoform-selectivity. The ability of the chiral linker in inhibitor binding modes may be the reason for the creation of a novel HDAC8i.

Overall, the research findings reveal that all the synthesized compounds were effective towards all the screened activities. The structural features required to enhance the activity are also revealed. These novel analogs may be designed or predicted by taking our title compounds as a lead for future drug discovery and development process.

CONCLUSION

Targeted therapy offers the medical community and patients an opportunity to vastly improve treatment and potentially cure disease. Targeted therapies provide an exciting time to utilize compiled information of the human genome along with the number of novel drug discovery technologies in order to create innovative medicines. Drugs that can specifically bind to a disease target and suppress its associated pathway to relieve patients from morbidity and decrease disease-associated mortalities. The concept of targeted therapy has been around for > 2 decades yet the concept of understanding the potential benefits of targeted therapy have never been nearer. Computational methods are emerged as a powerful toolbox for target identification, discovery and optimization of drug candidate molecules.

Currently, in the discovery of molecular targeted therapies, treatment strategies depend on the accuracy of molecular and genetic profiling of the cancer cells. Hence, it is very much essential to have precise knowledge of genes and underlying mechanistic pathways of a pathophysiological profile of a diseased condition to develop effective targeted therapeutics.

HDAC8 inhibitors are attractive candidates for a large number of diseases such as influenza (Yamauchi *et al.,* 2011), helminth worm infections and alzheimer's diseases (Martin *et al.,* 2013; Stolfa *et al.,* 2014). In conclusion, computational approach will witness a boom of research in the future years with many novel roles of HDAC8 yet to be discovered.

Understanding targeted proteins in the milieu of their enzymatic and scaffolding functions in terms of their interactions in complexes with proteins delineates the outlook of epigenetic interventional therapies for cancer. Obviously, the biology of HDACs and HDAC-related proteins will continue to afford exhilarating opportunities for the study of enzyme structure-mechanism and structure-inhibition rapports for several years in near future.

REFERENCES

Al-Hussaini, M., & DiPersio, J. F. (2014). Small Molecule Inhibitors in Acute Myeloid Leukemia: From the Bench to the Clinic. *Expert Review of Hematology*, *7*(4), 439–464. doi:10.1586/17474086.2014.932687 PMID:25025370

Alper, P. B., Hendrix, M., Sears, P., & Wong, C. (1998). Probing the Specificity of Aminoglycoside–Ribosomal RNA Interactions with Designed Synthetic Analogs. *Journal of the American Chemical Society*, *120*(9), 1965–1978. doi:10.1021/ja972599h

Anderson, V. R., & Perry, C. M. (2007). Fludarabine: A review of its use in non-Hodgkin's lymphoma. *Drugs*, *67*(11), 1633–1655. doi:10.2165/00003495-200767110-00008 PMID:17661532

Andrew, L. H., & Colin, R. G. (2002). The druggable genome. *Nature Reviews. Drug Discovery*, *1*(9), 727–730. doi:10.1038/nrd892 PMID:12209152

Bakheet, T. M., & Doig, A. J. (2009). Properties and identification of human protein drug targets. *Bioinformatics (Oxford, England)*, *25*(4), 451–457. doi:10.1093/bioinformatics/btp002 PMID:19164304

Balasubramanian, S., Ramos, J., Luo, W., Sirisawad, M., Verner, E., & Buggy, J. J. (2008). A novel histone deacetylase 8 (HDAC8)-specific inhibitor PCI-34051 induces apoptosis in T-cell lymphomas. *Leukemia*, *22*(5), 1026–1034. doi:10.1038/leu.2008.9 PMID:18256683

Baldwin, E. L., & Osheroff, N. (2005). Etoposide, topoisomerase II and cancer. *Current Medicinal Chemistry. Anti-Cancer Agents*, *5*(4), 363–372. doi:10.2174/1568011054222364 PMID:16101488

Barabasi, A. L., Gulbahce, N., & Loscalzo, J. (2011). Network medicine: A network-based approach to human disease. *Nature Reviews. Genetics*, *12*(1), 56–68. doi:10.1038/nrg2918 PMID:21164525

Beeler, A.B., Porco, J.A., Ingham, O.J. & Bradner, J.E. (2014). *Selective histone deacetylase 8 inhibitors*. PCT/ US2014/012968.

Bemporad, D., Luttmann, C., & Essex, J. W. (2005). Behaviour of small solutes and large drugs in a lipid bilayer from computer simulations. *Biochimica et Biophysica Acta Biomembranes*, *1718*(1-2), 1–21. doi:10.1016/j.bbamem.2005.07.009 PMID:16321606

Bieliauskas, A. V., & Pflum, M. K. H. (2008). Isoform-selective histone deacetylase inhibitors. *Chemical Society Reviews*, *37*(7), 1402–1413. doi:10.1039/b703830p PMID:18568166

Birnbaumer, L., Abramowitz, J., & Brown, A. M. (1990). Receptor-effector coupling by G proteins. *Biochimica et Biophysica Acta Biomembranes*, *1031*(2), 163–224. doi:10.1016/0304-4157(90)90007-Y PMID:2160274

Bolden, J. E., Peart, M. J., & Johnstone, R. W. (2006). Anticancer activities of histone deacetylase inhibitors. *Nature Reviews. Drug Discovery*, *5*(9), 769–784. doi:10.1038/nrd2133 PMID:16955068

Brooks, B. R., Bruccoleri, R. E., Olafson, B. D., States, D. J., Swaminathan, S., & Karplus, M. (1983). CHARMM: A program for macromolecular energy, minimization and dynamics calculations. *Journal of Computational Chemistry*, *4*(2), 187–217. doi:10.1002/jcc.540040211

Brooks, W. H., Guida, W. C., & Daniel, K. G. (2011). The significance of chirality in drug design and development. *Current Topics in Medicinal Chemistry*, *11*(7), 760–770. doi:10.2174/156802611795165098 PMID:21291399

Buchan, N. S., Rajpal, D. K., Webster, Y., Alatorre, C., Gudivada, R. C., Sanseau, P., & … . (2011). The role of translational bioinformatics in drug discovery. *Drug Discovery Today*, *16*(9-10), 426–434. doi:10.1016/j.drudis.2011.03.002 PMID:21402166

Buggy, J. J., Sideris, M. L., Mak, P., Lorimer, D. D., McIntosh, B., & Clark, J. M. (2000). Cloning and characterization of a novel human histone deacetylase, HDAC8. *The Biochemical Journal*, *350*(1), 199–205. doi:10.1042/bj3500199 PMID:10926844

Burgess, A., Ruefli, A., Beamish, H., Warrener, R., Saunders, N., Johnstone, R., & Gabrielli, B. (2004). Histone deacetylase inhibitors specifically kill nonproliferating tumour cells. *Oncogene*, *23*(40), 6693–6701. doi:10.1038j.onc.1207893 PMID:15235588

Cavasotto, C. N., & Phatak, S. S. (2009). Homology modeling in drug discovery: Current trends and applications. *Drug Discovery Today*, *14*(13-14), 676–683. doi:10.1016/j.drudis.2009.04.006 PMID:19422931

Centerwatch. (2007). *Drugs approved by the FDA*. Retrieved from http://www.centerwatch.com/patient/drugs/druglist.html

Chen, Z., Li, H. L., Zhang, Q. J., Bao, X. G., Yu, K. Q., Luo, X. M., ... Jiang, H. (2009). Pharmacophore-based virtual screening versus docking-based virtual screening: A benchmark comparison against eight targets. *Acta Pharmacologica Sinica*, *30*(12), 1694–1708. doi:10.1038/aps.2009.159 PMID:19935678

Choi, S. E., & Pflum, M. K. H. (2012). The structural requirements of histone deacetylase inhibitors: Suberoyl anilide hydroxamic acid analogs modified at the C6 position. *Bioorganic & Medicinal Chemistry Letters*, *22*(23), 7084–7086. doi:10.1016/j.bmcl.2012.09.093 PMID:23089527

Choi, S. E., Weerasinghe, S. V. W., & Pflum, M. K. H. (2011). The structural requirements of histone deacetylase inhibitors: Suberoyl anilide hydroxamic acid analogues modified at the C3 position display isoform selectivity. *Bioorganic & Medicinal Chemistry Letters*, *21*(20), 6139–6142. doi:10.1016/j.bmcl.2011.08.027 PMID:21889343

Copeland, R. A. (2013). Why Enzymes as Drug Targets? In *Evaluation of Enzyme Inhibitors in Drug Discovery: A Guide for Medicinal Chemists and Pharmacologists* (2nd ed.). Hoboken, NJ: John Wiley & Sons, Inc.; doi:10.1002/9781118540398.ch1

Dai, Y., Guo, Y., Curtin, M. L., Li, J., Pease, L. J., Guo, J., ... Michaelides, M. R. (2003). A novel series of histone deacetylase inhibitors incorporating hetero aromatic ring systems as connection units. *Bioorganic & Medicinal Chemistry Letters*, *13*(21), 3817–3820. doi:10.1016/j.bmcl.2003.07.012 PMID:14552787

David, E. G. (2008). Gerber Targeted Therapies: A New Generation of Cancer Treatments. *American Family Physician*, *77*(3), 311–319. PMID:18297955

Davidson, B. L., & McCray, P. B. Jr. (2011). Current prospects for RNA interference based therapies. *Nature Reviews. Genetics*, *12*(5), 329–340. doi:10.1038/nrg2968 PMID:21499294

Davies, M. N., Secker, A., Freitas, A. A., Mendao, M., Timmis, J., & Flower, D. R. (2007). On the hierarchical classification of G protein-coupled receptors. *Bioinformatics (Oxford, England)*, *23*(23), 3113–3118. doi:10.1093/bioinformatics/btm506 PMID:17956878

Delcuve, G. P., Khan, D. H., & Davie, J. R. (2013). Targeting class I histone deacetylases in cancer therapy. *Expert Opinion on Therapeutic Targets*, *17*(1), 29–41. doi:10.1517/14728222.2013.729042 PMID:23062071

DiMasi, J. A., Hansen, R. W., & Grabowski, H. G. (2003). The price of innovation: New estimates of drug development costs. *Journal of Health Economics*, *22*(2), 151–185. doi:10.1016/S0167-6296(02)00126-1 PMID:12606142

Doman, T. N., McGovern, S. L., Witherbee, B. J., Kasten, T. P., Kurumbail, R., Stallings, W. C., ... Shoichet, B. K. (2002). Molecular docking and high-throughput screening for novel inhibitors of protein tyrosine phosphatase-1B. *Journal of Medicinal Chemistry*, *45*(11), 2213–2221. doi:10.1021/jm010548w PMID:12014959

Dowling, D. P., Gantt, S. L., Gattis, S. G., Fierke, C. A., & Christianson, D. W. (2008). Structural studies of human histone deacetylase 8 and its site-specific variants complexed with substrate and inhibitors. *Biochemistry*, *47*(51), 13554–13563. doi:10.1021/bi801610c PMID:19053282

Drews, J. (2000). Drug discovery: A historical perspective. *Science*, *287*(5460), 1960–1964. doi:10.1126cience.287.5460.1960 PMID:10720314

Durst, K. L., Lutterbach, B., Kummalue, T., Friedman, A. D., & Hiebert, S. W. (2003). The inv (16) fusion protein associates with corepressors via a smooth muscle myosin heavy-chain domain. *Molecular and Cellular Biology*, *23*(2), 607–619. doi:10.1128/MCB.23.2.607-619.2003 PMID:12509458

Duvic, M., Talpur, R., Ni, X., Zhang, C., Hazarika, P., Kelly, C., ... Frankel, S. R. (2007). Phase 2 trial of oral vorinostat (suberoylanilide hydroxamic acid, SAHA) for refractory cutaneous T-cell lymphoma (CTCL). *Blood*, *109*(1), 31–39. doi:10.1182/blood-2006-06-025999 PMID:16960145

Ecker, D. J., & Griffey, R. H. (1999). RNA as a small-molecule drug target: Doubling the value of genomics. *Drug Discovery Today*, *4*(9), 420–429. doi:10.1016/S1359-6446(99)01389-6 PMID:10461152

Estiu, G., West, N., Mazitschek, R., Greenberg, E., Bradner, J. E., & Wiest, O. (2010). On the inhibition of histone deacetylase 8. *Bioorganic & Medicinal Chemistry*, *18*(11), 4103–4110. doi:10.1016/j.bmc.2010.03.080 PMID:20472442

Falkenberg, K. J., & Johnstone, R. W. (2014). Histone deacetylases and their inhibitors in cancer, neurological diseases and immune disorders. *Nature Reviews. Drug Discovery*, *13*(9), 673–691. doi:10.1038/nrd4360 PMID:25131830

Galletti, P., Quintavalla, A., Ventrici, C., Giannini, G., Cabri, W., Penco, S., ... Giacomini, D. (2009). Azetidinones as zinc-binding groups to design selective HDAC8 inhibitors. *ChemMedChem*, *4*(12), 1991–2001. doi:10.1002/cmdc.200900309 PMID:19821480

Galperin, M. Y., & Koonin, E. V. (1999). Searching for drug targets in microbial genomes. *Current Opinion in Biotechnology*, *10*(6), 571–578. doi:10.1016/S0958-1669(99)00035-X PMID:10600691

Gentles, A. J., & Gallahan, D. (2011). Systems biology: Confronting the complexity of cancer. *Cancer Research*, *71*(18), 5961–5964. doi:10.1158/0008-5472.CAN-11-1569 PMID:21896642

Ghanemi, A., He, L., & Yan, M. (2013). New factors influencing G protein coupled receptors' system functions. *Alexandria Journal of Medicine*, *49*(1), 1–5. doi:10.1016/j.ajme.2012.10.002

Glenn, M. P., Kahnberg, P., Boyle, G. M., Hansford, K. A., Hans, D., Martyn, A. C., ... Fairlie, D. P. (2004). Antiproliferative and phenotype-transforming antitumor agents derived from cysteine. *Journal of Medicinal Chemistry*, *47*(12), 2984–2994. doi:10.1021/jm030222i PMID:15163181

Gryder, B. E., Sodji, Q. H., & Oyelere, A. K. (2012). Targeted cancer therapy: Giving histone deacetylase inhibitors all they need to succeed. *Future Medicinal Chemistry*, *4*(4), 505–524. doi:10.4155/fmc.12.3 PMID:22416777

Haider, S., Joseph, C. G., Neidle, S., Fierke, C. A., & Fuchter, M. J. (2011). On the function of the internal cavity of histone deacetylase protein 8: R37 is a crucial residue for catalysis. *Bioorganic & Medicinal Chemistry Letters*, *21*(7), 2129–2132. doi:10.1016/j.bmcl.2011.01.128 PMID:21320778

Hajduk, P. J., Huth, J. R., & Fesik, S. W. (2005). Druggability indices for protein targets derived from NMR-based screening data. *Journal of Medicinal Chemistry*, *48*(7), 2518–2525. doi:10.1021/jm049131r PMID:15801841

Haq, I. (2002). Thermodynamics of drug-DNA interactions. *Archives of Biochemistry and Biophysics*, *403*(1), 1–15. doi:10.1016/S0003-9861(02)00202-3 PMID:12061796

Hardy, L. W., & Malikayil, A. (2003). The impact of structure-guided drug design on clinical agents. *Feature*, 15-20. Retrieved from https://pdfs.semanticscholar.org/8685/8146bca4c33c19fc7b31ed0bd5b4ff1835fb.pdf

Hasegawa, H., Yamada, Y., Tsukasaki, K., Mori, N., Tsuruda, K., Sasaki, D., ... Kamihira, S. (2011). LBH589, a deacetylase inhibitor, induces apoptosis in adult T-cell leukemia/ lymphoma cells via activation of a novel RAIDD-caspase-2 pathway. *Leukemia*, *25*(4), 575–587. doi:10.1038/leu.2010.315 PMID:21242994

Havelka, A. M., Berndtsson, M., Olofsson, M. H., Shoshan, M. C., & Linder, S. (2007). Mechanisms of action of DNA-damaging anticancer drugs in treatment of carcinomas: Is acute apoptosis an "off-target" effect? *Mini-Reviews in Medicinal Chemistry*, *7*(10), 1035–1039. doi:10.2174/138955707782110196 PMID:17979806

Holmes, M. A., & Matthews, B. W. (1981). Binding of hydroxamic acid inhibitors to crystalline thermolysin suggests a pentacoordinate zinc intermediate in catalysis. *Biochemistry*, *20*(24), 6912–6920. doi:10.1021/bi00527a026 PMID:7317361

Hopkins, H. L., & Groom, C. R. (2002). The druggable genome. *Nature Reviews. Drug Discovery*, *1*(9), 727–730. doi:10.1038/nrd892 PMID:12209152

Hu, E., Dul, E., Sung, C. M., Chen, Z., Kirkpatrick, R., & Zhang, G. F. (2003). Identification of novel isoform-selective inhibitors within class I histone deacetylases. *The Journal of Pharmacology and Experimental Therapeutics*, *307*(2), 720–728. doi:10.1124/jpet.103.055541 PMID:12975486

Huang, W. J., Wang, Y. C., Chao, S. W., Yang, C. Y., Chen, L. C., Lin, M. H., ... Chang, C.-I. (2012). Synthesis and biological evaluation of orthoaryl N-hydroxycinnamides as potent histone deacetylase (HDAC) 8 isoform-selective inhibitors. *ChemMedChem*, *7*(10), 1815–1824. doi:10.1002/cmdc.201200300 PMID:22907916

Huynen, M. A., Diaz-Lazcoz, Y., & Bork, P. (1997). Differential genome display. *Trends in Genetics*, *13*(10), 389–390. doi:10.1016/S0168-9525(97)01255-9 PMID:9351339

Insinga, A., Monestiroli, S., Ronzoni, S., Gelmetti, V., Marchesi, F., Viale, A., ... Pelicci, P. G. (2005). Inhibitors of histone deacetylases induce tumor-selective apoptosis through activation of the death receptor pathway. *Nature Medicine*, *11*(1), 71–76. doi:10.1038/nm1160 PMID:15619634

Irwin, J. J., Sterling, T., Mysinger, M. M., Bolstad, E. S., & Coleman, R. G. (2012). ZINC: A free tool to discover chemistry for biology. *Journal of Chemical Information and Modeling*, *52*(7), 1757–1768. doi:10.1021/ci3001277 PMID:22587354

Ivanov, A. S., Veselovsky, A. V., Dubanov, A. V., & Skvortsov, V. S. (2006). Bioinformatics platform development: From gene to lead compound. *Methods in Molecular Biology (Clifton, N.J.)*, *316*, 389–431. PMID:16671411

Kahnberg, P., Lucke, A. J., Glenn, M. P., Boyle, G. M., Tyndall, J. D. A., Parsons, P. G., & Fairlie, D. P. (2006). Design, synthesis, potency and cytoselectivity of anticancer agents derived by parallel synthesis from α- amino suberic acid. *Journal of Medicinal Chemistry*, *49*(26), 7611–7622. doi:10.1021/jm050214x PMID:17181145

Kim, S., Thiessen, P. A., Bolton, E. E., Chen, J., Fu, G., Gindulyte, A., ... Bryant, S. H. (2015). Pubchem substance and compound databases. *Nucleic Acids Research*, *44*(D1), D1202–D1213. doi:10.1093/nar/gkv951 PMID:26400175

Knox, C., Law, V., Jewison, T., Liu, P., Ly, S., Frolkis, A., ... Wishart, D. S. (2011). Drug Bank 3.0: A comprehensive resource for 'omics' research on drugs. *Nucleic Acids Research*, *39*(Database), 1035–1041. doi:10.1093/nar/gkq1126 PMID:21059682

Krennhrubec, K., Marshall, B. L., Hedglin, M., Verdin, E., & Ulrich, S. M. (2007). Design and evaluation of 'Linkerless' hydroxamic acids as selective HDAC8 inhibitors. *Bioorganic & Medicinal Chemistry Letters*, *17*(10), 2874–2878. doi:10.1016/j.bmcl.2007.02.064 PMID:17346959

Kulkarni, A., & Wilson, D. M. III. (2008). The involvement of DNA-damage and -repair defects in neurological dysfunction. *American Journal of Human Genetics*, *82*(3), 539–566. doi:10.1016/j.ajhg.2008.01.009 PMID:18319069

Kunze, M. B. A., Wright, D. W., Werbeck, N. D., Kirkpatrick, J., Coveney, P. V., & Hansen, D. F. (2013). Loop interactions and dynamics tune the enzymatic activity of the human histone deacetylase 8. *Journal of the American Chemical Society*, *135*(47), 17862–17868. doi:10.1021/ja408184x PMID:24171457

Lagerstrom, M. C., & Schioth, H. B. (2008). Structural diversity of G protein-coupled receptors and significance for drug discovery. *Nature Reviews. Drug Discovery*, *7*(4), 339–357. doi:10.1038/nrd2518 PMID:18382464

Larry, W.H. & Antony, M. (2003). The impact of structure-guided drug design on clinical agents. *Current Drug Discovery*, 15-20.

Liang, J., Edelsbrunner, H., & Woodward, C. (1998). Anatomy of protein pockets and cavities: Measurement of binding site geometry and implications for ligand design. *Protein Science*, *7*(9), 1884–1887. doi:10.1002/pro.5560070905 PMID:9761470

Ma, P., & Zemmel, R. (2002). Value of Novelty? *Nature Reviews. Drug Discovery*, *1*(8), 571–572. doi:10.1038/nrd884 PMID:12402497

Martin, M., Srinivasaraghavan, K., Alexander-Thomas, H., Marina, M. M., Stephanie, C., & Vincent, C. (2013). Structural basis for the inhibition of histone deacetylases 8 (HDAC8), a key epigenetic player in the blood fluke Schistosomamansoni. *PLoS Pathogens*, *9*(9), e1003645. doi:10.1371/journal.ppat.1003645 PMID:24086136

Martinez-Mancilla, M., Rosa, Z. G., & Gomez, R. E. (2006). Molecular haemoto-oncology and new specific treatment strategies for leukemia. *Gaceta Medica de Mexico*, *142*, 145–150. PMID:16711549

Mc Guire, J. J. (2003). Anticancer antifolates: Current status and future directions. *Current Pharmaceutical Design*, *9*(31), 2593–2613. doi:10.2174/1381612033453712 PMID:14529544

Melesina, J., Robaa, D., Pierce, R. J., Romier, C., & Sippl, W. (2015). Homology modeling of parasite histone deacetylases to guide the structure-based design of selective inhibitors. *Journal of Molecular Graphics & Modelling*, *62*, 342–361. doi:10.1016/j.jmgm.2015.10.006 PMID:26595183

Mihaylova, M. M., & Shaw, R. J. (2013). Metabolic reprogramming by class I and II histone deacetylases. *Trends in Endocrinology and Metabolism*, *24*(1), 48–57. doi:10.1016/j.tem.2012.09.003 PMID:23062770

Milne, J. R., Hellestrand, K. J., Bexton, R. S., Burnett, P. J., Debbas, N. M., & Camm, A. J. (1984). Class 1 antiarrhythmic drugs characteristic electrocardiographic differences when assessed by atrial and ventricular pacing. *European Heart Journal*, *5*(2), 99–107. doi:10.1093/oxfordjournals.eurheartj.a061633 PMID:6723689

Moazed, D., & Noller, H. F. (1987). Interaction of antibiotics with functional sites in 16S ribosomal RNA. *Nature*, *327*(6121), 389–394. doi:10.1038/327389a0 PMID:2953976

Oehme, I., Oehme, I., Deubzer, H. E., Wegener, D., Pickert, D., Linke, J. P., & ... . (2009). Histone deacetylase 8 in neuro blasto matumorigenesis. *Clinical Cancer Research*, *15*(1), 91–99. doi:10.1158/1078-0432.CCR-08-0684 PMID:19118036

Olson, D. E., Wagner, F. F., Kaya, T., Gale, J. P., Aidoud, N., Davoine, E. L., ... Holson, E. B. (2013). Discovery of the first histone deacetylase 6/8 dual inhibitors. *Journal of Medicinal Chemistry*, *56*(11), 4816–4820. doi:10.1021/jm400390r PMID:23672185

Ononye, S. N., Heyst, M. V., Falcone, E. M., Anderson, A. C., & Wright, D. L. (2012). Toward isozyme-selective inhibitors of histone deacetylase as therapeutic agents for the treatment of cancer. *Pharmaceutical Patent Analyst*, *1*(2), 207–221. doi:10.4155/ppa.12.21 PMID:24163736

Ortore, G., Colo, F. D., & Martinelli, A. (2009). Docking of hydroxamic acids into HDAC1 and HDAC8: A rationalization of activity trends and selectivities. *Journal of Chemical Information and Modeling*, *49*(12), 2774–2785. doi:10.1021/ci900288e PMID:19947584

Overington, J. P., Al-Lazikani, B., & Hopkins, A. L. (2006). How many drug targets are there? *Nature Reviews. Drug Discovery*, *5*(12), 993–996. doi:10.1038/nrd2199 PMID:17139284

Peter, I., Christian, S., & Achim, M. (2006). Drugs, their targets and the nature and number of drug targets. *Nature Reviews. Drug Discovery*, *5*(10), 821–834. doi:10.1038/nrd2132 PMID:17016423

Rask-Andersen, M., Almen, M. S., & Schioth, H. B. (2011). Trends in the exploitation of novel drug targets. *Nature Reviews. Drug Discovery*, *10*(8), 579–590. doi:10.1038/nrd3478 PMID:21804595

Salisbury, C. M., & Cravatt, B. F. (2007). Activity-based probes for proteomic profiling of histone deacetylase complexes. *Proceedings of the National Academy of Sciences of the United States of America*, *104*(4), 1171–1176. doi:10.1073/pnas.0608659104 PMID:17227860

Shaikh, S. A., Jain, T., Sandhu, G., Latha, N., & Jayaram, B. (2007). From drug target to leads--sketching a physicochemical pathway for lead molecule design in silico. *Current Pharmaceutical Design*, *13*(34), 3454–3470. doi:10.2174/138161207782794220 PMID:18220783

Singh, S., Malik, B. K., & Sharma, D. K. (2006). Molecular drug targets and structure based drug design: A holistic approach. *Bioinformation*, *1*(8), 314–320. doi:10.6026/97320630001314 PMID:17597912

Slovakova, A., & Hutt, A. J. (1999). Chiral compounds and their pharmacologic effects [in Slovak]. *Ceska a Slovenska Farmacie*, *48*, 107–112. PMID:10422348

Smil, D. V., Manku, S., Chantigny, Y. A., Leit, S., Wahhab, A., Yan, T. P., ... Déziel, R. (2009). Novel HDAC6 isoform selective chiral small molecule histone deacetylase inhibitors. *Bioorganic & Medicinal Chemistry Letters*, *19*(3), 688–692. doi:10.1016/j.bmcl.2008.12.045 PMID:19111466

Somoza, J. R., Skene, R. J., Katz, B. A., Mol, C., Ho, J. D., Jennings, A. J., ... Tari, L. W. (2004). Structural snapshots of human HDAC8 provides insights into the class I histone deacetylases. *Structure (London, England)*, *12*(7), 1325–1334. doi:10.1016/j.str.2004.04.012 PMID:15242608

Song, J., Noh, J. H., Lee, J. H., Eun, J. W., Ahn, Y. M., Kim, S. Y., ... Nam, S. W. (2005). Increased expression of histone deacetylase 2 is found in human gastric cancer. *APMIS*, *113*(4), 264–268. doi:10.1111/j.1600-0463.2005.apm_04.x PMID:15865607

Sreenivasa Reddy, P. E., Sreenivasulu Reddy, T., & Krushna, G. S. (2011). Advantages of Bio and Cheminformatics tools in drug design. *Current Research in Drug Targeting*, *1*(2), 6–17.

Stewart, B., & Wild, C. P. (2014). *World Cancer Report*. Lyon, France: International Agency for Research on Cancer.

Stolfa, D. A., Marek, M., Lancelot, J., Hauser, A. T., Walter, A., Leproult, E., ... Jung, M. (2014). Molecular basis for the antiparasitic activity of a mercaptoacetamide derivative that inhibits histone deacetylase 8 (HDAC8) from the human pathogen Schistosomamansoni. *Journal of Molecular Biology*, *426*(20), 3442–3453. doi:10.1016/j.jmb.2014.03.007 PMID:24657767

Sumithira, G., & Sujatha, M. (2013). Drug chirality & its clinical significance evident, future for the development/separation of single enantiomer drug from racemates - The chiral switch. *International Journal of Advanced Pharmaceutical Genuine Research*, *1*(1), 1–19.

Suzuki, T., Muto, N., Bando, M., Itoh, Y., Masaki, A., Ri, M., ... Miyata, N. (2014). Design, synthesis, and biological activity of NCC149 derivatives as histone deacetylase 8-selective inhibitors. *ChemMedChem*, *9*(3), 657–664. doi:10.1002/cmdc.201300414 PMID:24403121

Tang, W. P., Luo, T. P., Greenberg, E. F., Bradner, J. E., & Schreiber, S. L. (2011). Discovery of histone deacetylase 8 selective inhibitors. *Bioorganic & Medicinal Chemistry Letters*, *21*(9), 2601–2605. doi:10.1016/j.bmcl.2011.01.134 PMID:21334896

Terstappen, G. C., Schlüpen, C., Raggiaschi, R., & Gaviraghi, G. (2007). Target deconvolution strategies in drug discovery. *Nature Reviews. Drug Discovery*, *6*(11), 891–903. doi:10.1038/nrd2410 PMID:17917669

Tessier, P., Smil, D. V., Wahhab, A., Leit, S., Rahil, J., Li, Z., ... Besterman, J. M. (2009). Diphenylmethylenehydroxamic acids as selective class IIa histone deacetylase inhibitors. *Bioorganic & Medicinal Chemistry Letters*, *19*(19), 5684–5688. doi:10.1016/j.bmcl.2009.08.010 PMID:19699639

Tintori, C., Manetti, F., & Botta, M. (2010). Pharmacophoric models and 3D QSAR studies of the adenosine receptor ligands. *Current Topics in Medicinal Chemistry*, *10*(10), 1019–1035. doi:10.2174/156802610791293118 PMID:20370655

Umamaheswari, A., Irfan, N., & Puratchikody, A. (2015). *In silico* molecular interaction studies of chiral heterocyclic analogs of SAHA as selective histone deacetylase 8 inhibitors. *Letters in Drug Design & Discovery*, *12*(9), 711–727. doi:10.2174/1570180812666150326004848

Ungerstedt, J. S., Sowa, Y., Xu, W. S., Shao, Y., Dokmanovic, M., Perez, G., ... Marks, P. A. (2005). Role of thioredoxin in the response of normal and transformed cells to histone deacetylase inhibitors. *Proceedings of the National Academy of Sciences of the United States of America*, *102*(3), 673–678. doi:10.1073/pnas.0408732102 PMID:15637150

Vannini, A., Volpari, C., Gallinari, P., Jones, P., Mattu, M., Carfí, A., ... Di Marco, S. (2007). Substrate bindingto histone deacetylases as shown by the crystal structure of the HDAC8-substrate complex. *The EMBO Journal*, *8*(9), 879–884. doi:10.1038j.embor.7401047 PMID:17721440

Vaughan Williams, E. M. (1984). Subgroups of class 1 antiarrhythmic drugs. *European Heart Journal*, *5*(2), 96–98. doi:10.1093/oxfordjournals.eurheartj.a061632 PMID:6373262

Vijayakumar, B., Umamaheswari, A., Puratchikody, A., & Velmurugan, D. (2011). Selection of an improved HDAC8 inhibitor through structure-based drug design. *Bioinformation*, *7*(3), 134–141. doi:10.6026/97320630007134 PMID:22125384

Waltregny, D., Glenisson, W., Tran, S. L., North, B. J., Verdin, E., Colige, A., & Castronovo, V. (2005). Histone deacetylase HDAC8 associates with smooth muscle alpha-actin and is essential for smooth muscle cell contractility. *Federation of American Societies for Experimental Biology Journal*, *19*(8), 966–968. doi:10.1096/fj.04-2303fje PMID:15772115

Wang, X., Wei, X., Thijssen, B., Das, J., Lipkin, S. M., & Yu, H. (2012). Three-dimensional reconstruction of protein networks provides insight into human genetic disease. *Nature Biotechnology*, *30*(2), 159–164. doi:10.1038/nbt.2106 PMID:22252508

Wang, Y., Shaikh, S. A., & Tajkhorshid, E. (2010). Exploring transmembrane diffusion pathways with molecular dynamics. *Physiology (Bethesda, MD)*, *25*(3), 142–154. doi:10.1152/physiol.00046.2009 PMID:20551228

Whalen, E. J., Rajagopal, S., & Lefkowitz, R. J. (2011). Therapeutic potential of beta-arrestin and G protein-biased agonists. *Trends in Molecular Medicine*, *17*(3), 126–139. doi:10.1016/j.molmed.2010.11.004 PMID:21183406

Whitehead, L., Dobler, M. R., Radetich, B., Zhu, Y., Atadja, P. W., Claiborne, T., ... Stams, T. (2011). Human HDAC isoform selectivity achieved via exploitation of the acetate release channel with structurally unique small molecule inhibitors. *Bioorganic & Medicinal Chemistry*, *19*(15), 4626–4634. doi:10.1016/j.bmc.2011.06.030 PMID:21723733

Witt, O., Deubzer, H. E., Milde, T., & Oehme, I. (2009). HDAC family: What are the cancer relevant targets? *Cancer Letters*, *277*(1), 8–21. doi:10.1016/j.canlet.2008.08.016 PMID:18824292

Yamauchi, Y., Boukari, H., Banerjee, I., Sbalzarini, I. F., Horvath, P., & Helenius, A. (2011). Histone deacetylase 8 is required for centrosome cohesion and influenza A virus entry. *PLoS Pathogens*, *7*(10), e1002316. doi:10.1371/journal.ppat.1002316 PMID:22046129

Yan, W., Liu, S., Xu, E., Zhang, J., Zhang, Y., Chen, X., & Chen, X. (2012). Histone deacetylase inhibitors suppress mutant p53 transcription via histone deacetylase 8. *Oncogene*, *32*(5), 599–609. doi:10.1038/onc.2012.81 PMID:22391568

Yan-Fen, D., & Xing-Ming, Z. (2015). *A Survey on the Computational Approaches to Identify Drug Targets in the Postgenomic Era*. BioMed Research International.

Yoh, D., Akiteru, G., Maiko, K., & Tomoyuki, N. (2012). Molecularly Targeted Therapy: Past, Present and Future. *Chemotherapy*, *1*, 105.

Yuhong, X., Liang, Z., & Zhuoyong, Z. (2012). QSAR and Docking studies on different series of histone deacetylase inhibitors (HDACIs). *Letters in Drug Design & Discovery*, *9*(4), 367–378. doi:10.2174/157018012799860033

Zhao, S., & Li, S. (2010). Network-based relating pharmacological and genomic spaces for drug target identification. *PLoS One*, *5*(7), e11764. doi:10.1371/journal.pone.0011764 PMID:20668676

Zheng, P. P., Li, J., & Kros, J. M. (2017). Breakthroughs in modern cancer therapy and elusive cardiotoxicity: Critical research-practice gaps, challenges, and insights. *Medicinal Research Reviews*, *00*, 1–49. PMID:28862319

Zhu, P., Martin, E., Mengwasser, J., Schlag, P., Janssen, K. P., & Gottlicher, M. (2004). Induction of HDAC2 expression upon loss of APC in colorectal tumorigenesis. *Cancer Cell*, *5*(5), 455–463. doi:10.1016/S1535-6108(04)00114-X PMID:15144953

Zhu, Y., Li, H. F., Lu, S., Zheng, Y. X., Wu, Z., Tang, W. F., ... Lu, T. (2010). Investigation on the isoform selectivity of histone deacetylase inhibitors using chemical feature based pharmacophore and docking approaches. *European Journal of Medicinal Chemistry*, *45*(5), 1777–1791. doi:10.1016/j.ejmech.2010.01.010 PMID:20153566

Chapter 8
Molecular Modelling Studies of Novel COX-2 Inhibitors

A. Puratchikody
Anna University, India

A. Umamaheswari
Anna University, India

Navabshan Irfan
Anna University, India

Dharmaraj Sriram
Birla Institute of Technology and Sciences, India

ABSTRACT

Molecular modelling uses theoretical and computational chemistry, which offers insight into the nature of molecular systems. This chapter highlights the theoretical explanation of molecular modelling methods and describes the designing of novel tyrosine COX-2 inhibitors using molecular modelling as an example. As a first step, fragment-based drug design is used to design the novel tyrosine analogues and ligand-based drug design such as QSAR, and pharmacophore was used to identify the descriptors, ensemble of steric and electronic features, which is responsible for the selective COX-2 inhibition. The next step, structure-based drug design, was used to analyses intra- and intermolecular interactions in the drug receptor system to improve the binding affinity and pharmacokinetic properties. Finally, the pharmacokinetic and toxicity properties were predicted quantitatively using rationalization of observed structure-activity relationships and the results are reported.

INTRODUCTION

COX-2 Inhibitors

The design of new anti-inflammatory agents (COX-2 inhibitors) continues to be a tough task due to complexity of the inflammatory process. Production of prostaglandins, the inflammatory mediators depend on the enzyme cyclooxygenases (COX-1 and COX-2). Cyclooxygenases catalyse the oxygenation

DOI: 10.4018/978-1-5225-7326-5.ch008

of biologically active C20 metabolites of arachidonic acid (AA) to produce inflammatory eicosanoids namely, prostaglandins and thromboxane. These key regulatory enzymes facilitate a range of physiological and pathophysiological functions in variety of cells within the body (Blobaum & Marnett, 2007).

The discovery of nonsteroidal anti-inflammatory drugs (NSAIDs) inhibiting prostaglandin synthesis in guinea pig lung and human platelets established COX-1 as an inflammatory target for the ancient class of drugs (Vane, 1971; Smith &Willis, 1971; Ferreria et al. 1971). The subsequent discovery of COX-2 in 1991 during inflammation, recommended that this form of the enzyme signifies the molecular target for the anti-inflammatory effects of NSAIDs (Xie et al., 1991; Fu et al. 1990; Kujubu et al. 1991; Patel et al. 2009). The primary form of COX-1 expressed in the gastrointestinal (GI) tract directed to the search for selective COX-2 inhibitors as potential anti-inflammatory drugs. The new finding of COX-2 inhibitors unveil the reduced GI side effects when compared to gastric side effects exhibited by traditional NSAIDs (Kawai et al. 2005; Al-Hourani et al. 2011; Pairet et al., 1996). As a result, some highly selective COX-2 inhibitors were introduced in the market vizcelecoxib, rofecoxib, valdecoxib, etoricoxib, and lumiracoxib (Prasit & Riendeaue, 1997; Talley, 1999; Talley et al., 1999; Chan et al., 1999; Esser et al., 2005; Marnett et al., 2009). Later on, researchers in United States and Europe conducted long-term placebo-controlled studies that revealed the existence of cardiac side effects in the above cited COX-2 inhibitors. It led to withdrawal of valdecoxib and rofecoxib from the market. These risks until now are assumed to be due to the presence of COX-2 in blood vessels. Later on, it was reported that COX-2 is in fact largely absent in major blood vessels (Ahmetaj-Shala et al., 2015; Hochstrasser, 20017; Liu et al., 2012). This critical information on role of COX-2 in chronic inflammatory disease paved the way to the researchers for rational design of selective COX-2 inhibitors with devoid of cardiovascular and GI events.

On review of literature, abundant information on structural activity relationship of different COX-2 inhibitors was studied. Sing et al. (2004) reported that substitution of methane sulfonamide at various positions of 1, 5-diaryl pyrazole influences the COX-2 inhibiting activity. In particular, introduction of 4-methanesulfonamide group at position-4 of the C-5 phenyl ring of 1, 5-diaryl pyrazoles induced the COX-2 inhibitory activity. This report is on par with the studies of Penning et al., (1997), who found that the most effective COX-2 inhibitor, nimesulide possesses methane sulfonamide group at para position of phenyl ring. Further, Zargi et al (2011) have reported a series of 1,3-diaryl urea and it possess methane sulphonyl functional group at the para position of N-1 phenyl ring and addition of diverse substituents viz -H, -F, -Cl, -Me and -OMe at the para-position of N-3 phenyl ring which enhances COX-2 selective inhibition. During the search of literature, we excavated out that the majority of the research reported so far possess similar pharmacophores with enhanced COX-2 selectivity (Chaudhary et al, 2010; Bali et al, 2012).

The authors of this chapter have taken tyrosine as their core nucleus to design a series of selective COX-2 inhibitors. In this concern, an investigation was made on tyrosine scaffold from the natural sources, since it possesses sterically more complex structure and exhibit advanced binding characteristics compared with synthetic tyrosine compounds (Lahlou, 2013). These quite distinct structural characters may enhance the non-existence of cardiovascular side effects and direct towards COX-2 selectivity. It is found that the complex structures of bioactive dibromotyrosine derivatives obtained from natural sources have proven to possess anti-inflammatory activity (Peng & Hamann, 2005). Therefore, tyrosine scaffolds derived from natural sources are of great interest as candidate COX-2 inhibitor with negligible side effects.

This novel tyrosine skeleton is a proof of principle to be further developed by substituting methane sulphonyl group at p-position of tyrosine moiety along with electron donating groups for enhancing COX-2 inhibiting activity. It is understood from the literature that substitutions of different alkyl, aryl and heteroaryl groups at –OH position of tyrosine nucleus inhibited angiogenesis, growth and development of malignant cells and their migration into the surrounding tissues with negligible toxicity on the living cells (Sallam et al, 2010). It is speculated that substitution of alkyl and aryl groups at –OH position of tyrosine nucleus may eliminate the cardiovascular problems exhibited by COX-2 inhibitors.

Herein, we report how we virtually improved the selectivity of designed tyrosine molecules towards the enzyme COX-2 in order to reduce the risk of cardiovascular events by computational molecular modelling approaches. The section 2 explains various methods adopted in our studies for designing a series of COX-2 inhibitors.

MOLECULAR MODELLING

Molecular modelling may be defined as simplified or idealised description of a system used to model or mimic the behaviour of molecules and molecular system (Andrew, 2001). These methods are applied to study molecular systems ranging from small molecules to large biological molecules and material assemblies. It is particularly applicable in the fields of computational chemistry, drug design, computational biology and materials science etc.

In this chapter, we have described three molecular modelling methods which are more essential to design and identify the novel drug molecules

1. Fragment based drug design When the protein information only available this methoed is selected for design novel ligands
2. Ligand based drug design Only ligand information known, this method is selected for activity pridiction studies
3. Structure-based drug design This method selected when the 3D secondary structure and ligand information available

Fragment-Based Ligand Design: LUDI

De Novo ligand design (Ludi) identifies potential new ligands by analysing a library of small molecules to find those that are complementary to a target receptor. Complementarity is defined as an appropriate spatial orientation of hydrogen-bonding and hydrophobic functional groups. Molecules that cannot be mapped without suffering van der Waals clashes or electrostatic repulsions are screened out during the search process. De Novo methods uses the Ludi algorithm which works in three steps.

1. Interaction sites within a defined search sphere inside the target receptor are calculated. Typically, the search sphere definition is based on the location of a set of known ligands which bind within the receptor cavity.
2. Ludi-formatted libraries are examined for fragments that can map inside the binding site sphere while forming favourable interactions with the interaction sites.
3. An alignment or linking for the fragments is proposed.

To generate the interaction map site, Ludi uses a some of non- bonded contact rules that are intended to cover the wide-ranging range of energetically favourable orientations for hydrophobic and hydrogen bonds interactions.

Aligning Fragments With Partially Built Ligands

Ludi simply positions the fragment onto the active sites and simultaneously linking the fragments to a ligand link site. A link site is a hydrogen atom that can be replaced by a suggested fragment. The specific link site can be selected either manually or by allowing Ludi to assume that all the hydrogen atoms of the positioned ligand are link sites. It is notable that Ludi does not actually create the ligand-fragment bond(s). Ludi aligns the fragment to multiple link sites on the existing ligand for multiple links. If the partially built ligand is composed of multiple pieces, Ludi may allow fragments to connect the bridges. Figure 1a shows a partially built ligand and a fragment aligned at one link site. Figure 1b shows two-link alignments and Figure 1c indicates three-link alignments. Merging and bonding the fragments and ligands is shown in the Figure 1.

Ligand-Based Drug Design

In the absence of receptor 3D information, lead identification and optimization depend on available pharmacologically relevant agents and their bioactivities (Stahura & Bajorath, 2004; Gunner et al., 2004; Hansch et al., 2004). The computational approaches include QSAR, pharmacophore modelling, and database mining (Parvy, 2003; Langer &Wolber, 2004; Dror et al., 2004).

Figure 1. Schematic representation of one (a), two (b), and three (c) linksites in Ludi

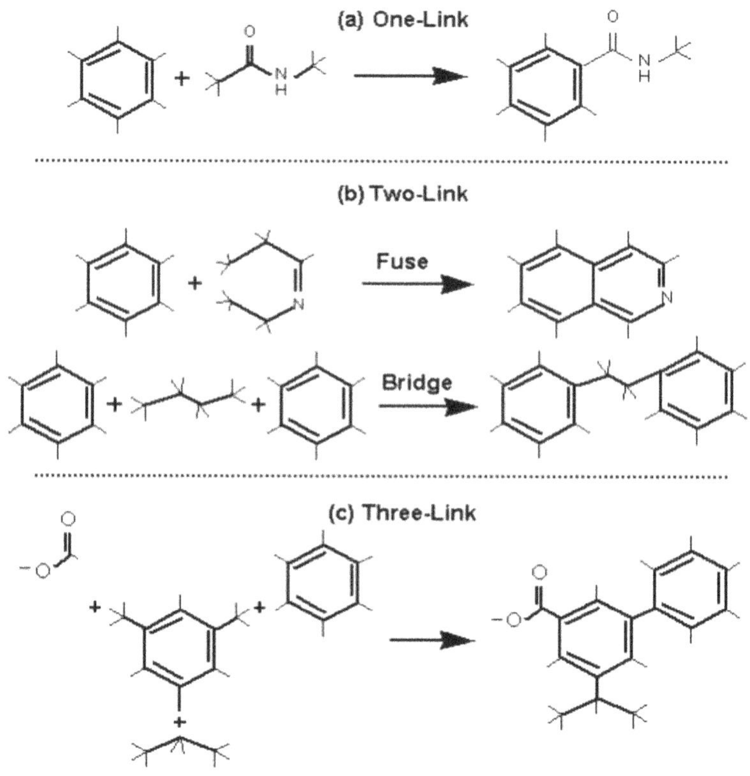

Pharmacophore Modelling

The concept of pharmacophore was introduced by Paul Ehrlich in the early 1900s while doing screening of biological activity of chemical dyes and other compounds for their corresponding chemotherapeutic activity. In the order of chromophores and toxophores, the term pharmacophore was developed by him to cite the molecular framework that carries (phoros) the essential features responsible to ensure the efficacy of the drug with a specific biological target and to trigger its biological response. Later on in 1977, Peter Gund comes out with a widely accepted definition "a set of structural features in a molecule that is recognised at the receptor site and is responsible for that molecule's biological activity". In reality, the modern definition completely tends to give minimal response to cover only specific, noncovalent interactions between a molecule and receptor. Therefore, a pharmacophore model is not associated with binding that occurs solely as a consequence of short-lived surface-to-surface hydrophobic interactions, nor does binding that involve the formation of covalent bonds. In fact, Pharmacophore methods be composed of a range of computer-aided approaches, including, but not limited to, automated pharmacophore perception, structure alignment (Perkin et al, 2003; Tropsha, 2001), identification and representation of sterically forbidden regions (Garg et al, 2003; Kier & Hall, 1993), 3D similarity based on pharmacophore fingerprints (Tetko et al, 1994; Ajay &Murcko, 1995; Bolis et al 1991; King et al 1992).

QSAR

Quantitative structure/ activity relationship (QSAR) modelling is a well-established method in the last fifty years of drug design and development research field. In the primary stages of drug design, when the geometry of the active site is not known, 3D-QSAR tends to be used for more accurate predictions of compound's activity. The QSAR methodologies used at earlier 1963 were relatively simple, employing a small number of physical-chemical descriptors and statistical methods such as multiple linear regression.

Since the late 1980s, the field has changed dramatically and fuelled by changes in the size, complexity, and availability of experimental data sets of biologically active compounds. These changes have been coincidental with the advances in chemometrics, resulting in a significant increase in the number of chemical descriptors as well as growing implementation of machine learning and advanced statistical modelling techniques available for QSAR studies.

3D-QSAR is a technique used to quantitatively predict the structural descriptors of a molecule and the pharmacological activity. The great advantage of 3D-QSAR is that the active site information of target receptor is not necessary to analyse the active compounds (David, 2009). It defines the properties of the active site without knowing the ligand's structure using mathematical designs. QSAR mainly compute the electrostatic and steric interactions by placing imaginary probe atom at various positions on a grid around the known active compound. In some cases, other interactions such as hydrogen bonding is also be included. After the interaction calculation for multiple active compounds, a partial least squares algorithm can be used to determine what spatial arrangement of features there could be in an active site that interacts with the known active molecules. In these two LBDD stages, pharmacophore searches tend to be more useful for quickly searching very large molecular structure databases, while 3D-QSAR tends to give more accurate activity predictions.

ADMET

ADMET stands for "Adsorption, Distribution, Metabolism, Excretion, and Toxicity." Recent years have seen a higher growth of computational ADMET prediction software tools and various methodologies. This is because of the majority of clinical trial failures have been due to ADMET issues, not from a lack of efficacy. The prediction of ADMET properties is incredibly very difficult task. As a compound moves from the digestive tract to the drug target, it will encounter tens of thousands of proteins, lipids, blood-borne compounds, etc. The present state of technology is not up to the task of predicting every potential interaction and the probability of that interaction occurring. Thus, most ADMET predictions are made by relatively simple data, such as compound size, lipophilicity, and functional groups present. There are QSAR programs designed specifically for creating ADMET prediction models, such as ADMET Predictor from Simulations Plus. Most of the ADMET QSAR equations are developed using the standard practice of finding correlations between the property to predict and descriptor values. One program that takes a somewhat different approach is TOPKAT from ACCELRYS Discovery Studio. The ADMET predictions produced by COSMO therm, such as blood-brain barrier permeability, are generated from a linear combination of the terms that went into the chemical potential calculation.

This chapter explains the molecular modelling theory with the example of analysing lead compound to treat inflammation based on the active site of COX-2, COX-1 and hERG by fragment-based de novo design approach to increase efficiency and reduce the toxicity of novel anti-inflammatory agents. De Novo ligand design identifies potential novel ligands by screening a library of small molecules to find those that are appropriate spatial orientation of hydrogen-bonding and hydrophobic functional groups. This final lead molecules recognised by fragment-based design aided the further design of 184 novel tyrosine derivatives based on the structural relationship studies. Consequently, the comparative molecular field analysis, drug-receptor interaction studies and toxicity studies were performed. Toxicity studies were performed by quantitative structural properties relationship method to know the oral absorption, carcinogenicity, mutagenicity and development of toxicity potential of these fragment-based drug designed molecules. CDOCKER was used to perform this study which is aCHARMm based interaction study tool (docking) using a rigid receptor and flexible ligand for docking.

Structure-Based Drug Design (SBDD)

SBDD has played as a most powerful tool in the drug lead discovery process (Reddy &Erion, 1998; Taylor et al., 2002). This approach requires knowledge of the three dimensional structure of the biological target to assess affinity of its ligand pair during interaction. The design of new ligands is possible, if the target 3D structure is known (Kuntz, Meng&Shoichet, 1994). The protein structural information is acquired either from X-ray crystallography, NMR or homology modelling. SBDD approaches are responsible for evaluating the molecular complementarities and predicting the possible binding modes and ability to interact between small molecules and their macromolecular receptors. The great potentials and success of SBDD have been well documented (Hardy &Malikayil, 2003; Maryanoff, 2004) and the *insilico* approaches vary widely in methodology, performance, protocol and speed. This approach is either capable of providing accurate binding modes or more suitable for fast searching of large databases (Chan et al., 2009; Du-Cunyet al., 2009; Mahadevanet al, 2008; Moses et al 2009; Zanget al, 2003). This is generally the preferred method of drug design where it has highest success rate. Success rate of this approach is relied on clear understanding of how the drug works, and how to improve efficacy, specificity, pharmacokinetics, etc. Herein, we will focus on the most frequently used strategies: molecular docking and scoring.

Molecular Docking

Molecular docking is to find the best matches between a protein and a ligand. It involves the forecast of ligand conformations and orientations (or posing) within a binding site and tries to place the ligand into binding site in proper configurations and conformations appropriate for interacting with the receptor (Kitchen et al., 2004). Docking methods can be divided into two categries such as matching and simulation studies. The former approach create a binding site model, typically including the favourable hydrogen binding and electostatic interactions, and then it attempt to dock the ligands into this model by geometrical conformations (Morris et al., 1999). Although early attempts of matching methods consider only the translational and orientational degrees of the ligand, most of newly developed approaches take into account the conformational flexibility of ligands and limited flexibility of the receptor (Halperin, Wolfson & Nussinoy, 2002). The examples of this class include C-Docker, DOCK (Makino & Kuntz, 1997; Shoichet & Kuntz, 1991), FlexX (Kramer et al. 1999; Goodsell et al., 1996), etc. On the other hand, simulation methods place a molecule into a binding site by exploring the translations, orientations, and conformations until an ideal binding mode is obtained.

Scoring

All the ligand poses are assessed and prioritised according to the Dock Score function. Two types of score are calculated. One is based on a forcefield approximation, the another is Piecewise Linear Potential function (PLP).

DockScore = - (ligand/receptor complex interaction energy + ligand internal energy) (1)

Dock Score (PLP) = - (PLP potential) (2)

Two energy terms are exposed in Equation 1, in Dock Score

The interaction energy is measured as the sum of the non-bonded interactions such as van der Waals energy and electrostatic energy. Here in, grid-based approximation of the ligand-receptor complex interaction energy is employed to reduce the time required for calculation of interaction energy. The van der Waals energy typically displays a sharp rise at short interatomic distances, which have values in the context of ligand-receptor docking. In specific, the mixture of receptor structure as rigid and limitation of ligand conformational space tends to superimpose penalise poses with “mild” short contacts between the complex, due to the “static” nature of the van der and Waals potential in standard forcefields. This inclination can be overcome by submitting an unstiffened (soften) form of the van der Waals potential with function of the Dock Score. To sustain a proper equilibrium between electrostatics and van der Waals, the electrostatic energy is also converted as softened to prevent it from leading the van der Waals energy at short separations. The internal molecular energy of the ligand is totalled when using the forcefield to avoid ligand conformations with bad internal nonbond clashes. By default, only the standard van der Waals energy is used for calculation of internal ligand energy.

MODELLING OF COX-2 INHIBITORS

Designing of Novel Tyrosine Derivatives

Structurally divergent 184 tyrosine-moieties have been designed based on the fragment-based drug design studies of COX-2 inhibitors. In this study, Ludi algorithm was used which formed interaction sites within a defined search sphere inside the target receptor. This algorithm uses the nature of active site amino acids spreading into account by creating an ensemble of interaction sites distributed around the area of suitable geometries. Molecules that cannot be fitted without incurring van der Waals clashes or electrostatic repulsions are withdrawn during the search process.

Eraser algorithm is used to define site sphere of the COX-2 enzyme and volume occupied by a known ligand poses already in an active site. Ludi models generate interaction sites from the functional group of COX-2 protein that can participate in a nonbonded contact (Figure 2). This set of interaction sites covers the range of appropriate positions for a ligand atom or functional group involved in the putative interaction. Initial fragment is grown to add interactions between the receptor and the ligand fragment. Further, tyrosine scaffolds are positioned in the target site and then theoretically connected to each other by linkers to produce a complete molecule that satisfies all the key interactions.

Ludi link identified the $-SO_2-CH_3$ and heterocyclic fragments that create the more affinity and geometrically fit active site amino acids of COX-2 protein. Further, De novo evaluation protocol covalently fused the electronegative group substituted tyrosine skeleton to the Ludi fragments to produce a collection of molecule with higher binding interaction score.

Wherein, 184 tyrosine molecules were generated by substituting different electronegative groups such as -Cl, -Br, -F, -I and $-OCH_3$ at R_1 and R_2 positions of tyrosine skeleton. In tyrosine moiety, each one hydrogen atom at $R_3$and R_4 positions were replaced by $-SO_2CH_3$ and diverse heterocyclic fragments respectively (Figure 3). These structures were drawn and the energies were minimised using ADS version 2.5. The energy minimised ligands were saved in structural data (.sd) for further studies. Further, the

Figure 2. Ludi hotspot generation and link fragment identification

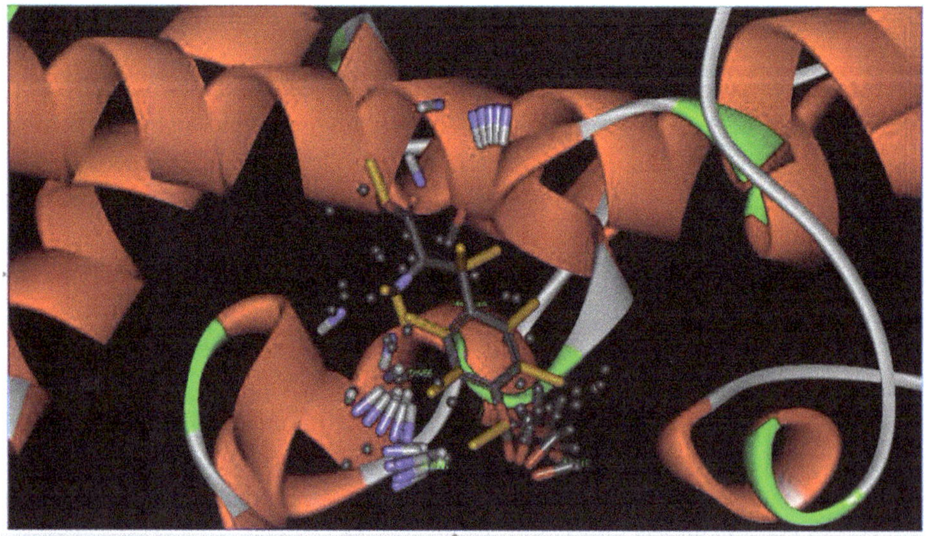

Figure 3. Pharmacophoric groups of (a) rofecoxib (b) celecoxib and (c) core tyrosine moiety with different substitution

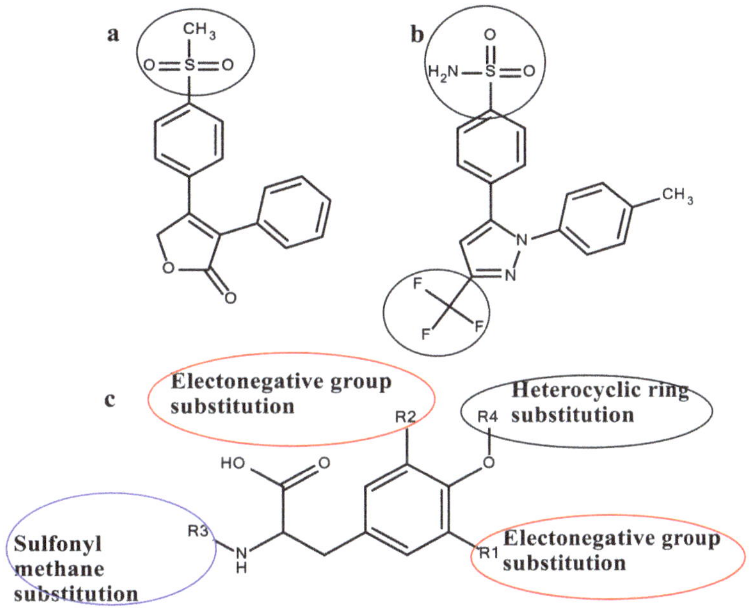

BEST / Flexible search method in Ligand Pharmacophore Mapping protocol was performed to identify hits that satisfy the chemical feature requirements and spatial orientation with corresponding features in the pharmacophoric query.

Pharmacophore Modelling

The pharmacophore models were developed with the most active training set compounds. 3D QSAR-based pharmacophore methodology was used to forecast the activity of newly designed compounds. A set of five pharmacophore models called Hypogen was generated by a training set containing 17 known COX-2 inhibitors. The result revealed that the pharmacophore model 1 (hypo 1) is found to have four features viz. One hydrogen bond acceptor (HBA), two hydrophobic regions (Hy) and one aromatic ring (RA) feature (Figure 4a-4c). These chemical features are essential for COX-2 inhibition as identified from the literature but other models are lacking these features. Hence, Hypo1 has been chosen as best pharmacophore model for further studies.

The five pharmacophore models possess total cost values which are ranged from 96.85 to 126.73 (Table 1). In principle, a best pharmacophore model should possess greater difference between null cost and total cost and it should be lesser between fixed cost and total cost values.

Hypo 1was developed with a fixed cost value of 107.15 and null cost value of 235.93 bits. Among the five pharmacophore models, Hypo 1 recorded the closest value (96.85) to the fixed cost value (107.15) than other models. The cost difference between total cost and null cost for the Hypo 1 was found to exhibit 139.08 bits. A cost difference value greater than 60 bits suggests that the pharmacophore model relates the predicted and experimental activity values more than 90%.

Figure 4. Comparative Pharmacophoric features map of standard drugs rofecoxib (a), celecoxib (b) and designed tyrosine core moiety (c)

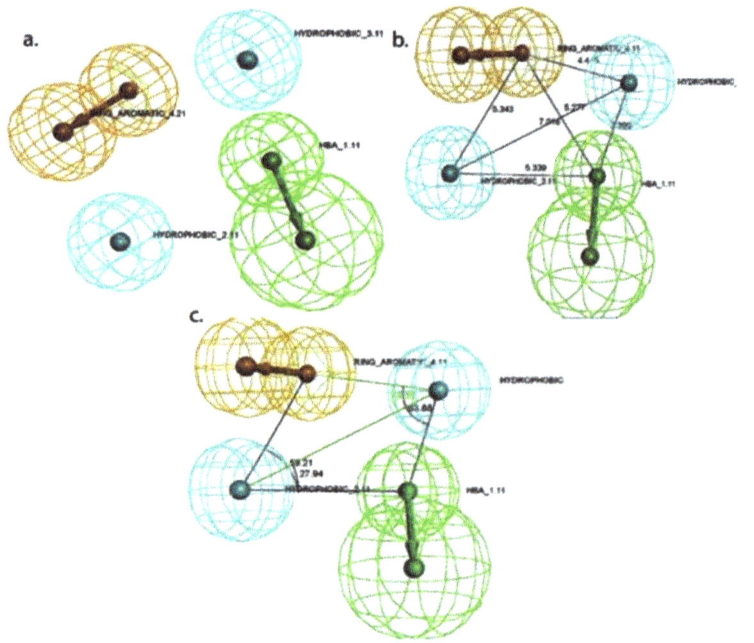

Table 1. Statistical significance and cost values for the 5 Hypogen models

Hypogen No	Total Cost (Bits)	Cost Difference[a]	RMS[b] (Å)	Correlation	Features[b]	Max Fit
Hypo 1	96.85	139.08	1.15	0.941	1HBA,2Hy,1RA	10.92
Hypo 2	116.65	119.28	1.69	0.906	1HBA lipid, 2Hy, 1RA	9.01
Hypo 3	123.65	112.27	1.51	0.920	1HBA lipid, 1Hy, 1RA	11.02
Hypo 4	124.21	111.71	1.80	0.897	1HBA lipid, 1Hy, 2RA	5.20
Hypo 5	126.73	109.19	1.86	0.893	1HBA, 1Hy, 1RA	5.27

[a] Cost difference between the null (235.925) and the total cost. [b] Abbreviation used for features: RMS, root mean square deviation; HBA, hydrogen bond acceptor; HBD, hydrogen bond donor, Hy, hydrophobic and RA, ring aromatic.

These five pharmacophore models were further evaluated by statistical methods viz. correlation coefficient and RMSD. The correlation values for the generated pharmacophore models were ranged between 0.893 - 0.941. Among the five models, Hypo 1 exposed the highest correlation coefficient value of 0.941. Moreover, RMSD values between the five pharmacophore models lie in the range of 1.15-1.86 and 1.15 for Hypo 1 depicts the minor deviation between predicted activity values from the experimental value than other four models. The results proved that, Hypo 1 was developed with improved statistical values, such as higher correlation coefficient, superior cost difference and smaller RMSD. Statistical methods verified the capability of the pharmacophore model (Hypo 1) to predict the activity of the training set compounds. Regression parameters of Hypo 1, further predict the activity of each training set compound. Based on the experimental activity (IC_{50}) values, training set and test set of 179 compounds were categorised in following three groups viz. Highly active (IC_{50}< 4.51 μM), moderately active (IC50

< 26.40 μM) and less active (IC_{50}< 78.25 μM). The pharmacophore mapping of high and low active compounds is shown in Figure5 (a-d). The most highly active compound (0.0036 μM) aligned all the features of Hypo 1 and the least active compound (67.62 μM) failed to notice hydrophobic and hydrogen bond acceptor features. The geometric fit values for every hit were determined by their map on the feature location. The greater activity of the most highly active compound articulates that the compound's geometric fit is better and its features map on well with Hypo 1. If the geometric fit is less, the activity can be predicted to be lesser in that particular compound which may be due to their lack of similarity owing to their inability to attain an energetically favourable conformation like other active compounds. It is concluded from the analysis that Hypo 1 was able to predict the activity of compounds to a high degree of accuracy relative to their experimental IC_{50} values. The Fisher's randomisation and test set are utilised to further validate the reliability and statistical significance of the best pharmacophore model.

Pharmacophore Model Validation

The rationale behind the evaluation of quantitative pharmacophore model is to determine its predictive ability to identify the active compounds. To explore the ability to estimate the activity of new compounds, the pharmacophore models should be statistically significant and retrieve active compounds from the database. Here, the selected pharmacophore model was further internally validated by Fisher's randomisation and externally cross-validated by test set method (Figure 5a - d).

For Fisher's randomisation test, 95% confidence level was chosen, and the 19 random spread sheets were formed to produce the hypothesis. The formula S=(1-19+X)/Y) ×100 was used to estimate the significance level of hypothesis at 95% (S), where X and Y indicate the total number of hypothesis

Figure 5. (a) and (b) Pharmacophore angle feature maps with most active and least active training set compounds. (c) and (d) Pharmacophore distance feature map with most active and least active training set compounds.

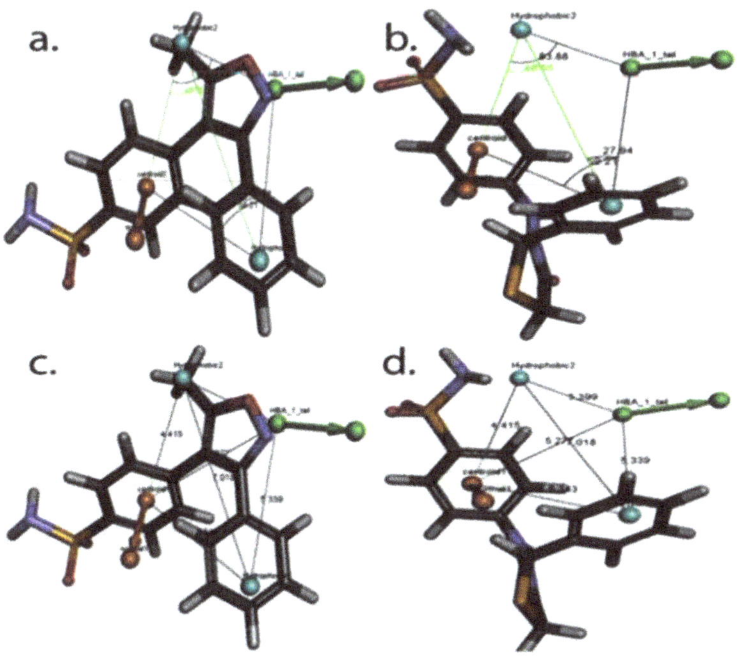

having a total cost value lower than the original hypothesis and the total number of Hypogen runs respectively. But, in this study, X = 0 and Y= (1+19), S can be calculated as (1- {(1+0) / (19+1)}) × 100. While comparing the total costs of 19 scrambled runs (118.93 - 381.49) with the best hypothesis, Hypo 1 (96.85), the later found to contain greater quality than the other 19 hypotheses. On the other hand, the correlation coefficient values of 19 scrambled runs (0.272 - 0.938) were found to be lower than the Hypo 1 (0.941). It ultimately, evidenced that the best pharmacophore Hypo 1 was not created by chance. Hence, this Hypo 1 is considered as the best hypothesis that possesses all the necessary chemical features to inhibit COX-2 activity.

Test set containing 162 diverse compounds were used to cross validate the best pharmacophore model, Hypo 1. The test set was used to verify whether the Hypo 1 was able to select molecules with orders of magnitude of activity on par with the active training set and to determine the strength of Hypo 1 in discriminating the potential COX-2 inhibitors from other compounds. Herein, Hypo 1 predicted good correlation coefficient of 0.921 between experimental and predicted COX-2 inhibitory activity of the test set, demonstrated remarkable consistency. Thus, we propose that generated Hypo 1 is able to estimate the activity of test set compounds to a high degree of accuracy relative to their experimental IC_{50} values (Figure 6).

Pharmacophore Mapping of Tyrosine Derivatives

The validated best predictive pharmacophore model, Hypo 1 was used as 3D structural search query to screen the designed 184 compounds in order to point out novel hit compounds. Search 3D Database protocol with Best search option was applied in database screening. The selected best model, Hypo 1, comprised of one HBA, two Hy and one RA with high a correlation value of 0.941. The results of search

Figure 6. Graph of the correlation between experimental activity and estimated activity by Hypo1

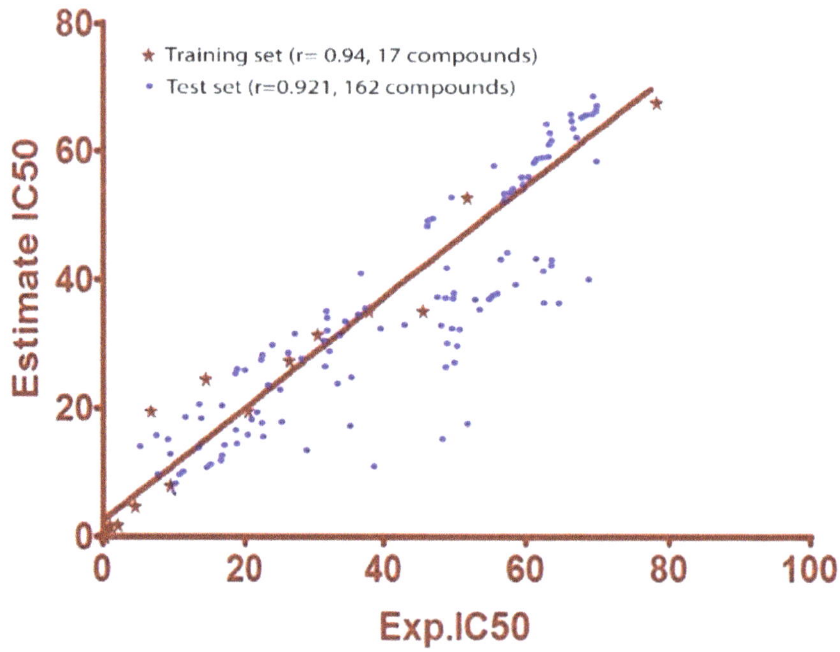

3D database protocol showed that 81 molecules were well aligned with the features of Hypo 1 with the fit value greater than 8. The Best/ Flexible search method revealed that the 3D constraints, features, shape and excluded volume of the 81 molecules (Figure 7). The resulted 81 well-mapped molecules were preferred for QSAR studies.

QSAR Model Generation

3D-QSAR studies emphasis on changes in 3D structural features like electrostatic distribution, hydrophobic distribution, hydrogen bond forming ability and impact of positioning of functional groups on biological activity predominantly. The Genetic Function Algorithm (GFA) uses a genetic algorithm to perform search for optimal QSAR models using LOF score to assess the fitness of each model. Table 2 lists the QSAR models derived for the training set compounds using the reported biological activity. The descriptors which gave the best models for all the training set compounds are 2D structural, thermodynamic, 3D molecular fractional polar surface area properties and semi-empirical QM properties. Among the five developed models, the r^2 value of models 1- 4 was found as 0.992 and model 5 exhibited 0.991. On the other hand, r^2(pred) values of generated models 1-5 were found to possess 0.794, 0.814, 0.790, 0.811 and 0.784 respectively Table 3. It signifies that the model 2 has good predictive ability since its r^2(pred) value is closer to r^2 compared to other models. In this chapter, QSAR model equation symbolised graphically by point plots of the experimental activity against the predicted activity value (IC_{50}) for the training set compounds as illustrated in Figure 8.

The best 3D-QSAR model (Model-2) developed to predict the COX-2 inhibiting activity of tyrosine analogues depicts a positive correlation with ALogP, Mean Polarizability, total energy and negative correlation with H-bond acceptors, and Extended Connectivity Finger Prints (ECFP) as outlined in Table 2.

The generated equations in each model were analyzed for goodness of fit and their corresponding predictive capability. GFA Model 2 showed greater correlation coefficient (r^2), lowest LOF and least

Figure 7. One of the designed tyrosine molecule mapping with the Hypo1 features

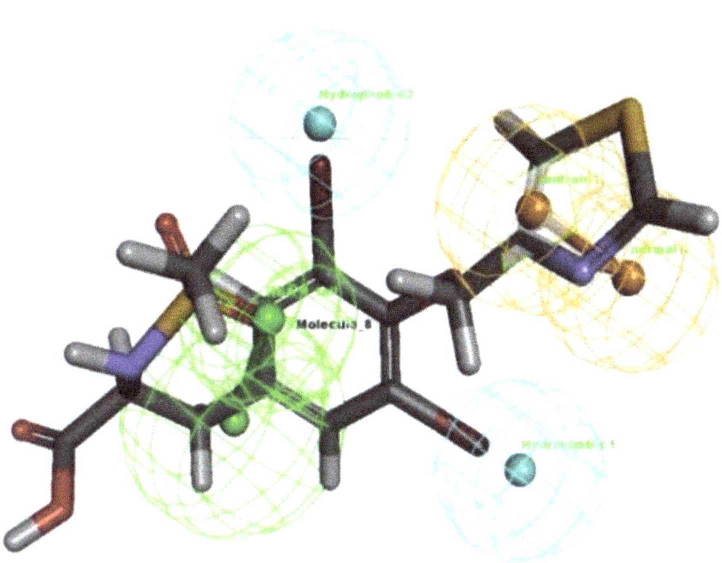

Figure 8. Experimental activity (X-axis) and predicted activity (Y-axis) values of training set compounds conferring to the QSAR equation

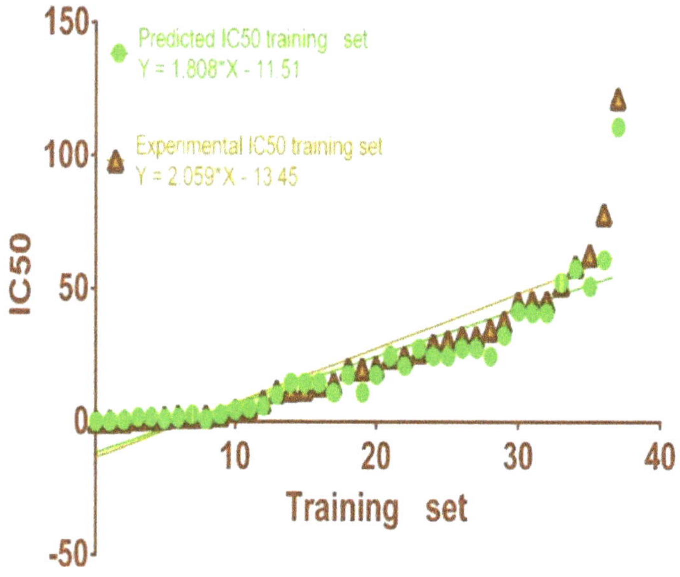

Table 2. Equations of generated 5 QSAR models

Generated GFA Model Equations
GFATempModel_1 = -0.5535 + 5.0595 × Count<ECFP 6:826878152> + 2.7496 × ALogP× Count<ECFP 6:-936157482> + 0.067192 × Count<ECFP 6:-1758752087>× Mean Polarizability VAMP + 0.0017663 × Count<ECFP 6:-936157482>× Total Energy VAMP + 1.0497 × <NumHAcceptors–6.122> + 0.70547 × <0.9464–Count<ECFP6:912478223>
GFATemp Model2 = - 0.4913 + 5.0706 Count < ECFP 6:826878152 > + 2.7572 × ALogP × Count <ECFP 6: -936157482> + 0.063525 × Count <ECFP 6: -758752087> × Mean Polarizability VAMP + 0.0017817 × Count <ECFP6: -936157482> × Total Energy VAMP + 0.98576 × <Num H Acceptors – 6.122> + 0.76123 × <0.9464 – Count <ECFP6:912478223>
GFATempModel_3 = 0.087724 + 4.9017 × Count<ECFP 6:826878152> + 2.7243 × ALogP× Count<ECFP_6: -936157482> + 0.067993 × Count<ECFP 6: -1758752087>× Mean Polarizability VAMP + 0.0018616 × Count<ECFP6: -936157482>× Total Energy VAMP + 1.0654 × <Num H Acceptors–6.122>
GFATempModel_4 = 0.21088 + 4.9002 × Count<ECFP6:826878152> + 2.7305 × ALogP× Count<ECFP6: -936157482> + 0.064062 × Count<ECFP_6: -1758752087>× Mean Polarizability VAMP + 0.0018867 × Count<ECFP6: -936157482>× Total Energy VAMP + 0.99699 × <NumHAcceptors–6.122
GFATempModel_5 = 0.23478 + 4.7448 × Count<ECFP 6:826878152> + 2.6756 × ALogP× Count<ECFP 6: -936157482> + 0.068959 × Count<ECFP 6:-1758752087>× Mean Polarizability VAMP + 0.0017587 × Count<ECFP_6:-936157482>× Total Energy VAMP + 1.048 × <NumHAcceptors–6.122>

Table 3. Generated QSAR models and its prediction values

Model	r^2	r^2(adj)	r^2(pred)	Friedman L.O.F.
GFATempModel_1	0.992	0.984	0.794	439.6
GFATempModel_2	0.992	0.985	0.814	231.7
GFATempModel_3	0.992	0.985	0.791	293.4
GFATempModel_4	0.992	0.985	0.811	224.1
GFATempModel_5	0.991	0.984	0.785	209.0

possible intervariable correlation comparatively was employed to estimate the activity. The predictive model thus obtained can readily be applied to large databases of drugs to identify active structures.

The structural descriptor viz. H-bonding acceptor is primarily an electrostatic interaction which depends on conformation. This was modelled by calculated atomic charges and molecular orbital energies. ECFP are circular topological fingerprints designed for molecular characterisation, similarity and structural activity modelling of training set compounds. It represents the molecule at different levels such as presence of a halogen and a large section of molecular structure.

Additional insight into the COX-2 inhibitory activity was obtained by visualising the QSAR model in the perspective of one or more ligands in the training set with varying activity. The most active (Figure 9a) and least active (Figure 9b) training set compounds were chosen for this study. Structural analysis of those compounds articulated that the HBA (Green), HBD (pink), orbital energies (HOMO and LUMO) and polarizability variables vitally influences the selective COX-2 inhibitory activity. Reduction of the selective COX-2 inhibitory activity in Figure 9b may be owing to the presence of more number of HBD (pink) in the aromatic ring system.

The HBD groups substitution diminishes the HOMO energy and escalates the LUMO energy of the molecules thus may lead to unfavourable binding of molecules inside the hydrophobic tunnel of COX-2 enzyme (Figure 10). In particular, the energy difference between the HOMO and LUMO is considered as an indicator of stability index. The most active training set molecule in this study contained the HOMO energy of -9.72787 and LUMO energy of -1.37253 kcal/mol. The energy gap between the orbitals of the most active molecule was found to be two-fold more (-8.3553) than the least active molecules (-4.6788) as indicated in Figure 9. It is evidenced that even the stable compounds can be predicted by the developed model 2.

Figure 9. (a) Structural surface view of most active training set compound F2 EJMC a6. (b) Lowest active training set compound F7 EJMC 3e.

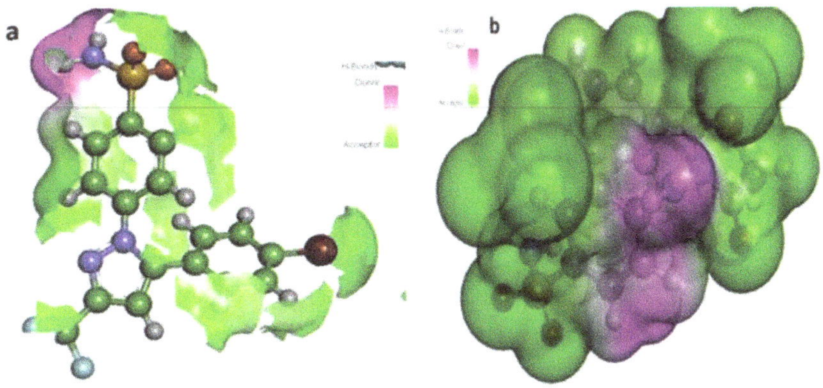

Figure 10. Comparison of different descriptors and activity relationships of training set compounds

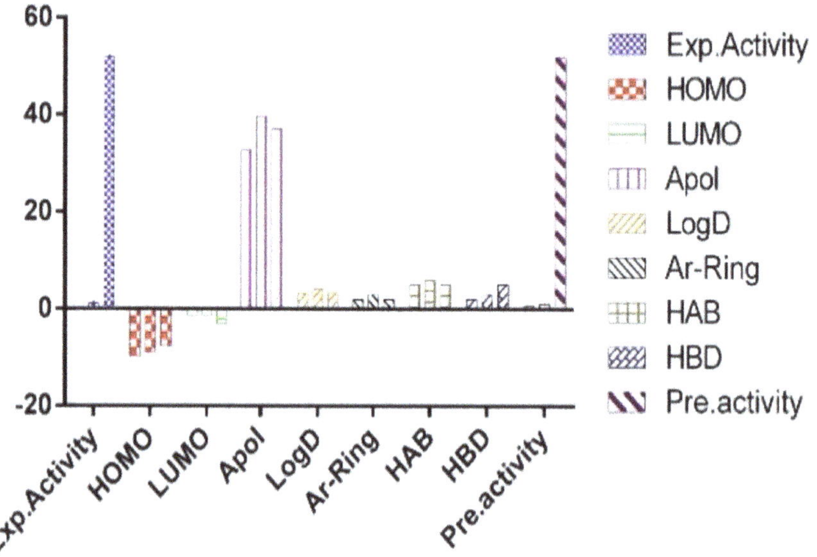

QSAR VALIDATION

Friedman's LOF Measure

The incorporation of Friedman's LOF error measure in GFA method estimates the most suitable number of features, resists overlay and allows control over the smoothness of fit. Such evolution of a population of randomly built models leads to the development of highly predictive QSARs. The Friedman's lack-of-fit (LOF) score of the generated QSAR model is described in the Table 3. The model 2 contain relatively less LOF score (231.7) compared to the rest of the models that indicates GFA model will fit the data.

Cross-Validation Analysis

Generated QSAR GFA models were cross-validated with 43 test set compounds by the 'leave one out' (LOO) scheme to identify the predictive capability of the model. The results of test set validation show high correlation coefficient, r^2(CV) of 0.982. The correlation point plot between experimental and predicted IC_{50} activity of test set is illustrated in Figure 11. It indicates that the developed model is an indicator of good external predictability as its value is larger than 0.525.

IC_{50} Prediction of Tyrosine Derivatives by GFA Model

In this study, the generated GFA model 2 was used to predict the probable COX-2 inhibitory activities (IC_{50}) of selected 81 tyrosine derivatives resulted from the pharmacophore screening. As a consequence, 55 molecules were selected based on their predicted IC_{50} values (Table 4) and the remaining molecules forecast as an outlier. Herein, the thermodynamic parameter, ALog P is considered to be an indication of bioavailability of the compounds which determines the amount of the compound that gets to the target

Figure 11. Linear regression line between the predicted and experimental activity of the Test set compounds by GFA model

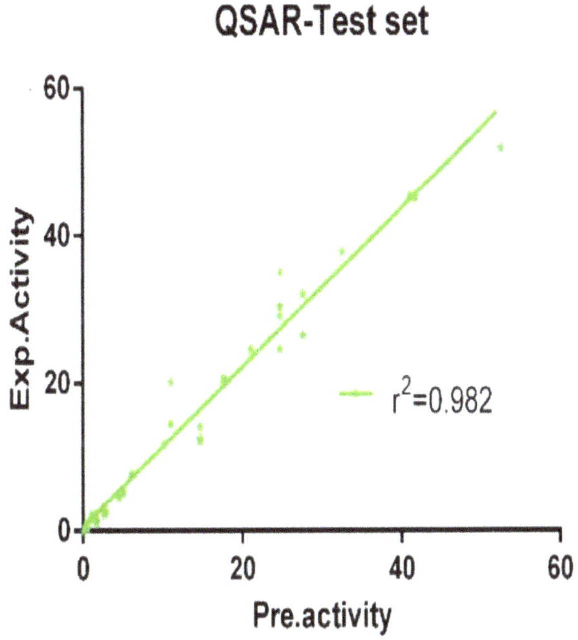

Table 4. Predicted IC_{50} value of the screened 55 Tyrosine derivative hits

Designed Tyrosine Molecules	Predicted IC_{50}	Designed Tyrosine Molecules	Predicted IC_{50}	Designed Tyrosine Molecules	Predicted IC_{50}
Molecule 21	0.00114647	Molecule 144	0.0458897	Molecule 15	0.272933
Molecule 26	0.00219316	Molecule 152	0.0718502	Molecule 103	0.326176
Molecule 17	0.00270044	Molecule 57	0.0081972	Molecule 146	0.340769
Molecule 6	0.00389357	Molecule 142	0.0883014	Molecule 102	0.346229
Molecule 14	0.00507229	Molecule 116	0.125113	Molecule 52	0.366704
Molecule 7	0.00550285	Molecule 112	0.127005	Molecule 10	0.37001
Molecule 9	0.0056096	Molecule 118	0.140002	Molecule 11	0.425391
Molecule 110	0.00615055	Molecule 23	0.141630	Molecule 115	0.440686
Molecule 12	0.00750067	Molecule 58	0.004266	Molecule 51	0.506685
Molecule 151	0.00837356	Molecule 20	0.0158626	Molecule 114	0.612637
Molecule 8	0.00109263	Molecule 117	0.161607	Molecule 54	0.640833
Molecule 111	0.0121545	Molecule 60	0.176103	Molecule 159	0.644601
Molecule 100	0.0124557	Molecule 141	0.182021	Molecule 104	0.712928
Molecule 59	0.0141984	Molecule 50	0.190438	Molecule 13	0.810522
Molecule 98	0.0157464	Molecule 24	0.195007	Molecule 67	0.8399
Molecule 19	0.0175583	Molecule 150	0.195656	Molecule 101	0.869527
Molecule 105	0.0194731	Molecule 122	0.207464	Molecule 154	1.45545
Molecule 143	0.0350068	Molecule 25	0.209826		
Molecule 107	0.0354119	Molecule 113	0.268979		

site. The Alog P value of selected 55 compounds are ranged between -2.05 and 4.366 reflecting a wide range of hydrophobicity that makes the tyrosine derivatives to pass through many membranes to reach the target site. One interpretation to account for the term polarizability is that highly polarizable molecules may enhance strong interaction with other molecules. The mean polarizability values relate the hydrophobicity and molar volume of the molecule with their corresponding biological activity. Herein, variations of anti-inflammatory activity among the 55 compounds were observed. This may owe to their bulk effects that can modify the structure of the COX-2 protein to which it is bound and thereby alter the nature of the substrate sites of the tyrosine derivatives on the protein. The binding affinity of the tyrosine analogues could be enhanced through charge transfer, possibly of an intramolecular nature and expected to perturb the structure of protein. The correlation of anti-inflammatory activity with electronic polarizability observed in this study tends to support suggestion that the bulky substituents on the 55 tyrosine derivatives may facilitate their anti-inflammatory COX-2 molecular recognition through various binding energies. Further, structural analysis revealed that the selected molecules possessed high HOMO energy (> -7.39343 kcal/mol) and low LUMO energy (< -2.0808 kcal/mol) which is directly correlated to the ionization potential, exemplifies the susceptibility of the molecule and more interaction towards electrophiles present in the COX-2 active site rather than nucleophiles. Here, the energy gap between HOMO-LUMO orbitals was found to be more that indicates stability of the selected molecules. Further, the presence of structural features namely HBA, HBD, hydrophobic and number of aromatic rings in the selected tyrosine molecules may enhance the formation of stable conformation inside the COX-2 catalytic site. It is postulated that selective COX-2 inhibitory activity of those compounds may be due to incorporation of heterocycles that confers various physical properties namely steric, electrostatic and hydrophobic parameters. This in turn fine-tunes chemical reactivity and plays a significant role in selective COX-2 inhibitory activity. These results confirm the utility of GFA Model 2 as a controlling tool in the search for new anti-inflammatory drugs.

COX-2 Interaction Studies

The docking results of COX-2 with tyrosine derivatives revealed that the selected 35 tyrosine derivatives among 55 possessed better binding affinities(–C-Docker energy)related to the standard celecoxib. Evaluation of the interaction finger prints of tyrosine analogue make clear that the molecule **8** have higher affinity (-78.7003)with COX-2 active site related to celecoxib(17.3339). This interaction energy is because of the 24th oxygen atom of the carboxylic group in tyrosine moiety forming the two site point interactions with the amino hydrogen of the analogue (arachidonic acid) binding site residue Arg^{120} and one hydrogen bond with the aromatic ring –OH group in Tyr^{355} residue. The oxygen atom (25th)of the molecule created one ligand point interaction with Arg^{120} residue which allows key interaction impression of the tyrosine molecules on COX-2 protein active site. Besides, aromatic ring of the tyrosine skeleton makes π-cationic interaction with Arg^{120}.

This interaction shaped stable conformation of the tyrosine molecule **8** in the hydrophobic active site of the COX-2 protein. The presence of hydrophobic canal in COX-2 is being the site of NSAIDS drug binding. Also, R_1 and R_2 bromine substitution had generated VDW interaction with Val^{523} and Phe^{518} that permitted the molecule **8** to access an extra side pocket amino acids which is more responsible for the COX-2 selectivity. The substitution of 1, 3-thiazole ring at R_4 position of tyrosine tempted the VDW and electrostatic interactions with the binding site amino acids. It created favorable chemical environment in the COX-2 binding site. Electronegative group substituted sulfonyl group at R_3 position enhanced the binding potential of the molecule by networking with Ser[353](Figure 12). It is inveterate from this study, the COX-2 specificity of the tyrosine analogue (molecule**8**) is higher than the standard celecoxib. The rest of 34 molecules were inspected and found to have more stability when compared to the standard.

Interaction studies of COX-1 protein explicated the COX-2 specificity of the 55 tyrosine derivatives. In this COX-1 docking study, the bulky nature of Ilu[523] amino acid residue and non-polar moieties of the His[513]of designed tyrosine analogue had not allowed to form appropriate conformation within the active site of COX-1 enzyme. The VDW space of the tyrosine derivativies in COX-1enzyme active site clatters with the essential receptor volume. This clash creates steric repulsion between electron density cloud of COX-1amino acids side chain and designed molecules. It strongly demonstrated that there is drop in the attraction of the designed tyrosine analogue with COX-1 when compared to the standard drugs. These results exposed that the designed tyrosine derivatives are more selective on COX-2than COX-1.

Ulcerogenic Interaction Studies of Designed Molecules

The ulcerogenicity of coxib derivatives is due to the drug molecules binding with the COX-1 protein. The interaction among designed tyrosine moiety and COX-1 protein assisted to identify the ulcerogenicity level of designed molecules. It was observed from the results of docking studies (C-Docker) that the designed tyrosine derivatives exhibited more binding energy which was in dissimilarity with the standard celecoxib. The standard drug formed one sigma-π, π-cationic and two hydrogen bond interactions with the Ile[523], Arg[120], Gln[192] and Lue[352] amino acids respectively. These bonds support the celecoxibto fit inside the cavity region of COX-1enzyme. On the other hand, the designed tyrosine derivatives formed hydrogen bonds with the Tyr[385] and Ser[530] (Figure 13) and there is no other additional interaction with the active site amino acids of COX-1 receptor. Also, the electronegative groups (-Br, -I) of the designed molecules forms intermolecular bumps which disfavors the binding capability of the molecules. This unstable conformation of the designed molecule proves their negligible ulcerogenic side effect.

Figure 12. Active site amino acids Interactions of molecule 8 with of COX-2

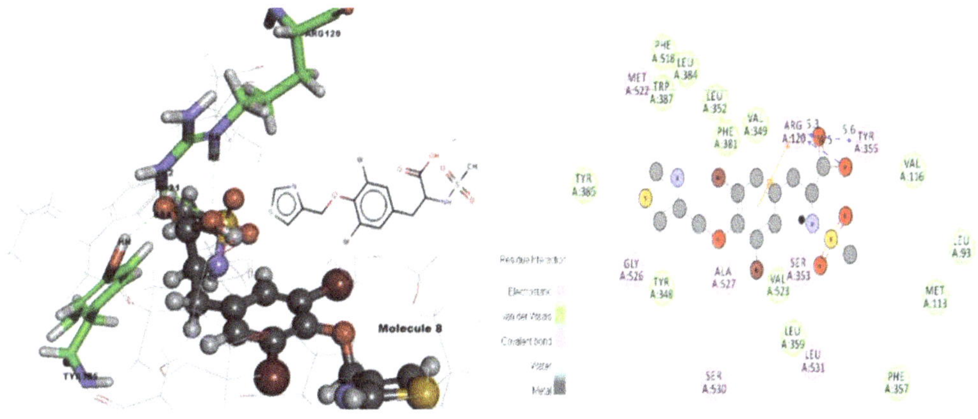

hERGprotein Interaction Studies

The hERG is the most answerable network involved in drug-induced Torsade de Pointes (TdP) arrhythmias. Extracellular application of standard celecoxib caused fast suppression of hERG channels which tempts the cardiac disturbances. Assessment of spatial orientation of the designed tyrosine scufold interactions with the hERG protein measure the cardiotoxicity level of molecules. The results of docking studies exposed that among the 55 designed molecules, 52 molecules influenced higher interaction energy against the standard. It exposed that these molecules are having weak binding interaction to the active site residues of the hERG protein. In standard celecoxib, the benzyl ring creates π interaction with the Tyr^{652}permitted to fit well into the hydrophobic pocket of COX-2 protein. On contrary, tyrosine derivatives did not form any π interactions and the electron density of the electronegative group substitutions in the R1 and R2 position which snub the tyrosine molecules to bind in the active site (Figure 14). Hence, the cardiotoxicity level of the designed molecules was lighter amount when compared to standard celecoxib.

Figure 13. Celecoxib interaction map with the COX-1 protein (a) 2D interaction showing non-bonded interactions (b) 3D interaction view

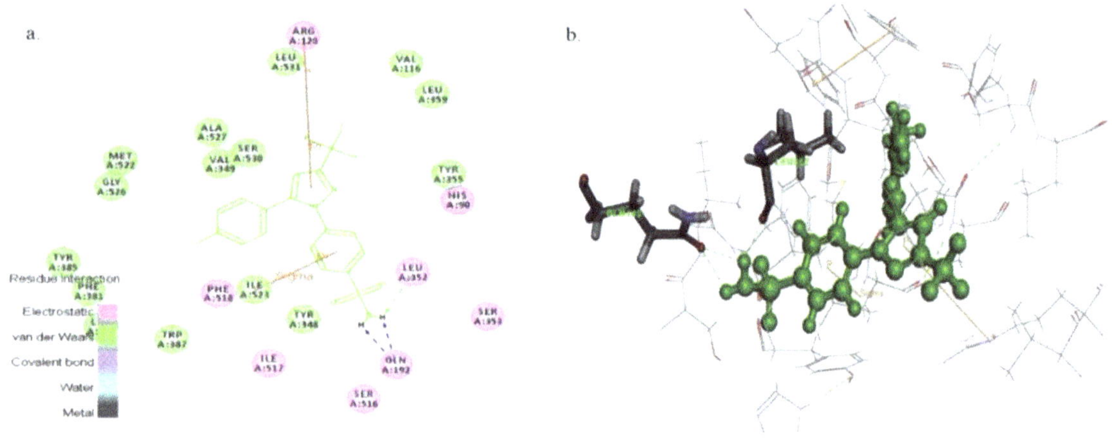

Figure 14. Tyrosine derivatives interaction map with the hERG protein (a) 2D interaction showing non-bonded interactions (b) 3D interaction view hERG protein interaction

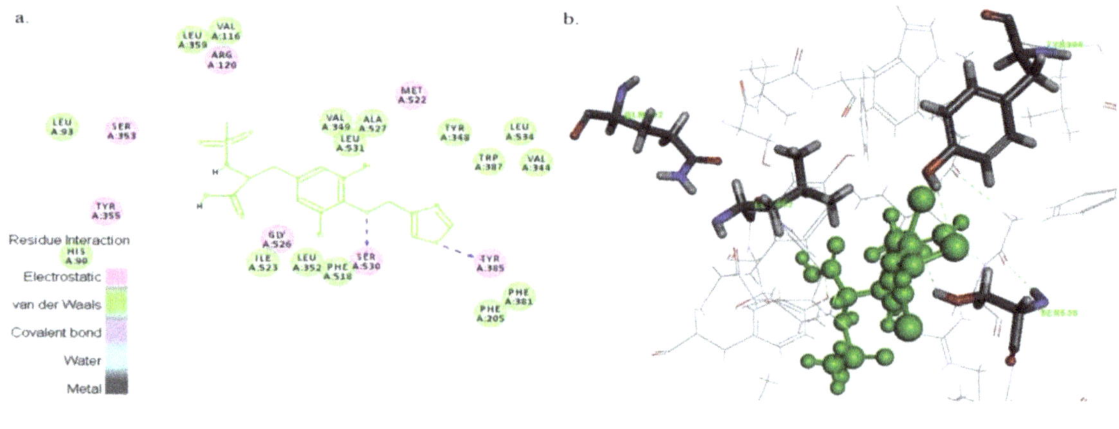

The selected 35 tyrosine molecules proved higher COX-2 selectivity, less COX-1 (ulcerogenic) and hERG(cardiotoxicity) binding affinity. Further, these molecules were examined using ADMET descriptors measurement and OSIRIS properties explorer to identify more safe molecule.

Docking Protocol Validation

The selected docking protocol was precisely distinguished the selective and nonselective COX-2 inhibitors. The docking results exhibited that C-Docker energy of selective COX-2 inhibitors found in the negative kcal/mol range and the nonselective drugs energies found in the range of positive kcal/mol. Further, the correlation result between the C-docker energy and the experimental IC_{50} value of the nonselective inhibitors was 0.835 (r^2). This correlation study strongly signifying that the docking protocol possessed good energy and interaction predicting ability as well as it distinguishes the selective and nonselective COX-2 inhibitors precisely.

ADMET Descriptors Study

In the present work, ADMET descriptors were used to filter the undesired pharmacokinetic and toxicity properties containing 35 selected tyrosine molecule. The six precalculated QSTR-ADMET models were used to predict pharmacokinetic properties of all the tyrosine molecules in ADS 2.5 software. The 95% and 99% confidence ellipse for the Human Intestinal Absorption(HIA) and Blood Brain Barrier (BBB)models were generated in ADMET plot. This plot represents the zone of chemical space around the molecules having excellent absorption through cell membrane.

These selected tyrosine analogue as well as celecoxib drug fall in the 99% and 95% confidence ellipse for both HIA and BBB (Figure 15). The HIA of the tyrosine derivatives have ranged from good absorption (0) to moderate absorption (1) level. It highlights the good bioavailability of designed tyrosine molecules to produce desired therapeutic activity. BBB penetration of the designed molecules has

Figure 15. The 95% and 99% confidence limit ellipses corresponding to the BBB and HIA models for tyrosine derivatives

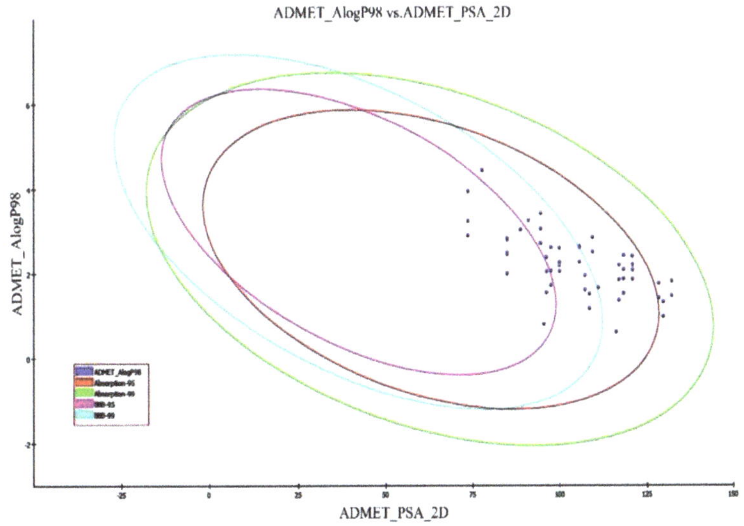

shown approximate low penetration, except the molecule 141 whereas celecoxib exhibited moderate penetration to the BBB. The aqueous solubility plays a dynamic role in the bioavailability of the drug. The Table 5referred designed tyrosine derivatives solubility in the range of 2 (low soluble) to 3 (soluble). The hepatotoxicity level displayed, the toxic liver nature of the molecule. Likewise, all the molecules were noninhibitors of the metabolic enzyme CYPD2D6, it suggested that the tyrosine derivatives are safe to develop as a drug molecule.

The Plasma Protein Binding (PPB) prediction denotes that selected molecules have binding affinity ≤ 90%, clearly revealing that the molecules have good bioavailability and not likely bound to carrier proteins in the blood. Eventually, 19 designed tyrosine compounds which possessed safety profile and potency was chosen for synthesis and the Table 6 showed the structure of safe potent tyrosine COX-2 inhibitors.

Integrating Different Approaches and Future Directions

The use of molecular modelling and computational chemistry is extensive and continuing to expand spectrum) in drug discovery and development. There remain major deficiencies in understanding and ability to model certain processes well, but substantial progress is being made. The goal of drug repurposing is to expose new links between drugs and diseases, most commonly *via* targets. As illustrated in the previous segments, computational predictions followed by experimental assessment have been successfully used to identify new drug repurposing possibilities. All computational approach has its own advantages and boundaries. In fact none of these methods alone will be sufficiently able to unveil the complex interplay between drugs, targets and diseases. Therefore, we are left with using one or more computational approaches to "navigate" through the wealth of available information and "clues" are solid enough to rationalize a repurposing hypothesis worth of experimental investigation. The choice of the most suitable method(s) selection will depend on the nature of the problem to solve and quantity of information available about that problem in the literature or public or proprietary databases. Unfortunately, information is often fragmented, and reflects only a single or few aspects of a much more complicated story. Future efforts should be more systematically directed toward disclosing centers and relations of the complex network that relates drugs, targets and diseases. Assimilating the vast and heterogeneous volume of existing chemical, biological, and structural data into a unified workflow is obviously a challenging task. In this respect, the integration and usage of various *insilico* approaches, as revealed above, will provide valuable opportunities to extend the field of applicability of each technique exploit information imminent from different sources. Likewise, this will greatly advantage from better combination of multidisciplinary work. Changes in the fields were observed, correlated with movements in charged residues on the rim of the active site. This or other ways of analysing the effects of molecular motions on molecular fields are an important area of future study. The improvement in understanding of the relationship between chemical structure and biological activity, in which the analysis of molecular fields plays a major role, is responsible for the development of molecular modelling from being a primarily descriptive to an increasingly predictive activity. A network-based method built upon these considerations will likely provide new directions to navigate through all the potential links between drugs and diseases, thus making new chances for drug repurposing and drug discovery in general.

Table 5. ADMET predictions of 35 tyrosine molecules and celecoxib

Name of the Molecule	Absorption Level	PSA 2D	BBB Level	Solubility Level	Hepatotoxicity Level	CYP 2D6	PPB Level
Molecule_6	0	109.513	4	2	0	0	0
Molecule_8	0	105.719	4	2	0	0	0
Molecule_9	0	118.273	4	3	1	0	0
Molecule_10	1	129.534	4	3	0	0	0
Molecule_11	0	120.689	4	2	0	0	0
Molecule_12	0	120.774	4	3	1	0	0
Molecule_13	0	118.273	4	2	1	0	0
Molecule_14	1	132.035	4	2	0	0	0
Molecule_15	0	94.458	3	2	1	0	0
Molecule_17	0	109.513	4	2	1	0	0
Molecule_20	0	118.273	4	3	0	0	0
Molecule_21	1	129.534	4	3	0	0	0
Molecule_23	0	120.774	4	2	0	0	0
Molecule_24	0	118.273	4	3	0	0	0
Molecule_25	1	132.035	4	3	0	0	0
Molecule_26	0	94.458	3	2	1	0	0
Molecule_50	0	105.719	4	3	0	0	0
Molecule_51	0	116.98	4	3	0	0	0
Molecule_54	0	116.198	4	3	0	0	0
Molecule_58	0	105.719	3	3	0	0	0
Molecule_67	0	116.98	4	3	0	0	0
Molecule_99	0	90.972	3	2	1	0	0
Molecule_102	0	108.662	3	3	1	0	0
Molecule_103	0	99.817	3	2	1	0	0
Molecule_113	0	108.662	3	3	1	0	0
Molecule_115	0	99.902	3	2	1	0	0
Molecule_117	0	111.163	4	3	1	0	0
Molecule_141	0	73.586	2	2	1	1	0
Molecule_146	0	95.326	3	3	1	0	0
Molecule_154	0	99.817	3	3	1	0	0
Molecule_7	0	120.774	4	2	0	0	0
Molecule_52	1	128.241	4	3	1	0	0
Molecule_57	0	94.458	3	2	0	0	0
Molecule_59	0	116.98	4	3	0	0	0
Molecule_60	1	128.241	4	3	1	0	0
Celecoxib	0	77.75	2	1	1	0	1

Table 6. Selected 19 safe potent tyrosine COX-2 inhibitors

Molecule number	Chemical Structure	Molecular Formula	Molecular weight g/mol
6	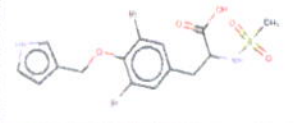	$C_{15}H_{16}Br_2N_2O_5S$	496.171
7	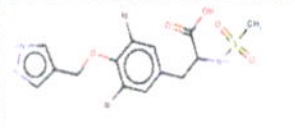	$C_{15}H_{17}Br_2N_3O_4S$	495.186
8	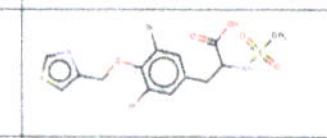	$C_{15}H_{16}Br_2N_2O_4S_2$	512.237
10	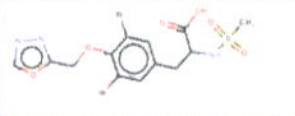	$C_{13}H_{15}Br_2N_3O_6S$	501.148
11	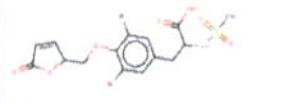	$C_{15}H_{15}Br_2NO_7S$	513.155
13	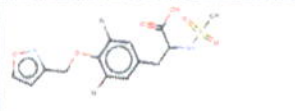	$C_{14}H_{14}Br_2N_2O_6S$	498.144
14	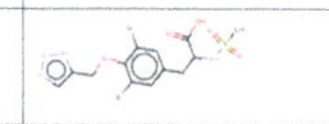	$C_{13}H_{14}Br_2N_4O_5S$	498.147
20	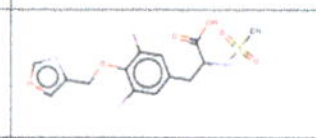	$C_{14}H_{14}I_2N_2O_6S$	592.145
21	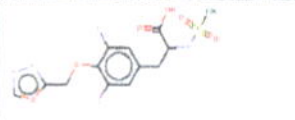	$C_{13}H_{13}I_2N_3O_6S$	593.133
23	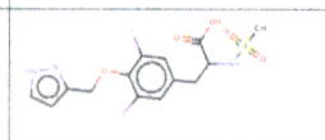	$C_{14}H_{15}I_2N_3O_5S$	591.16
24	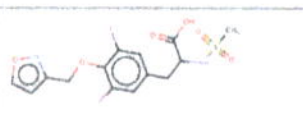	$C_{14}H_{14}I_2N_2O_6S$	592.145
25	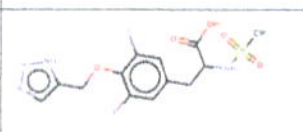	$C_{13}H_{14}I_2N_4O_5S$	592.148
50	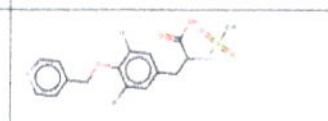	$C_{16}H_{16}Br_2N_2O_5S$	508.182
51	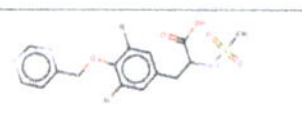	$C_{15}H_{15}Br_2N_3O_5S$	509.17
54	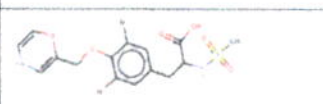	$C_{15}H_{16}Br_2N_2O_6S$	509.909
57	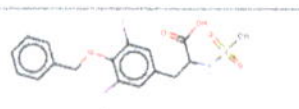	$C_{17}H_{17}I_2NO_5S$	600.891
58	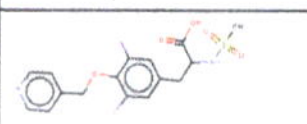	$C_{16}H_{16}I_2N_2O_5S$	602.183
59	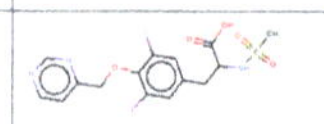	$C_{15}H_{15}I_2N_3O_5S$	603.171
67	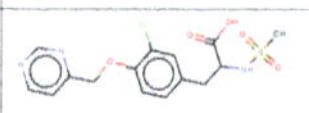	$C_{15}H_{16}Cl N_3O_5S$	385.823

CONCLUSION

This whole chapter explained the evidence based molecular modelling studies on novel tyrosine derivatives against COX-2 enzyme by incorporating FBDD, LBDD and SBDD methodologies. It concludes that the3D pharmacophore and QSAR for substituted tyrosines as COX-2 inhibitors were studied through a ligand-based computational approach. The descriptors chosen for the model appeared to be complementary to the COX–2 enzyme topology. An effort has been made to advance hypothetical features of inhibitor and enzyme interactions. The designed COX-2 inhibitors, owing to their greater bulkiness occupy exact volume of COX–2 binding site as in the case of known COX–2 inhibitors but may have different interactions with the active site residues. It is proven that the existence of small polarizable functional groups improved the COX–2 inhibitory potency. The findings of this study afford significant insight into the structure-activity relationship for efficient designing and screening of tyrosine derivatives with anti-inflammatory activity. The model could be used to screen compounds with numerous structures in quest of potent COX–2 inhibitory activity.

ACKNOWLEDGMENT

The authors are thankful to the D3 research group and Department of Science and Technology (DST-SERB), New Delhi for their financial support provided for this research (SR/S1/OC-48/2011 Dt: 14-05-2013).

REFERENCES

Ahmetaj-Shala, B., Kirkby, N. S., Knowles, R., Al'Yamani, M., Mazi, S., Wang, S. Z., ... Mitchell, J. A. (2015). Evidence That Links Loss of Cyclooxygenase-2 With Increased Asymmetric Dimethylarginine. *Circulation*, *131*(7), 633–642. doi:10.1161/CIRCULATIONAHA.114.011591 PMID:25492024

Ajay, A., & Murcko, M. A. (1995). Computational methods to predict binding free energy in ligand-receptor complexes. *Journal of Medicinal Chemistry*, *38*(26), 4953–4967. doi:10.1021/jm00026a001 PMID:8544170

Al-Hourani, B. J., Sharma, S. K., Mane, J. Y., Tuszynski, J., Baracos, V., Kniess, T., ... Wuest, F. (2011). Synthesis and evaluation of 1,5-diaryl-substituted tetrazoles as novel selective cyclooxygenase-2 (COX-2) inhibitors. *Bioorganic & Medicinal Chemistry Letters*, *21*(6), 1823–1826. doi:10.1016/j.bmcl.2011.01.057 PMID:21316237

Andrea, T. A., & Kalayeh, H. (1991). Applications of neural networks in quantitative structure-activity-relationships of dihydrofolate-reductase inhibitors. *Journal of Medicinal Chemistry*, *34*(9), 2824–2836. doi:10.1021/jm00113a022 PMID:1895302

Andrew, R. L. (2001). *Molecular Modelling Principles and Applications*. Pearson Education Limited.

Bali, A., Ohri, R., & Deb, P. K. (2012). Synthesis, evaluation and docking studies on 3-alkoxy-4-methanesulfonamido acetophenone derivatives as non-ulcerogenic anti-inflammatory agents. *European Journal of Medicinal Chemistry*, *49*, 397–405. doi:10.1016/j.ejmech.2012.01.018 PMID:22318166

Bolis, G., Dipace, L., & Fabrocini, F. (1991). A machine learning approach to computer-aided molecular design. *Journal of Computational Methods in Molecular Design*, *5*(6), 617–628. doi:10.1007/BF00135318 PMID:1818094

Chan, C. C., Boyce, S., Brideau, C., Charleson, S., Cromlish, W., Ethier, D., ... Riendeau, D. (1999). Rofecoxib(Vioxx, MK-0966; 4-(4′-methylsulfonylphenyl)-3-phenyl-2(5H)-furanone): A potent and orally active cyclooxygenase-2 inhibitor. Pharmacological and biochemical profiles. *The Journal of Pharmacology and Experimental Therapeutics*, *290*, 551–560. PMID:10411562

Chaudhary, P., Sharma, P. K., Sharma, A., & Varshney, J. (2010). Recent AdvancesIn Pharmacological Activity Of Benzothiazole Derivatives. *International Journal of Current Pharmaceutical Research*, *4*, 5–11.

Chen, L. S., Nowak, B. J., Ayres, M. L., Krett, N. L., Rosen, S. T., Zhang, S., & Gandhi, V. (2009). Inhibition of ATP synthase by chlorinated adenosine analogue. *Biochemical Pharmacology*, *78*(6), 583–591. doi:10.1016/j.bcp.2009.05.019 PMID:19477165

Cheng, A., & Dixon, S. L. (2003). In silico models for the prediction of dose-dependent human hepatotoxicity. *Journal of Computer-Aided Molecular Design*, *17*(12), 811–823. doi:10.1023/B:JCAM.0000021834.50768.c6 PMID:15124930

Cheng, A., & Merz, K. (2003). Prediction of aqueous solubility of a diverse set of compounds using quantitative structure-property relationships. *Journal of Medicinal Chemistry*, *46*(17), 3572–3580. doi:10.1021/jm020266b PMID:12904062

David, C. Y. (2009). *Computational Drug Design*. Hoboken, NJ: John Wiley & Sons.

Dror, O., Shulman-Peleg, A., Nussinov, R., & Wolfson, H. J. (2004). Predicting molecular interactions in silico: I. A guide to pharmacophore identification and its applications to drug design. *Current Medicinal Chemistry*, *11*(1), 71–90. doi:10.2174/0929867043456287 PMID:14754427

Du-Cuny, L., Son, Z., Moses, S., Powis, G., Mas, E. A., Meuillet, E. J., & Zhang, S. (2009). Computational MODELLING of novel inhibitors targeting the Aktpleckstrin homology domain. *Bioorganic & Medicinal Chemistry*, *17*(19), 6983–6992. doi:10.1016/j.bmc.2009.08.022 PMID:19734051

Egan, W. J., & Lauri, G. (2002). Prediction of intestinal permeability. *Advanced Drug Delivery Reviews*, *54*(3), 273–289. doi:10.1016/S0169-409X(02)00004-2 PMID:11922948

Egan, W. J., Merz, K. M., & Baldwin, J. J. (2000). Prediction of Drug Absorption Using Multivariate Statistics. *Journal of Medicinal Chemistry*, *43*(21), 3867–3877. doi:10.1021/jm000292e PMID:11052792

Esser, R., Berry, C., Du, Z., Dawson, J., Fox, A., Fujimoto, R. A., ... Marshall, P. J. (2005). Preclinical pharmacology of lumiracoxib: A novel selective inhibitor of cyclooxygenase-2. *British Journal of Pharmacology*, *144*, 538–550. Marnett, L. J. (2009). The COXIB experience: A look in the rear-view mirror. *Annual Review of Pharmacology and Toxicology*, *49*, 265–290.

Ferreira, S. H., Moncada, S., & Vane, J. R. (1971). Indomethacin and aspirin abolish prostaglandin release from the spleen. *Nature: New Biology*, *231*(25), 237–239. doi:10.1038/newbio231237a0 PMID:5284362

Fu, J. Y., Masferrer, J. L., Seibert, K., Raz, A., & Needleman, P. (1990). The induction and suppression of prostaglandin H2 synthase (cyclooxygenase) in human monocytes. *The Journal of Biological Chemistry*, *265*(28), 16737–16740. PMID:2120205

Garg, R., Kurup, A., Mekapati, S. B., & Hansch, C. (2003). Searching for allosteric effects via QSAR. Part II. *Bioorganic & Medicinal Chemistry*, *11*(4), 621–628. doi:10.1016/S0968-0896(02)00382-6 PMID:12538028

Goodsell, D. S., Morris, G. M., & Olson, A. J. (1996). Automated docking of flexible ligands: Applications of AutoDock. *Journal of Molecular Recognition*, *9*(1), 1–5. doi:10.1002/(SICI)1099-1352(199601)9:1<1::AID-JMR241>3.0.CO;2-6 PMID:8723313

Guner, O., Clement, O., & Kurogi, Y. (2004). Pharmacophore modelling and three-dimensional database searching for drug design using catalyst: Recent advances. *Current Medicinal Chemistry*, *11*(22), 2991–3005. doi:10.2174/0929867043364036 PMID:15544485

Halperin, I., Ma, B., Wolfson, H., & Nussinov, R. (2002). Principles of docking: An overview of search algorithms and a guide to scoring functions. *Proteins*, *47*, 409–443.

Hansch, C., Leo, A., Mekapati, S. B., & Kurup, A. (2004). QSAR and ADME. *Bioorganic & Medicinal Chemistry*, *12*(12), 3391–3400. doi:10.1016/j.bmc.2003.11.037 PMID:15158808

Hardy, L. W., & Malikayil, A. (2003). The impact of structure-guided drug design on clinical agents. *Current Drug Discovery*, *3*, 15–20.

Hochstrasser, R. M. (2007). Two-dimensional spectroscopy at infrared and optical frequencies. *Proceedings of the National Academy of Sciences of the United States*, *104*(36), 14190–14196. doi:10.1073/pnas.0704079104 PMID:17664429

Kawai, S., Kojima, F., & Kusunoki, N. (2005). Recent advances in nonsteroidal anti-inflammatory drugs. *Allergology International*, *54*(2), 209–215. doi:10.2332/allergolint.54.209

Kier, L. B., & Hall, L. H. (1993). The generation of molecular-structures from a graph-based Qsar equation. *Molecular Informatics*, *12*, 383–388.

King, R. D., Muggleton, S., Lewis, R. A., & Sternberg, M. J. E. (1992). Drug design by machine learning – the use of inductive logic programming to model the structure-activity relationships of trimethoprim analogues binding to dihydrofolate-reductase. *Proceedings of the National Academy of Sciences of the United States of America*, *89*(23), 11322–11326. doi:10.1073/pnas.89.23.11322 PMID:1454814

Kitchen, D. B., Decornez, H., Furr, J. R., & Bajorath, J. (2004). Docking and scoring in virtual screening for drug discovery: Methods and applications. *Nature Reviews. Drug Discovery*, *3*(11), 935–949. doi:10.1038/nrd1549 PMID:15520816

Kramer, B., Metz, G., Rarey, M., & Lengauer, T. (1999). Ligand docking and screening with FlexX. *Medicinal Chemistry Research*, *9*, 463–478.

Kujubu, D. A., Fletcher, B. S., Varnum, B. C., Lim, R. W., & Herschman, H. R. (1991). TIS10, a phorbol ester tumourpromoter-inducible mRNA from Swiss 3T3 cells, encodes a novel prostaglandin synthase. Cyclooxygenase homologue. *The Journal of Biological Chemistry*, *266*, 12866–12872.

Kuntz, I. D., Meng, E. C., & Shoichet, B. K. (1994). Structure-based molecular design. *Accounts of Chemical Research*, *27*(5), 117–123. doi:10.1021/ar00041a001

Lahlou, M. (2013). The Success of Natural Products in Drug Discovery. *Pharmacology & Pharmacy*, *4*(03), 17–31. doi:10.4236/pp.2013.43A003

Langer, T., & Wolber, G. (2004). Virtual combinatorial chemistry and in silico screening: Efficient tools for lead structure discovery? *Pure and Applied Chemistry*, *76*(5), 991–996. doi:10.1351/pac200476050991

Leo, A. J., & Hansch, C. (1999). Role of hydrophobic effects in mechanistic QSAR. *Perspectives in Drug Discovery and Design*, *17*, 1–25.

Liu, B., Luo, W., Zhang, Y., Li, H., Zhu, N., Huang, D., & Zhou, Y. (2012). Role of cyclooxygenase-1-mediated prostacyclin synthesis in endothelium-dependent vasoconstrictor activity of porcine interlobular renal arteries. *American Journal of Physiology. Renal Physiology*, *302*(9), F1133–F1140. doi:10.1152/ajprenal.00604.2011 PMID:22301626

Mahadevan, D., Powis, G., Mash, E. A., George, B., Gokhale, V. M., Zhang, S., ... Jana, U. (2008). Discovery of a novel class of AKT pleckstrin homology domain inhibitors. *Molecular Cancer Therapeutics*, *7*(9), 2621–2632. doi:10.1158/1535-7163.MCT-07-2276 PMID:18790745

Makino, S., & Kuntz, I. D. (1997). Automated flexible ligand docking method and its application for database search. *Journal of Computational Chemistry*, *18*(14), 1812–1825. doi:10.1002/(SICI)1096-987X(19971115)18:14<1812::AID-JCC10>3.0.CO;2-H

Maryanoff, B. E. (2004). Inhibitors of serine proteases as potential therapeutic agents: The road from thrombin totryptase to cathepsin G. *Journal of Medicinal Chemistry*, *47*(4), 769–787. doi:10.1021/jm030493t PMID:14761180

Morris, G. M., Goodsell, D. S., Halliday, R. S., Huey, R., Hart, W. E., Belew, R. K., & Olson, A. J. (1999). Automated docking using a Lamarckian genetic algorithm and an empirical binding free energy function. *Journal of Computational Chemistry*, *19*(14), 1639–1662. doi:10.1002/(SICI)1096-987X(19981115)19:14<1639::AID-JCC10>3.0.CO;2-B

Moses, S. A., Ali, M. A., Zuohe, S., Du-Cuny, L., Zhou, L. L., Lemos, R., ... Meuille, E. J. (2009). In vitro and in vivo activity of novel small-molecule inhibitors targeting the pleckstrin homology domain of protein kinase B/AKT. *Cancer Research*, *69*(12), 5073–5081. doi:10.1158/0008-5472.CAN-08-3839 PMID:19491272

Pairet, M., Churchill, L., Trummlitz, G., & Engelhardt, G. (1996). Differential inhibition of cyclooxygenase-1(COX-1) and –2 (COX2) by NSAIDS: Consequences on anti-inflammatory activity versus gastric and renal safety. In Side Effects of Anti-Inflammatory Drugs IV (pp. 223-232). Kluwer Academic Publishers.

Parvu, L. (2003). QSAR – a piece of drug design. *Journal of Cellular and Molecular Medicine*, *7*(3), 333–335. doi:10.1111/j.1582-4934.2003.tb00235.x PMID:14594559

Patel, C. K., &Sen, D. J. (2009). COX-1 and COX-2 inhibitors: Current status and prospects over COX-3 inhibitors. *International Journal of Drug Development and Research*, 136-145.

Peng, J., Li, J., & Hamann, M. (2005). The Marine Bromotyrosine Derivatives. *The Alkaloids. Chemistry and Biology*, *6*, 59–262. doi:10.1016/S1099-4831(05)61002-4 PMID:16173400

Penning, T. D., Talley, J. J., Bertenshaw, S. R., Carter, J. S., Collins, P. W., Docter, S., ... Isakson, P. C. (1997). Synthesis and Biological Evaluation of the 1,5-Diarylpyrazole Class of Cyclooxygenase-2 Inhibitors: Identification of 4-[5-(4-Methylphenyl)-3- (trifluoromethyl)-1 *H* -pyrazol-1-yl]benzenesulfonamide (SC-58635, Celecoxib). *Journal of Medicinal Chemistry*, *40*(9), 1347–1365. doi:10.1021/jm960803q PMID:9135032

Perkins, R., Fang, H., Tong, W. D., & Welsh, W. J. (2003). Quantitative structure-activity relationship methods: Perspectives on drug discovery and toxicology. *Environmental Toxicology and Chemistry*, *2*(8), 1666–1679. doi:10.1897/01-171 PMID:12924569

Prasit, P., & Riendeau, D. (1997). Selective cyclooxygenase-2 inhibitors. In Annual Reports in Medicinal Chemistry (pp. 211-220). Elsevier Publishing.

Rarey, M., Kramer, B., Lengauer, T., & Klebe, G. (1996). A fast-flexible docking method using an incremental construction algorithm. *Journal of Molecular Biology*, *261*(3), 470–489. doi:10.1006/jmbi.1996.0477 PMID:8780787

Reddy, M. R., & Erion, M. D. (1998). Structure-based drug design approaches for predicting binding affinities of HIV1 protease inhibitors. *Journal of Enzyme Inhibition*, *14*(1), 1–14. doi:10.3109/14756369809036542 PMID:10520756

Sallam, A. A., Ramasahayam, S., Meyer, S. A., & El Sayed, K. A. (2010). Design, synthesis, and biological evaluation of dibromotyrosine analogues inspired by marine natural products as inhibitors of human prostate cancer proliferation, invasion, and migration. *Bioorganic & Medicinal Chemistry*, *18*(21), 7446–7457. doi:10.1016/j.bmc.2010.08.057 PMID:20884214

Shoichet, B. K., & Kuntz, I. D. (1991). Protein docking and complementarity. *Journal of Molecular Biology*, *221*(1), 327–346. doi:10.1016/0022-2836(91)80222-G PMID:1920412

Singh, S. K., Saibaba, V., Ravikumar, V., Rudrawar, S. V., Daga, P., Rao, C. S., ... Rao, Y. K. (2004). Synthesis and biological evaluation of 2,3-diarylpyrazines and quinoxalines as selective COX-2 inhibitors. *Bioorganic & Medicinal Chemistry*, *12*(8), 1881–1893. doi:10.1016/j.bmc.2004.01.033 PMID:15051057

Smith, J. B., & Willis, A. L. (1971). Aspirin selectively inhibits prostaglandin production in human platelets. *Nature: New Biology*, *231*(25), 235–237. doi:10.1038/newbio231235a0 PMID:5284361

Stahura, F. L., & Bajorath, J. (2004). Virtual screening methods that complement HTS. *Combinatorial Chemistry & High Throughput Screening*, *7*(4), 259–269. doi:10.2174/1386207043328706 PMID:15200375

Talley, J. J. (1999). 5 Selective inhibitors of cyclooxygenase-2 (COT-2). *Progress in Medicinal Chemistry*, *36*, 201–234. doi:10.1016/S0079-6468(08)70048-1 PMID:10818674

Talley, J. J., Bertenshaw, S. R., Brown, D. L., Carter, J. S., Graneto, M. J., Koboldt, C. M., ... Seibert, K. (1999). 4,5-Diaryloxazole inhibitors of cyclooxygenase-2 (COX-2). *Medicinal Research Reviews*, *19*(3), 199–208. doi:10.1002/(SICI)1098-1128(199905)19:3<199::AID-MED1>3.0.CO;2-7 PMID:10232649

Taylor, R. D., Jewsbury, P. J., & Essex, J. W. (2002). A review of protein-small molecule docking methods. *Journal of Computer-Aided Molecular Design*, *16*(3), 151–166. doi:10.1023/A:1020155510718 PMID:12363215

Tetko, I. V., Tanchuk, V. Y., Chentsova, N. P., Antonenko, S. V., Poda, G. I., Kukhar, V. P., & Luik, A. I. (1994). Hiv-1 reverse-transcriptase inhibitor design using artificial neural networks. *Journal of Medicinal Chemistry*, *37*(16), 2520–2526. doi:10.1021/jm00042a005 PMID:7520081

Tropsha, A., & Zhang, W. F. (2001). Identification of the descriptor pharmacophoresusing Variable selection QSAR: Applications to database mining. *Current Pharmaceutical Design*, *7*, 599–612.

Vane, J. R. (1971). Inhibition of prostaglandin synthesis as a mechanism of action for aspirin-like drugs. Nature (London). *Nature: New Biology*, *231*(25), 232–235. doi:10.1038/newbio231232a0 PMID:5284360

Votano, J. R., Parham, M., Hall, L. M., Hall, L. H., Kier, L. B., Oloff, S., & Tropsha, A. (2006). QSAR Modelling of Human Serum Protein Binding with Several Modelling Techniques Utilizing Structure? Information Representation. *Journal of Medicinal Chemistry*, *49*(24), 7169–7181. doi:10.1021/jm051245v PMID:17125269

Wu, G., Robertson, D. H., Brooks, C. L., & Vieth, M. (2003). Detailed Analysis of Grid-Based Molecular Docking: A Case Study of CDOCKER - ACHARMm-Based MD Docking Algorithm. *Journal of Computational Chemistry*, *24*(13), 1549–1562. doi:10.1002/jcc.10306 PMID:12925999

Xia, X., Maliski, E. G., Gallant, P., & Rogers, D. (2004). Classification of kinase inhibitors using a Bayesian model. *Journal of Medicinal Chemistry*, *47*(18), 4463–4470. doi:10.1021/jm0303195 PMID:15317458

Xie, W. L., Chipman, J. G., Robertson, D. L., Erikson, R. L., & Simmons, D. L. (1991). Expression of a mitogen-responsive gene encoding prostaglandin synthase is regulated by mRNA splicing. *Proceedings of the National Academy of Sciences of the United States*, *88*(7), 2692–2696. doi:10.1073/pnas.88.7.2692 PMID:1849272

Zarghi, A., & Arfaei, S. (2011). Selective COX-2 Inhibitors: A Review of Their Structure-Activity Relationships. *Iranian Journal of Pharmaceutical Research*, *10*, 655–683. PMID:24250402

Zhang, S., Ying, W. S., Siahaan, T. J., & Jois, S. D. S. (2003). Solution structure of a peptide derived from the beta subunit of LFA-1. *Peptides*, *4*, 827–835. PMID:12948834

KEY TERMS AND DEFINITIONS

BBB: The blood-brain barrier is composed of high-density cells restricting passage of substances from the bloodstream much more than do the endothelial cells in capillaries elsewhere in the body.

Cyclo-Oxygenase: An enzyme that catalyzes the conversion of arachidonic acid to prostaglandins and that has two isoforms of which one is involved in the creation of prostaglandins which mediate inflammation and pain.

Hepatotoxicity: Implies chemical-driven liver damage. Drug-induced liver injury is a cause of acute and chronic liver disease. The liver plays a central role in transforming and clearing chemicals and is susceptible to the toxicity from these agents.

Molecular Descriptor: The molecular descriptor is the final result of a logic and mathematical procedure which transforms chemical information encoded within a symbolic representation of a molecule into a useful number or the result of some standardized experiment.

Molecular Modelling: Molecular modelling is a technique for deriving, representing and manipulating the structures and reactions of molecules, and those properties that are dependent on these three-dimensional structures.

Pharmacophore: A set of structural features in a molecule that is recognized at the receptor site and is responsible for that molecule's biological activity.

QSAR: Quantitative structure-activity relationship models are regression or classification models used in the chemical and biological sciences and engineering. Like other regression models, QSAR regression models relate a set of "predictor" variables(X) to the potency of the response variable (Y), while classification QSAR models relate the predictor variables to a categorical value of the response variable.

Solubility: Amount of a substance (called the solute) that dissolves in a unit volume of a liquid substance (called the solvent) to form a saturated solution under specified conditions of temperature and pressure. Solubility is usually expressed as moles of solute per 100 grams of solvent.

Chapter 9
Construction and Analysis of Protein–Protein Interaction Network:
Role in Identification of Key Signaling Molecules Involved in a Disease Pathway

Divya Dasagrandhi
Bharathidasan University, India

Arul Salomee Kamalabai Ravindran
Bharathidasan University, India

Anusuyadevi Muthuswamy
Bharathidasan University, India

Jayachandran K. S.
Bharathidasan University, India

ABSTRACT

Understanding the mechanisms of a disease is highly complicated due to the complex pathways involved in the disease progression. Despite several decades of research, the occurrence and prognosis of the diseases is not completely understood even with high throughput experiments like DNA microarray and next-generation sequencing. This is due to challenges in analysis of huge data sets. Systems biology is one of the major divisions of bioinformatics and has laid cutting edge techniques for the better understanding of these pathways. Construction of protein-protein interaction network (PPIN) guides the modern scientists to identify vital proteins through protein-protein interaction network, which facilitates the identification of new drug target and associated proteins. The chapter is focused on PPI databases, construction of PPINs, and its analysis.

DOI: 10.4018/978-1-5225-7326-5.ch009

INTRODUCTION

Several decades of research in analyzing the mechanism of a disease progression, still cannot unravel complete signaling pathways. This is due to complexity in the mechanism of signal transduction. Proteins are the complex functional units that plays vital role in cellular metabolism. Proteins interact with other proteins to perform every task involved in cellular protection and death. Interaction of proteins determines the fate and acts molecular machines. Activity of proteins depends on its amino acid sequence, structure, chemical modifications, folding and active sites. All these together makes a protein to perform biochemical reactions and diverse functions based on the surrounding environmental milieu in both cellular and organ system levels. Physiochemical properties of proteins vary based on the levels of expression and localization.

Protein interactions stood for all the biological functions such as DNA replication, transcription, translation, cell division, growth and metabolism (Haque *et al.,* 2018) . It is challenging to identify all the mechanisms and getting a clue about vital proteins that aggravates the pathogenesis of the disease either by *in vivo* or *in vitro* experiments as large set of proteins are involved. A critical step was laid in the field of bioinformatics to analyze large set of proteins by constructing Protein-Protein interaction network that helps in decoding molecular basis of a disease and molecular machinery of cells. Identifications of key proteins involved in a disease not only help in understanding disease mechanism but also play a best role in identifying best therapeutic targets for drug discovery with little or no side effects (Ashraf *et al.,* 2018; Tsai *et al.,* 2009).

Protein-Protein Interactions

How a cell decides its biological function? The decision made by cells depends on the coordination of protein interactions. Isolated protein is not functional but more than 80% of proteins interact with other to become functional (Keskin *et al.,* 2016). The different regulatory behavior depends on different pathway interactions based on protein structure, dynamics and conformational change. The synthetic biology elucidates the different behaviors of protein in the complex system.

PPI are defined as the physical interactions between two or more proteins that help to process different functions of the cell. The interactions are either stable or unstable and depend on the environment, signaling from other molecular complexes and time. The interactions of these proteins are either in subcellular or extracellular regions. The complete set of PPI in a cell or an organism is known as interactome. Proteins in the interactome depend on the cell types as expressions of proteins vary in distinct cell types.

The interactions are said to be direct, if there is a molecular contact between two proteins and indirect, if two proteins interact by means of an intermediate (Zhang *et al.,* 2015). Permanent PPI are strong and irreversible and transient PPI are either weak or strong based on oligomeric state (Perkins *et al.,* 2010). Analyzing transient interactions is a challenging task as they are not stable. Fine-tuned technologies are required to analyze these as they have key role in biological network. PPI are not always seen in the same way as the presence of proteins vary based on cellular location, organ, cellular stage, environment, post translational modifications and protein folding. Alterations in these interactions cause disease or malfunction of the metabolic process.

PPI can be determined experimentally by yeast two-hybrid system, Nuclear Magnetic Resonance spectroscopy, co-immuno precipitation and phage display etc. (Rao *et al.,* 2014) But computational analysis of the PPI network can analyze the huge data and helps to understand the role of proteins.

Figure 1. Various methods to analyze protein-protein interactions using in vivo, in vitro and in silico methods.

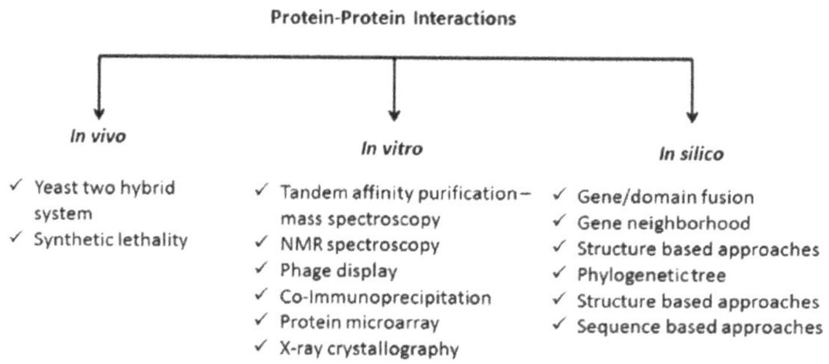

PROTEIN-PROTEIN INTERACTION DATABASES

High throughput technologies made possibility in unraveling several protein-protein interactions and interactome scale is constantly increasing. For the complete understanding of protein pathways and their contribution in cellular function, several PPI databases that store the interaction information are created to retrieve data for the easy access to the research community. They describe biological process of proteins that involved in various signaling pathways. But all the databases may not focus on similar kind of information, hence, cross validation is necessary to improve the efficiency and accuracy of analysis (Klingstrom and Plewczynski, 2011).

Database of Interacting Proteins (DIP)

Database of Interacting Proteins (DIP) is one of the biological databases that helps in identification and analysis of interacting proteins. It is operated from Howard Hughes Medical Institute, UCLA-DOE Institute for Genomics and Proteomics, US. This database contains data from experimentally determined protein-protein interactions in biological processes collected from peer reviewed publications(Xenarios, 2000). Apart from the computational data analysis, this database provides manual analysis and correction of the obtained results. They designed an algorithm, which judges whether the inputs are from biologically proven or system generated, provides larger correlation with experimentally confirmed results. DIP provides information of interacting proteins from many organisms. The database is maintained both manually by expert biologists and automatically using computational approaches. The input may be protein name, gene name, UniProt ID and GenBank accession number. Currently, DIP contains 28,826 proteins, 81,762 interactions from 843 organisms("DIP Home," n.d.).

Molecular INTeraction Database (MINT)

MINT is a relational database, operated from University of Rome, Italy, and it provides experimentally validated protein interaction information in binary and complex representation. MINT also performs sequence similarity search (BLAST) to find homologous partners to the query sequence. Protein query can be given as protein/gene names or unique identifiers from, databases like UniProt, PDB Ensembl, FlyBase, SGD, WormBase, OMIM, HUGE, PubMed and Reactome (Chatr-aryamontri *et al.,* 2007). It

Figure 2. Screen shot of DIP database and protein interaction information provided for NOTCH1

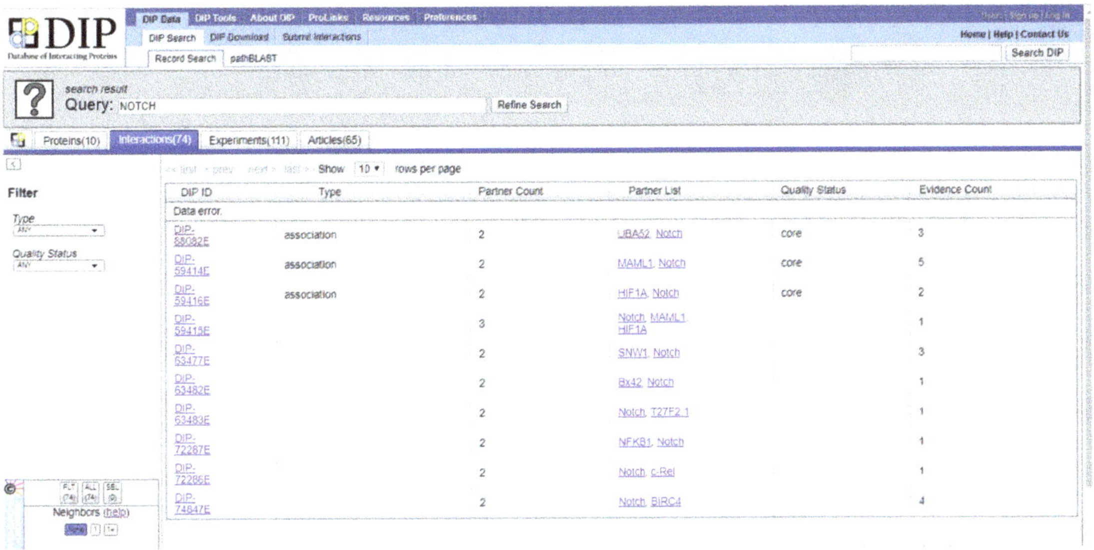

provides species specific information. Currently MINT consists of 61,001 interactions, 15953 interactors in 457 organisms ("The Molecular INTeraction Database – An ELIXIR Core Resource," n.d.). MINT also has another incorporation called HomoMINT, a database representing the human protein interaction network where, interaction determined in model organisms are mapped to its corresponding human orthologs.

Human Protein Reference Database (HPRD)

HPRD is a diverse source of human protein-protein interactions, post translational modifications (PTM), enzyme/substrate relationships, disease associations, tissue expression, and subcellular localization (Goel *et al.*, 2012). This is maintained by institute of Bioinformatics in Bangalore, India and the Pandey lab at Johns Hopkins University in Baltimore, USA. The data will be obtained manually through literature search and from unpublished data by skilled biologists. This is highly focused on interactive domains and provides complete information for the query protein. This also includes PhosphoMotif Finder and signaling pathway resource called NetPath to identify likely proteins. PhosphoMotif helps in searching for the presence of any phosphorylation-based motif for the query proteins and NetPath will provide information about protein interactions, catalytic reactions and protein translocation.

Biological General Repository for Interaction Datasets (BioGRID)

This database provides high quality information regarding protein-protein interactions. Compared to other databases, BioGRID not only provides PPI information, but also gene interactions, post translational modifications and chemical interactions. The entire data set can be downloaded and available in multiple formats (Stark, 2006). It provides function of the genes, localization and biological process it involved. BioGRID is a member of the International Molecular Exchange (IMEx) consortium which is a network of public databases.

Figure 3. Screen shot of MINT database and protein interaction information provided for NOTCH1 with interaction network

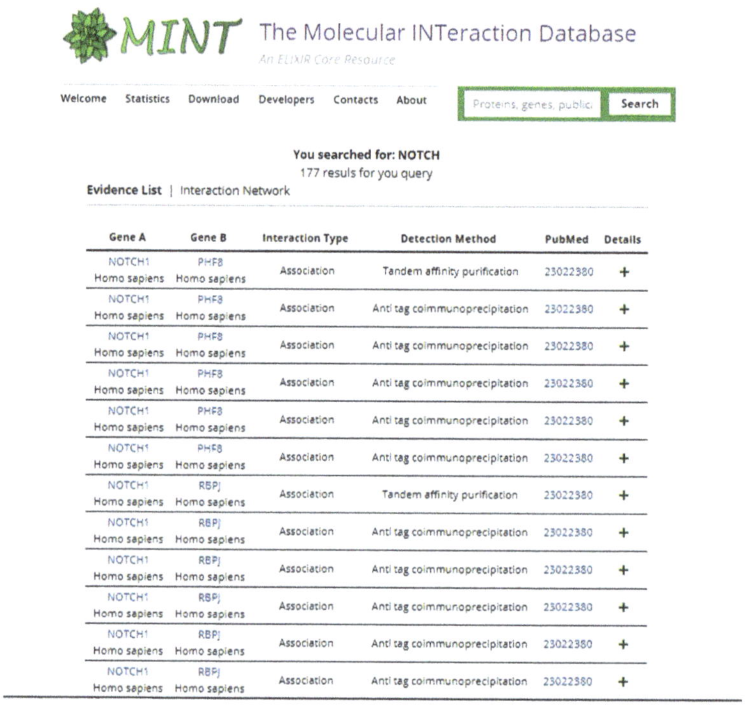

Figure 4. Screen shot of HPRD database and protein interaction information provided for NOTCH1 with interacting domains and motifs

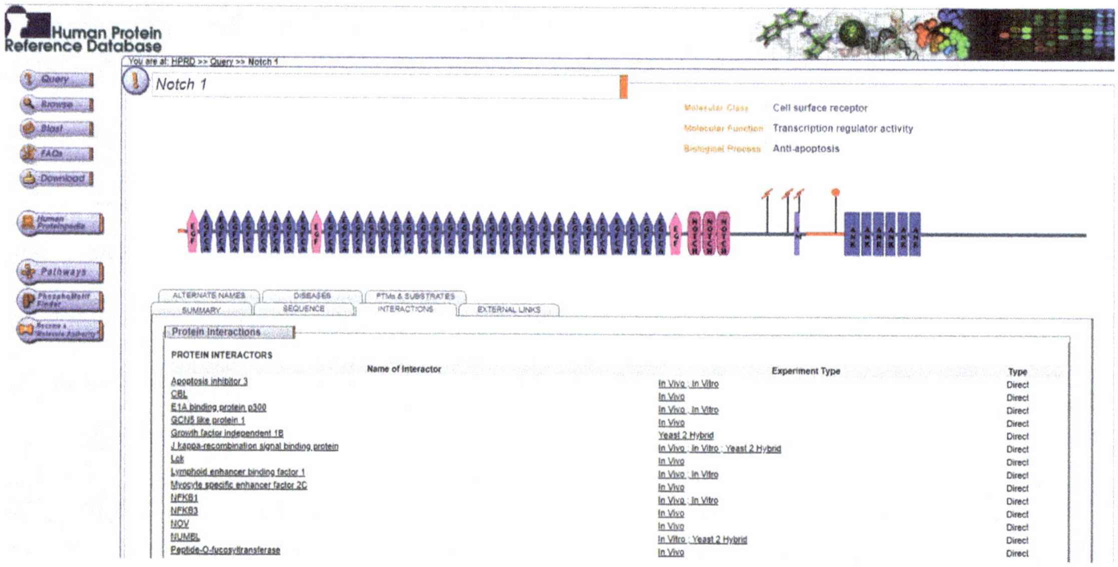

HitPredict

In this database PPI from the other sources such as BioGRID, MINT, HPRD, DIP and IntAct were combined and annotated. Input to HitPredict can be a keyword, Uniprot ID, Entrez ID or Ensembel ID. The reliability score, interaction score, annotation score, confidence, interactive proteins and gene ontology information is provided. The dataset contains, 3,98,696 physical interactions between 70,808 proteins from 105 species. Percentage of accuracy is high in this database as it provides statistical values (López *et al.,* 2015). Since its introduction, HitPredict has been constantly updated and maintained.

IntAct

This database belongs to IMEx Consortium and maintains IMEx standards. It contains information of interactors, interactions, method of interaction analysis and also provides interaction network. The new protein interactions are frequently updated and maintained properly. The data can be downloaded in different file formats for further analyses (Hermjakob, 2004; Kerrien *et al.,* 2012). The database contains simple URLs for the easy accession of protein interactions and their linked external resources. Cytoscape is also linked with IntAct for clear visualization of the networks. This provides 2,75,000 binary interactions from 10,000 curated experiments ("OpenHelix: IntAct protein interaction database," n.d.)

Biomolecular Interaction Network Database (BIND)

BIND provides information regarding biomolecular interactions, complexes and pathways. It is operated by the University of Pittsburgh, Penisulveniya. It provides information regarding interactive domains, biochemical and genetic networks (Bader *et al.,* 2003). Currently BIND is inactive.

Figure 5. Screen shot of BioGRID database and protein interaction information provided for NOTCH1.

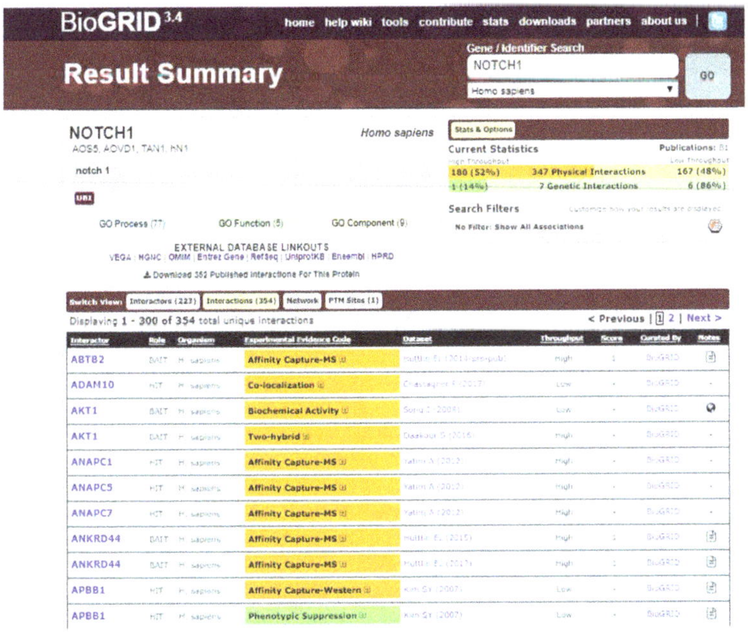

Figure 6. Screen shot of HitPredict database and protein interaction information provided for NOTCH1 of homosapiens.

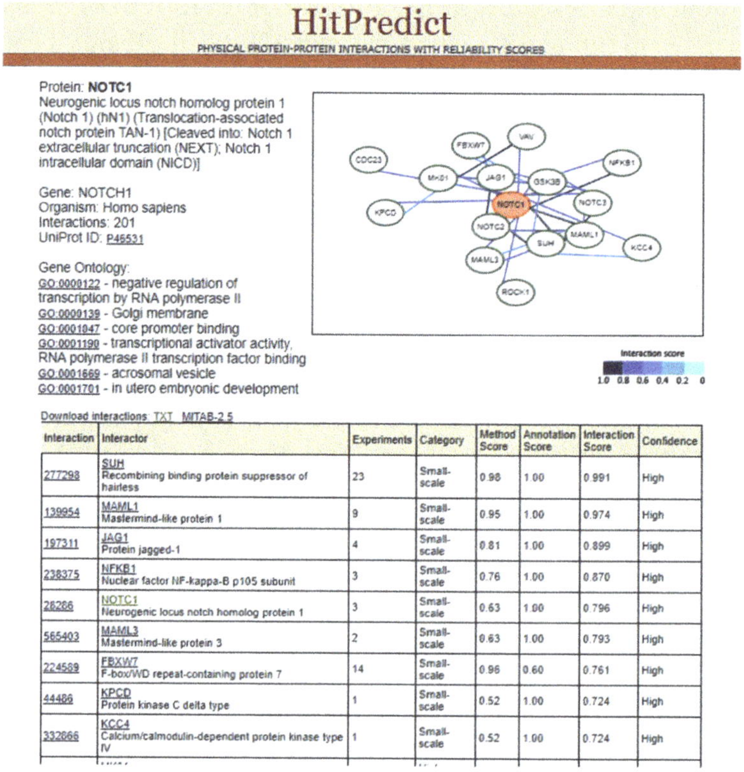

Figure 7. Screen shot of IntAct database and protein interaction information provided for NOTCH1.

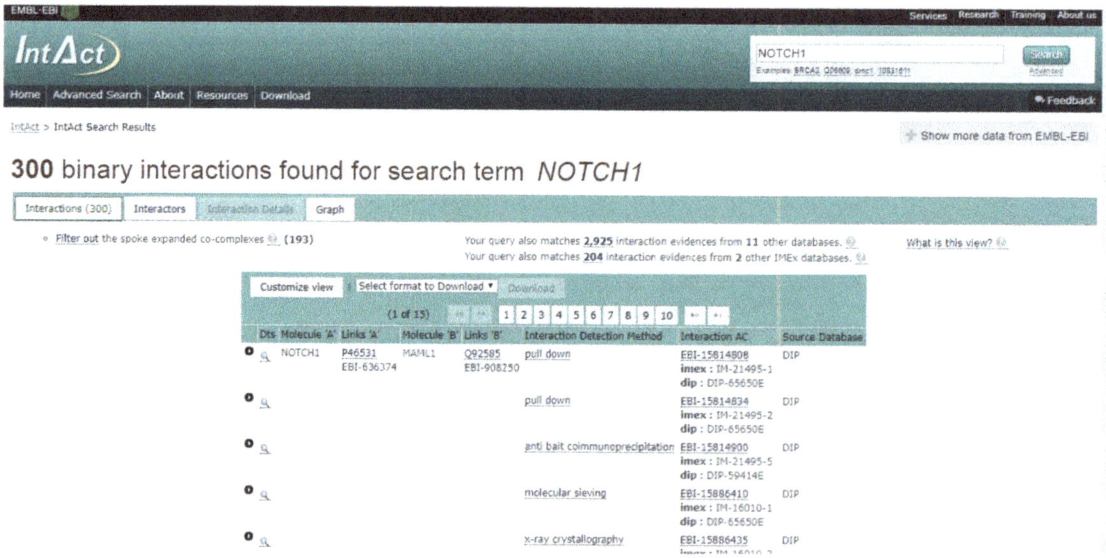

Kyoto Encyclopedia of Genes and Genomes (KEGG)

KEGG is one of the world's largest and known database for the systems biology applications, it integrates systemic and cellular functions. It provides mapping of large scale data, integration and analysis. It contains the gene catalogs for the species whose genome was completely sequenced. KEGG provides wider modules to analyse signaling pathway, metabolic pathway and disease pathway etc. [20, 21]. The main task of this is to discover best drug targets and therapeutics for a disease. KEGG provides various information such as pathway maps, hierarchies and tables, orthologs, genomic and proteomic information, compounds, biochemical reactions, enzyme nomenclature, disease related network, drugs and health information resource. It also supplements organism specific information. In addition to this KEGG provides various analysis tools such as KEGG Mapper, BLAST/FASTA for sequence similarity search and SIMCOMP for chemical structure similarity search etc.

REACTOME

This is a pathway database containing different pathway data of homosapiens. This helps in analysis of huge data such as microarray and provides information regarding protein localization and respective gene ontology, signaling pathways in which the query protein was involved and its analysis (Vastrik *et al.,* 2007). The information is shared among the various databases. This is mainly used for visualization, interpretation and pathway enrichment analysis ("What is Reactome ? - Reactome Pathway Database,"). This includes 2,216 pathways, 11,754 reactions, 10,762 proteins and 1,867 molecules.

Though there are several PPI databases, few databases are not up to date or active. The data reported in all the PPI databases are not similar as it depends on the understanding of the curator(Lehne and Schlitt, 2009). Hence, currently PPI databases are exchanging data in between them to maintain accuracy and to improve the quality and quantity of data.

PROTEIN-PROTEIN INTERACTION NETWORK CONSTRUCTION AND VISUALIZATION

Coordinated function of systematic proteins is responsible for most of the cellular function and the interaction of proteins is highly regulated. Alterations in regular signaling pathways are the prime cause of disease initiation and progression. But analyzing the complex and huge data is very challenging. Hence, systems biology laid an approach to decipher the interrelationship between complex protein interactions, using computational loom by designing multifaceted biological networks. Transition of biology from molecular to system level provides better understanding of regulatory systems and gives novel opportunities for its application (Kitano, 2002).

Protein-Protein interaction network (PPIN) is a graphical representation of PPI. The interaction networks helps to draft biological function of a protein and its significance in signaling pathways at various environments. Interestingly, a single protein with limited active surface interacts with tons of proteins due to presence of more binding sites and conformational changes. Interacting partners are represented

Figure 8. Screen shot of KEGG database and protein interaction information provided for NOTCH1

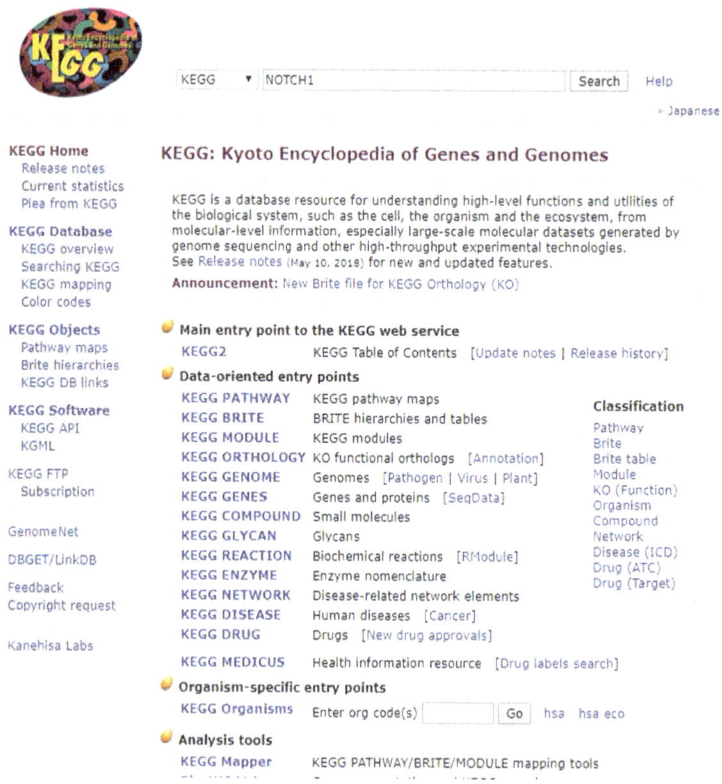

Figure 9. Screen shot of Reactome database and protein interaction information provided for NOTCH1

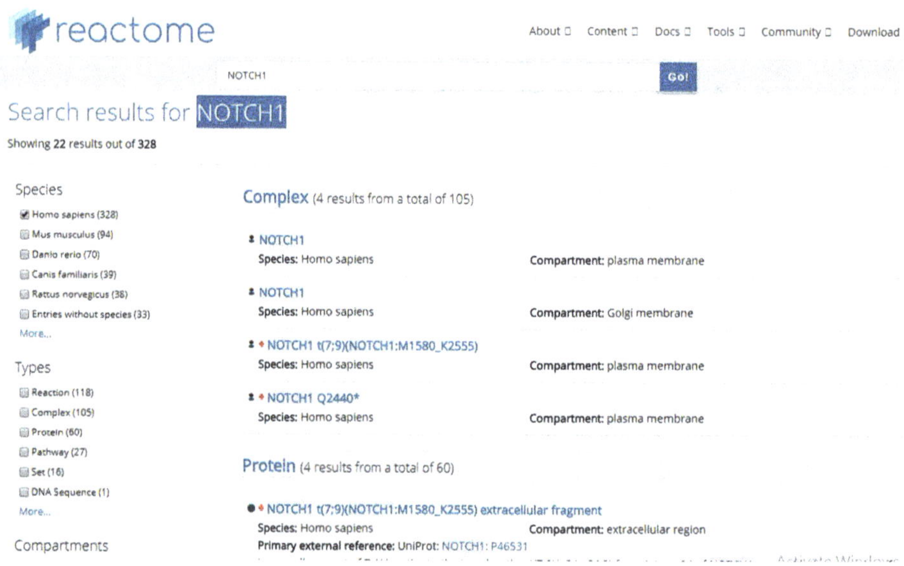

Table 1. Details of protein-protein interaction and pathway databases and its websites

S.No.	PPI database	Website
1	Database of Interacting Proteins (DIP)	http://dip.mbi.ucla.edu/dip/
2	Molecular INTeraction database (MINT)	https://mint.bio.uniroma2.it/
3	Human Protein Reference Database (HPRD)	http://www.hprd.org/
4	Biological General Repository for Interaction Datasets (BioGRID)	https://thebiogrid.org/
5	HitPredict	http://hintdb.hgc.jp/htp/
6	IntAct	https://www.ebi.ac.uk/intact/
7	Kyoto Encyclopedia of Genes and Genomes (KEGG)	http://www.genome.jp/kegg/
8	REACTOME	https://reactome.org/

as nodes and each node in the network signifies all the protein products of a single gene and depicts the collection of proteins where the structural confirmations may vary (Halakou *et al.,* 2017; Tsai *et al.,* 2009). The highly interacting proteins in a PPI network are known as hubs(He and Zhang, 2006). These hubs will have vital role in signaling pathway and can act as best drug targets. The interactions are represented in the form of edges that connect nodes with lines (Koh *et al.,* 2012).

Network Construction

Current research signifies that the signal transduction pathways are interconnected rather linear (Safari-Alighiarloo *et al.,* 2014). PPINs are scale free, few nodes have larger number of interactions and few have little. There are several platforms available to construct PPIN using data collected from various databases. Initial seed proteins can be collected either from literature or by text mining. These proteins can be used further to derive binary interactions using the PPI databases listed in the above section.

Step1: Collection of Proteins

The proteins can be collected from the review of literature by text mining and PubMed databases such as gene expression omnibus (GEO).

Step 2: Derivation of Interactions

Figure 11.

Step 3: Network Construction by Search Tool for the Retrieval of Interacting Genes/Proteins (STRING)

Functional associations of proteins can be determined widely using STRING (Szklarczyk *et al.,* 2015). This derives the information from different databases and literature and increases reliability of protein interactions (Halakou *et al.,* 2017). This also inspects interaction evidence from text mining, co-expression analyses, neighborhood, gene fusion and co-occurrence (Jensen *et al.,* 2009).

Figure 10. Schematic representation of PPI network construction, visualization and analysis

Collection of seed proteins from the literature (Using text mining/polysearch)

↓

Identify UniProt ID for the collected seed proteins

↓

Spot the binary interactions of the proteins using PPI databases such as HPRD, BioDRID and IntAct

↓

Construct PPI network using STRING/ PINa

↓

Derive the number of nodes and interactions with better confidence score

↓

Visualize the network using tools such as Cytoscape (advanced version :3.6.1)

↓

Cytoscape is used to analyze the PPI network to find major parameters such as degree, betweenness centrality and closeness centrality.

↓

Various analysis such as topological analysis, gene ontology can be performed by using different plugins in Cytoscape

↓

Determine the hub genes that have bottleneck effect and this can be hypothesized as best drug targets

Table 2. Details of seed or query proteins collected from literature, used to derive interactions

S.No	Protein name	Uni Prot ID	Gene name
1	Fibroblast growth factor 12	P61328	FGF12
2	Vascular cell adhesion protein 1	P19320	VCAM1
3	Plasminogen activator inhibitor 1	P05121	SERPINE1
4	C-C motif chemokine 2	P13500	CCL2
5	Interleukin-8	P10145	CXCL8
6	C-C chemokine receptor type 2	P41597	CCR2
7	Macrophage colony-stimulating factor 1 receptor	P07333	CSF1R
8	Granulocyte colony-stimulating factor receptor	Q99062	CSF3R
9	Toll-like receptor 2	O60603	TLR2
10	Tumor necrosis factor	P01375	TNF

Based on the level of confidence score from IntAct 10% of high priority proteins are selected and used as input in STRING version: 10.5 for the network construction. PPIN has to be constructed by selecting better confidence score. The network shows more the 1500 proteins with greater interactions. The data from STRING is downloaded in tab delimited format and can be further used to visualize and analyse the network using Cytoscape 3.6.1

Figure 11. Screen shot of interactors and interactions derived from IntAct database

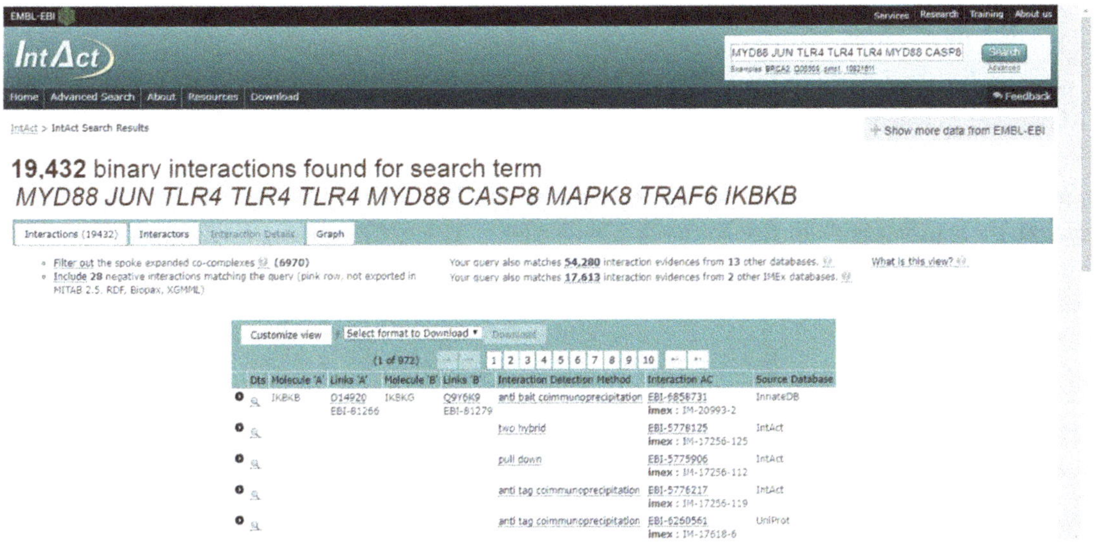

Figure 12. PPIN construction using STRING version 10.5 with the value of basic parameters

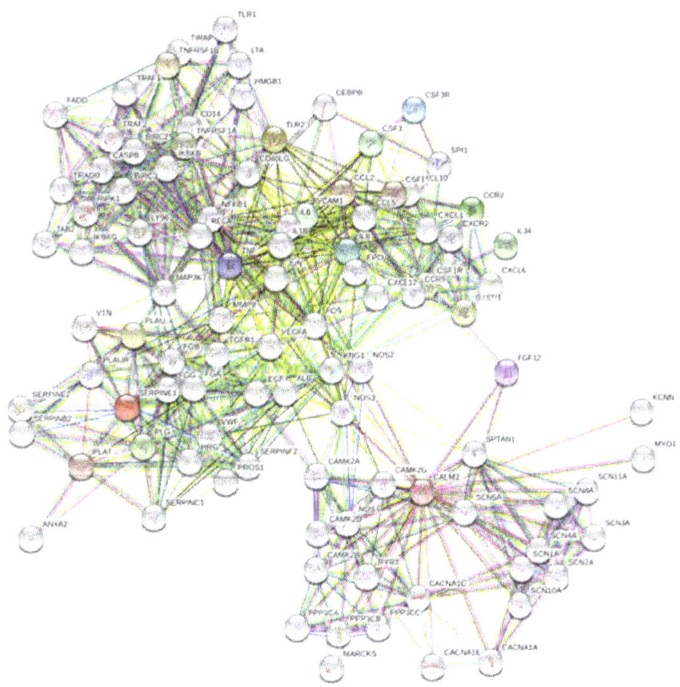

Number of nodes: 100
Number of edges: 756
Average node degree:15.1
Avg. local clustering coefficient:0.696
PPI enrichment p-value:< 1.0e-16

Network Visualization

Visualization is very important for the clear understanding of the pathway or PPIN and also simplifies the complexity of the pathway. Network can be visualized using Cytoscape with advanced version 3.6.1.Cytoscape is an open source software for analysis of protein and gene interactions, data integration and generation of network. Cytoscape provides several plugins that can be used for various analyses such as gene enrichment, module detection Network can be validated based on closeness centrality, betweenness centrality and degree. Network can also be visualized in various forms such as tree layout, circular layout and hierarchy layout etc. (Agapito *et al.,* 2013; Saito *et al.,* 2012). Nodes and edges can be colored or edited based on the requirement.

Figure 13. Network visualization from Cytoscape depicting Toll-like receptor signaling pathway derived using seed proteins. Network is visualized bases on degree layout (highest interacting proteins are represented in bigger font size)

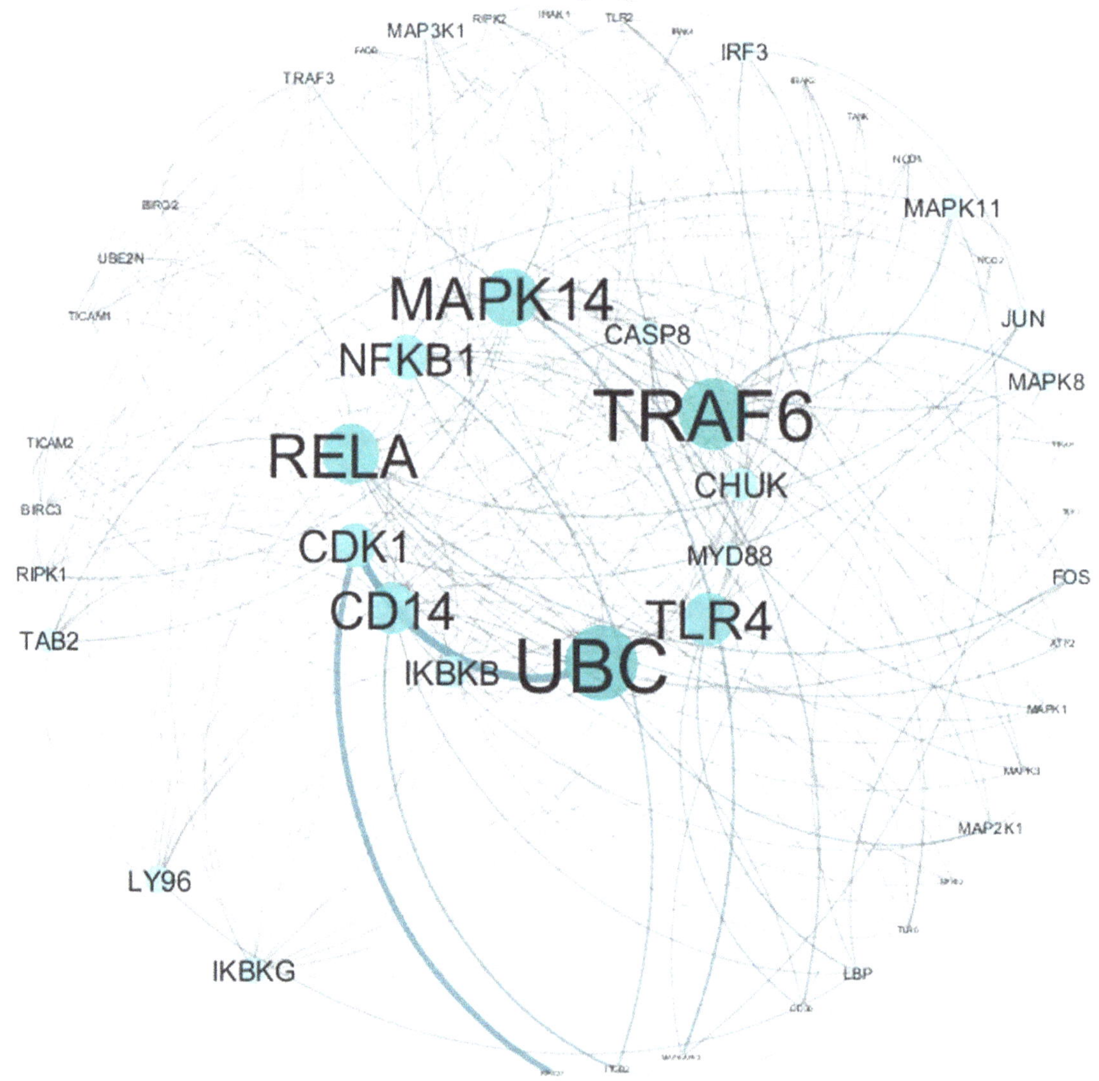

Network Analysis

Using Cytoscape several parameters can be easily analyzed using different plugins. PPINs are highly complex and difficult to analyze and interpret. Network analysis is performed in the Cytoscape using network analyzer. The STRING data is given as input for the analysis. The statistical analysis of PPIN constructed in the STRING is as follows.

Figure 14. Network analysis: A) Basic statistical parameters analyzed in the Cytoscape for PPIN constructed in STRING; B) Graph represents betweenness centrality vs number of neighbors C) Graph represents closeness centrality vs number of neighbors D) Graph represents number of nodes vs degree

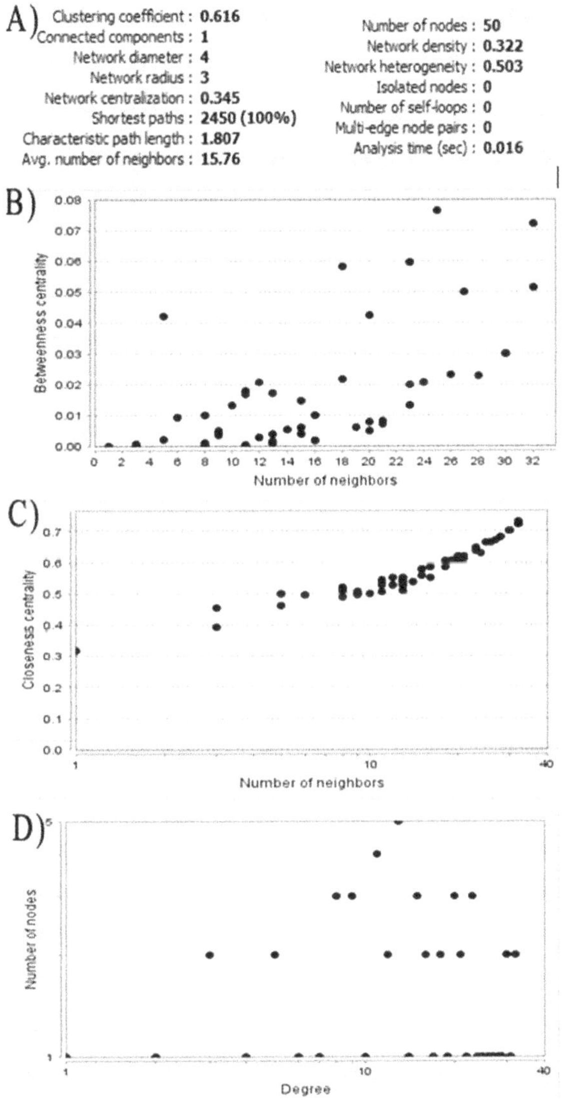

CONCLUSION

The systems biology era has opened up the identification and analysis of larger protein interactions, which is not performed so far. The hub proteins are the vital proteins that have highest number of interactions which means that, they influence several signaling pathways. These are easily identified with the help of PPI networks. This information is nearly a milestone in the biological research, because, most of the disease mechanisms are connected with several upstream and downstream signaling. In few instances, drug discovery is executed without the prior knowledge of associated proteins of disease target, which may play a lethal role in the development of toxicity and hypersensitivity. These kinds of errors can be avoided by using the PPI networks, where most of the associated proteins and genes identified and analyzed for a stated disease. Experimental methods have limitation in analyzing huge set of proteins. It involves longer time, extensive expertise and highly expensive. Computational analysis of PPI network may not provide data with 100% accuracy, but gives better clue regarding where to start laboratory experiments and also provide the missing interactions. It is feasible for better understanding of disease mechanisms using PPINs. Identification of crucial proteins from the network will help in choosing best drug targets and further for drug discovery.

REFERENCES

Agapito, G., Guzzi, P., & Cannataro, M. (2013). Visualization of protein interaction networks: Problems and solutions. *BMC Bioinformatics*, *14*(Suppl 1). doi:10.1186/1471-2105-14-S1-S1 PMID:23368786

Ashraf, M. I., Ong, S. K., Mujawar, S., Pawar, S., More, P., Paul, S., & Lahiri, C. (2018). A side-effect free method for identifying cancer drug targets. *Scientific Reports*, 8. PMID:29703908

Bader, G. D., Betel, D., & Hogue, C. W. V. (2003). BIND: The Biomolecular Interaction Network Database. *Nucleic Acids Research*, *31*(1), 248–250. doi:10.1093/nar/gkg056 PMID:12519993

Chatr-aryamontri, A., Ceol, A., Palazzi, L. M., Nardelli, G., Schneider, M. V., Castagnoli, L., & Cesareni, G. (2007). MINT: The Molecular INTeraction database. *Nucleic Acids Research*, *35*(Database), D572–D574. doi:10.1093/nar/gkl950 PMID:17135203

Goel, R., Harsha, H. C., Pandey, A., & Prasad, T. S. K. (2012). Human Protein Reference Database and Human Proteinpedia as resources for phosphoproteome analysis. *Molecular BioSystems*, *8*(2), 453–463. doi:10.1039/C1MB05340J PMID:22159132

Halakou, F., Kilic, E. S., Cukuroglu, E., Keskin, O., & Gursoy, A. (2017). Enriching Traditional Protein-protein Interaction Networks with Alternative Conformations of Proteins. *Scientific Reports*, 7. PMID:28775330

Haque, M., Sarmah, R., & Bhattacharyya, D. K. (2018). A common neighbor based technique to detect protein complexes in PPI networks. *Journal of Genetic Engineering and Biotechnology*, *16*(1), 227–238. doi:10.1016/j.jgeb.2017.10.010

He, X., & Zhang, J. (2006). Why Do Hubs Tend to Be Essential in Protein Networks? *PLOS Genetics*, *2*(6), e88. doi:10.1371/journal.pgen.0020088 PMID:16751849

Hermjakob, H. (2004). IntAct: An open source molecular interaction database. *Nucleic Acids Research, 32*(90001), 452D–455. doi:10.1093/nar/gkh052 PMID:14681455

HomeD. I. P. (n.d.). Retrieved from http://dip.mbi.ucla.edu/dip

Jensen, L. J., Kuhn, M., Stark, M., Chaffron, S., Creevey, C., Muller, J., ... von Mering, C. (2009). STRING 8--a global view on proteins and their functional interactions in 630 organisms. *Nucleic Acids Research, 37*(Database), D412–D416. doi:10.1093/nar/gkn760 PMID:18940858

Kanehisa, M. (2004). The KEGG resource for deciphering the genome. *Nucleic Acids Research, 32*(90001), 277D–280. doi:10.1093/nar/gkh063 PMID:14681412

Kanehisa, M., Goto, S., Sato, Y., Furumichi, M., & Tanabe, M. (2012). KEGG for integration and interpretation of large-scale molecular data sets. *Nucleic Acids Research, 40*(D1), D109–D114. doi:10.1093/nar/gkr988 PMID:22080510

Kerrien, S., Aranda, B., Breuza, L., Bridge, A., Broackes-Carter, F., Chen, C., ... Hermjakob, H. (2012). The IntAct molecular interaction database in 2012. *Nucleic Acids Research, 40*(D1), D841–D846. doi:10.1093/nar/gkr1088 PMID:22121220

Keskin, O., Tuncbag, N., & Gursoy, A. (2016). Predicting Protein–Protein Interactions from the Molecular to the Proteome Level. *Chemical Reviews, 116*(8), 4884–4909. doi:10.1021/acs.chemrev.5b00683 PMID:27074302

Kitano, H. (2002). Systems Biology: A Brief Overview. *Science, 295*(5560), 1662–1664. doi:10.1126cience.1069492 PMID:11872829

Klingstrom, T., & Plewczynski, D. (2011). Protein-protein interaction and pathway databases, a graphical review. *Briefings in Bioinformatics, 12*(6), 702–713. doi:10.1093/bib/bbq064 PMID:20851835

Koh, G. C. K. W., Porras, P., Aranda, B., Hermjakob, H., & Orchard, S. E. (2012). Analyzing Protein–Protein Interaction Networks. *Journal of Proteome Research, 11*(4), 2014 2031. doi:10.1021/pr201211w PMID:22385417

Lehne, B., & Schlitt, T. (2009). Protein-protein interaction databases: Keeping up with growing interactomes. *Human Genomics, 3*, 291–297. PMID:19403463

López, Y., Nakai, K., & Patil, A. (2015). HitPredict version 4: Comprehensive reliability scoring of physical protein–protein interactions from more than 100 species. *Database, 2015*, bav117. doi:10.1093/database/bav117 PMID:26708988

OpenHelix. (n.d.). *IntAct protein interaction database.* Retrieved from http://www.openhelix.com/tutorialInfo.cgi?id=55

Perkins, J. R., Diboun, I., Dessailly, B. H., Lees, J. G., & Orengo, C. (2010). Transient Protein-Protein Interactions: Structural, Functional, and Network Properties. *Structure (London, England), 18*(10), 1233–1243. doi:10.1016/j.str.2010.08.007 PMID:20947012

Rao, V. S., Srinivas, K., Sujini, G. N., & Kumar, G. N. S. (2014). Protein-Protein Interaction Detection: Methods and Analysis. *International Journal of Proteomics, 2014*, 1–12. doi:10.1155/2014/147648 PMID:24693427

Safari-Alighiarloo, N., Taghizadeh, M., Rezaei-Tavirani, M., Goliaei, B., & Peyvandi, A. A. (2014). Protein-protein interaction networks (PPI) and complex diseases. *Gastroenterology and Hepatology from Bed To Bench, 7*, 17–31. PMID:25436094

Saito, R., Smoot, M. E., Ono, K., Ruscheinski, J., Wang, P. L., Lotia, S., ... Ideker, T. (2012). A travel guide to Cytoscape plugins. *Nature Methods, 9*(11), 1069–1076. doi:10.1038/nmeth.2212 PMID:23132118

Stark, C. (2006). BioGRID: A general repository for interaction datasets. *Nucleic Acids Research, 34*(90001), D535–D539. doi:10.1093/nar/gkj109 PMID:16381927

Szklarczyk, D., Franceschini, A., Wyder, S., Forslund, K., Heller, D., Huerta-Cepas, J., ... von Mering, C. (2015). STRING v10: Protein–protein interaction networks, integrated over the tree of life. *Nucleic Acids Research, 43*(D1), D447–D452. doi:10.1093/nar/gku1003 PMID:25352553

The Molecular INTeraction Database. (n.d.). *An ELIXIR Core Resource*. Retrieved from https://mint.bio.uniroma2.it/

Tsai, C. J., Ma, B., & Nussinov, R. (2009). Protein–protein interaction networks: How can a hub protein bind so many different partners? *Trends in Biochemical Sciences, 34*(12), 594–600. doi:10.1016/j.tibs.2009.07.007 PMID:19837592

Vastrik, I., D'Eustachio, P., Schmidt, E., Joshi-Tope, G., Gopinath, G., Croft, D., ... de. (2007). Reactome: A knowledge base of biologic pathways and processes. *Genome Biology, 8*(3), R39. doi:10.1186/gb-2007-8-3-r39 PMID:17367534

What is Reactome? (n.d.). *Reactome Pathway Database*. Retrieved from https://reactome.org/what-is-reactome

Xenarios, I. (2000). DIP: The Database of Interacting Proteins. *Nucleic Acids Research, 28*(1), 289–291. doi:10.1093/nar/28.1.289 PMID:10592249

Zhang, X. F., Ou-Yang, L., Hu, X., & Dai, D. Q. (2015). Identifying binary protein-protein interactions from affinity purification mass spectrometry data. *BMC Genomics*, 16. PMID:26438428

Chapter 10
Quality by Design in Pharmaceutical Formulation

Sundaramurthy Vivekanandan
Bluefish Pharmaceuticals Pvt. Ltd, India

ABSTRACT

Quality by design (QbD) is a systematic, scientific, risk-based approach to product development and manufacturing process to consistently deliver the quality product. In this chapter, application, benefits, opportunities, regulatory requirements involved in quality by design of pharmaceutical products are discussed. In quality by design approach, during development, the developer defines quality target product profile (QTPP) and identifies critical quality attributes (CQA). Critical process parameters (CPP) of unit operations which impacts critical quality attributes need to be identified to understand the impact of critical material attributes (CMA) on quality attributes of the drug product. Quality by design approach is defined in ICH guidelines Q8 – Pharmaceutical Development, Q9 – Quality Risk Management, Q10 – Pharmaceutical Quality System. This chapter describes the implementation of new concepts in quality by design like design of experiments to achieve design space, control strategy to consistently manufacture quality product throughout the product lifecycle.

INTRODUCTION

Quality by design is a systematic approach to product and process design, development that begins with predefined objectives and emphasizes product and process understanding and process control, based on sound science and quality risk management (ICH Q8(R2)).

FDA had provided detailed description to Quality by Design in 2004 via 'pharmaceutical cGMPs for 21st century – a risk based approach'

FDA faced issue of increase in number of regulatory variations to registered New Drug Applications (NDAs) and Abbreviated New Drug Applications (ANDA's) in 2007. FDA had observed that, the applicants had focused more in chemistry section of dossier and least priority provided to manufacturing process and product development. Hence, FDA decided that, more controls were required on drug product manufacturing process and the qualitative, quantitative composition. In 2005 FDA had insisted the applicants to submit chemistry manufacturing control (CMC) section with an application of QbD as part of New Drug Application and Abbreviated New Drug Application (Patricia Van Arnum *et al.*, 2007).

DOI: 10.4018/978-1-5225-7326-5.ch010

IMPORTANCE OF QUALITY BY DESIGN APPROACH

Quality must be built in drug product development as well as during manufacturing process (ICH Q8(R2) 2017; Robert A. Lionberger, Sau Lawrence Lee, LaiMing Lee, Andre Raw, and Lawrence X. Yu 2008). Quality can not be improved by testing finished product or by performing in-process tests. In traditional pharmaceutical manufacturing process, the manufacturing process controlled through fixed parameters or range with additional in-process testing at different process stages. Whereas Quality by Design approach defines design space and control strategy to maintain design space to ensure quality of finished product (Lan Zhang, Shirui Mao *et. al.,* 2017; Jaiprakash N. Sangshetti Mrinmayee Deshpande Zahid Zaheer Devanand B.Shinde Rohidas Arote. e*t al.,* 2017). This infers that, QbD approach helps to develop quality product through consistent, robust process. The same is depicted in Figure 1.

QbD ultimately helps to implement ICH Q8, Q9 and Q10. ICH released 'Q8(R2) Pharmaceutical Development' in 2009, 'Q9 Quality Risk Management' in 2005 and 'Q10 Pharmaceutical Quality System Guidelines' in 2008 (Rathore *et. al.,* 2009). ICH released Q8/Q9/Q10 Questions & Answers (R4) in 2010 to emphasis details about design space, real-time release testing and control strategy (ICH Q&A 2010). Now FDA has increased implementation of QbD concepts in drug product development made by the applicants from January 2013 (Jaiprakash N. Sangshetti Mrinmayee Deshpande Zahid Zaheer Devanand B.Shinde Rohidas Arote. e*t al.,* 2017).

ELEMENTS OF QUALITY BY DESIGN IN PHARMACEUTICAL DEVELOPMENT

Various elements of Quality by Design system (Vemuri Pavan Kumar, N. Vishal Gupta 2015; Jaiprakash N. Sangshetti Mrinmayee Deshpande Zahid Zaheer Devanand B.Shinde Rohidas Arote. e*t al.,* 2017; Lawrence X.Yu *et. al.,* 2008) are listed below and the same is shown in Figure 2.

1. **QTPP:** Identify the Quality Target Product Profile (QTPP) by defining desired drug product characteristics.
2. **CQA:** Identify Critical Quality Attributes (CQA's).
3. **CPP & CMA:** Identify Critical Process Parameters (CPP's) and Critical Material Attributes (CMA's).
4. **Risk Assessment:** Perform risk assessment by linking CMA's and CPP's to CQA's to assess impact of these parameters on QTPP.

Figure 1. Traditional system Vs QbD approach

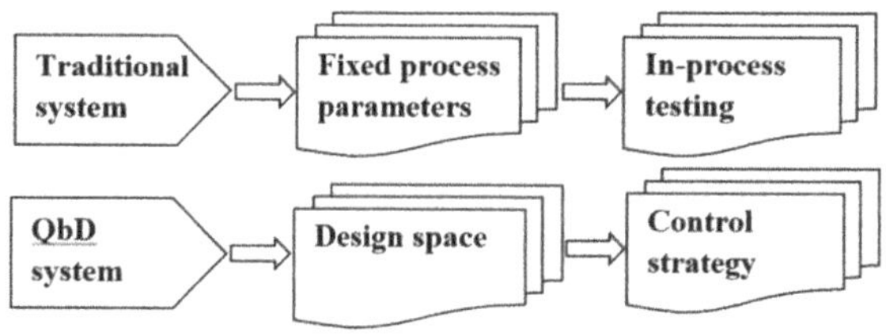

Figure 2. Elements of quality by Design

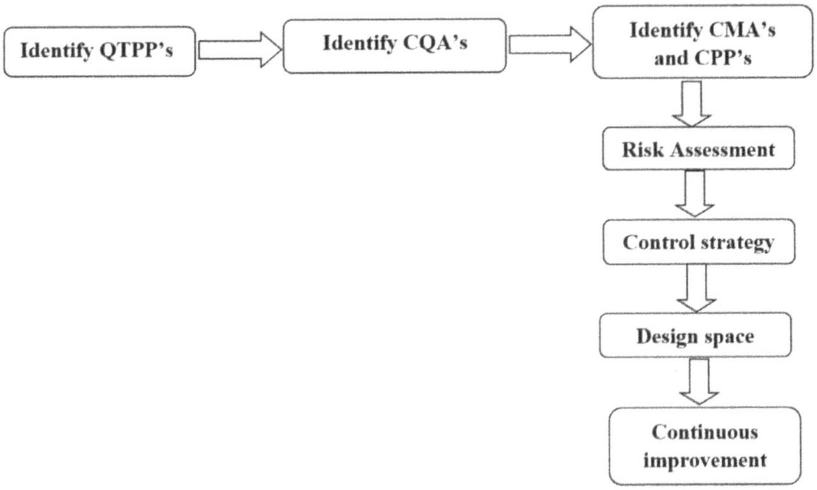

5. **Control Strategy:** Implement control strategy by controlling CMA's and CPP's through experimental design.
6. **Design Space:** Develop and assess design space to achieve finished product with desired QTPP.
7. **Continuous Improvement:** Continually monitor and improve the manufacturing process throughout lifecycle of product to ensure consistent quality of finished product.

IMPLEMENTATION OF QUALITY BY DESIGN IN PHARMACEUTICAL DEVELOPMENT

Quality by design approach in Pharmaceutical development implemented by performing detailed assessment of various elements of Quality by Design system as listed below.

Identification of Quality Target Product Profile (QTPP)

Quality Target Product Profile (QTPP) is "a prospective summary of the quality characteristics of a drug product that ideally will be achieved to ensure the desired quality of drug product, by considering safety and efficacy (ICH Q8(R2); QbD for ANDA's An example of IR dosage forms & An example for MR dosage forms)."

Quality Target Product Profile describes the design criteria for the drug product and hence, provides the basis for defining Critical Quality Attributes (CQA's), Critical Process Parameters (CPP's), Critical Material Attributes (CMA's) and control strategy (Delasko, J.M., Cocchetto, D.M., Burke. L.B., 2005).

The critical elements derived from the Quality Target Product Profile are assessed during development phase, and the Critical Quality Attributes (CQA's) are identified. For a generic drug product development, the Quality Target Product Profile (QTPP) were identified by reviewing the label, Summary of Product Characteristics (SPC's) of reference product as well as by analysis of the reference product for quality characteristics like dissolution and other aspects of product quality (ICH Q8 (R2)).

Target Product Profile (TPP) of drug product like oral, immediate release, tablet of specific strength, specific shelf life in particular container closure system is to ensure labelled use as well as to ensure safety and efficacy to patient.

As an example, QTPP for Warfarin 2mg Immediate Release Tablets is defined in Table 1.

Target Product Profile (TPP) can be further explained with an example by taking into consideration of one of the element of TPP – dosage strength.

An example of generic product development of Warfarin 2mg immediate release, oral solid tablets was considered. In this case, the labelled use is 2mg Warfarin tablets. In case the generic drug product is developed with higher dose of 5mg warfarin instead of 2mg Warfarin, that will be a deviation from product label. The same will be harmful for the safety of the patient, since the higher dose might exhibit toxic effects to the patient. Hence, the TPP element - dosage strength ensures safety and efficacy of drug product as labelled.

Quality Target Product Profile (QTPP) of drug product is to ensure safety and efficacy of drug product to patients by evaluating and controlling quality characteristics of drug product. Drug product quality characteristic parameter – Assay can ensure that, the drug product contains intended content of 2mg of Warfarin as mentioned in product label.

Analysing specific batches of drug product for quality characteristics like assay, related substances, dissolution, content uniformity etc., ensures the quality of drug product throughout it's shelf life in specific container closure system, which ensures safety and efficacy of drug product to patient.

Table 1. Quality Target Product Profile (Vemuri Pavan Kumar, N. Vishal Gupta 2015; ICH Q8(R2); QbD for ANDA's An example of IR dosage forms & An example for MR dosage forms)

QTPP elements	Target	Justification
Dosage form	Tablet	Same dosage form as per Pharmaceutical equivalence requirement
Dosage design	Immediate release	Same dosage design as per Pharmaceutical equivalence requirement
Route administration	Oral	Same route of administration as per Pharmaceutical equivalence requirement
Dosage strength	2mg	Same strength as per Pharmaceutical equivalence requirement
Pharmacokinetics	Immediate release enabling T_{max} occur about 1 to 9 hours after oral administration; Bioequivalent to reference product	Bioequivalence requirement to meet rate and extent of in-vivo drug release similar to that of reference product to ensure efficacy and safety.
Stability	At least 36 months shelf-life at room temperature	Equivalent to or better than reference product shelf-life
Drug product quality attributes	Physical attributes	Pharmaceutical equivalence requirement: must meet the same compendial or other applicable (quality) standards (i.e., identity, assay, purity and quality).
	Identification	
	Dissolution	
	Content uniformity	
	Assay	
	Related substances	
	Residual solvents	
	Microbial limits	
Container closure	60CC HDPE bottle with 33mm child resistant closure and 1g silica gel canister	Needed to achieve the target shelf-life and to ensure tablet integrity during shipping
Administration/ concurrence with labelling	Similar food effect as that of reference product	Food affect prothrombin time
Alternative methods of administration	None	None are listed in the reference product label.

Identification of Critical Quality Attributes (CQA's)

Critical Quality Attribute (CQA) is a physical, chemical, biological or microbiological property or characteristic that should be within appropriate limit, range or distribution to ensure the desired product quality (ICH Q8(R2); QbD for ANDA's An example of IR dosage forms & An example for MR dosage forms).

During drug product development, list out all applicable quality attributes of drug product. Identify the Critical Quality Attribute (CQA) based on severity of harm to the patient safety and efficacy resulting from failure to meet that quality attribute.

Critical quality attributes (CQA's) for an immediate capsule dosage form are assessed as depicted in Table 2 (ICH Q8(R2); QbD for ANDA's An example of IR dosage forms & An example for MR dosage forms).

Identification of Critical Process Parameters (CPP's)

A process parameter whose variability can have a impact on critical quality attribute of drug product and hence should be monitored or controlled to ensure that, the process produces the desired quality (HuiquanWu, Mobin Tawakkul Maury White Mansoor A.Khan 2009; QbD for ANDA's An example of IR dosage forms).

Identify the drug product CQA (Example: Content uniformity), identify intermediate CQA (Example: Blend uniformity) for each process step (Example: Blending process) as applicable. Identify the process parameter that may affect the intermediate CQA of process steps.

Consider illustrative example of CPP elements of Blending time, number of revolutions of blender in blending process of low dose drug formulation and assess it's impact on drug product CQA - Content Uniformity through intermediate CQA Blend uniformity.

As explained in above example, the Critical Process Parameters – Blending time and number of revolutions impacts the intermediate Critical Quality Attributes Blend uniformity and % RSD. Non uniform blend will lead to poor Uniformity of dosage unit of finished product, which is threat to patient safety and efficacy.

Identification of Critical Material Attributes (CMA's)

A physical, chemical, biological or microbiological property or characteristic of an input material that should be within appropriate limit, range or distribution to ensure the desired quality of drug product (QbD for ANDA's An example of IR dosage forms).

Identify the drug product CQA (Example: Content uniformity), identify intermediate CQA (Example: Blend uniformity) for each process step (Example: Blending process) as applicable. Identify the material attribute that may affect the intermediate CQA of process steps.

Consider illustrative example of CMA elements – Particle size distribution of drug substance as well as blend in low dose drug formulation and assess its impact on drug product CQA Content Uniformity through intermediate CQA Blend uniformity.

As mentioned in above example, the Critical Material Attributes – Particle size distribution of drug substance as well as Blend affects the intermediate Critical Quality Attribute Blend uniformity and % RSD. Non uniform blend will lead to poor Uniformity of dosage unit of finished product, which is threat to patient safety and efficacy.

Table 2. Critical quality attributes (CQA's) (ICH Q8(R2); QbD for ANDA's An example of IR dosage forms & An example for MR dosage forms)

Drug Product Quality Attributes		Target	Is This Critical?	Justification of Criticality
Physical attributes	Appearance (color and integrity)	White opaque hard capsule	Yes	Integrity (cracking) of the capsule may affect.
	Size	Size 4 capsule	No	The size may not affect the safety and efficacy of the product.
	Score configuration	Not applicable	No	The formulation is a capsule dosage form so there is no score configuration.
	Odour	No unpleasant odour	No	In general, a noticeable odour is not directly linked to safety and efficacy, but odour can affect patient acceptability. For this product, neither the drug substance nor the excipients have an unpleasant odor. No organic solvents will be used in the drug product manufacturing process.
	Friability	Not applicable	No	The formulation is a capsule dosage form there is no need for friability.
	Weight variation	NMT 10% m/m	Yes	Flow of the final blend will influence the weight variation in the capsule. The formulation and process variables will influence the flow of the blend. Therefore, this CQA will be monitored during development.
Identification		Positive for drug substance	Yes	Though identification is critical for safety and efficacy, this CQA can be effectively controlled by the quality management system and will be monitored at drug product release. Formulation and process variables do not impact identity. Therefore, this CQA will not be discussed during formulation and process development. However, the CQA remains a target element of the drug product profile and should be addressed accordingly.
Assay		95.0% m/m to 105.0% m/m	Yes	Assay variability will affect safety and efficacy. Product and Process variables may affect the assay of the drug product. Thus, assay will be evaluated throughout product and process development.
Related substances		Impurity 1 - Not more than 0.50% m/m Impurity 2 - Not more than 0.50% m/m Impurity 3 - Not more than 0.50% m/m *Impurity 4 - Not more than 1.00% m/m *Highest unknown impurity - Not more than 0.20% m/m Total impurities - Not more than 1.50% m/m	Yes	Related substances can impact safety and must be controlled based on compendia / International Conference on Harmonisation (ICH) requirements or Reference product characterization to limit patient exposure. The limit for total impurities is also based on Reference product characterisation. The target for any unknown impurity is set according to the ICH Q3B identification threshold for this drug product. Formulation and process variables can impact degradation products. Therefore, degradation products will be assessed during product and process development.
Water content		NMT 7.5% m/m	Yes	Water content in the formulation might increase the microbial growth and affect the safety to the patient.
Dissolution		NLT 80%(Q) at 30 minutes in 900 mL of 0.1 N HCl with using USP apparatus 1 at 100 rpm	Yes	Failure to meet the dissolution specification can impact bioavailability. Both formulation and process variables affect the dissolution profile. This CQA will be investigated throughout formulation and process development.
Residual solvents		USP <467> option 1	Yes*	Residual solvents can impact safety. However, no solvent is planned to use in drug product manufacturing process and the drug product complies with USP <467> Option 1. Therefore, formulation and process variables are unlikely to impact this CQA.
Content uniformity		Ph. Eur. <2.9.40>	Yes	As the drug load in the formulation is low this CQA is critical.
Microbial limits		Meets relevant pharmacopoeia criteria (Ph. Eur. 5.1.4)	Yes	Non-compliance with microbial limits will impact patient safety. In this case, the risk of microbial growth is very high because water is utilized for this product. Therefore, this CQA will be monitored during development.

Table 3. Critical Process Parameters assessment

Critical Process Parameters		Intermediate CQA		Remarks
Lubrication Blending time	Number of revolutions of blender	Blend uniformity result	% RSD of blend uniformity	
5 mins	10 RPM / minute	96 to 101%	2.8%	Acceptable
5 mins	20 RPM / minute	88 to 112%	5.5%	No satisfactory
10 mins	10 RPM / minute	90 to 112%	5.2%	No satisfactory

RISK ASSESSMENT AND CONTROL STRATEGY

Risk assessment is commonly used tool in QbD. Other tools include Design of Experiments (DoE) and Process Analytical Technology (PAT). Quality risk management is a systematic process for the assessment, control, communication and review of risks to the quality of the drug (medicinal) product across the product lifecycle (Patricia Van Arnum 2007; Vemuri Pavan Kumar, N. Vishal Gupta 2015).

CONTROL STRATEGY

Control strategy is determined set of controls derived from current understanding of product and process that assures process performance and product quality.

The control strategy are parameters and attributes related to material attributes like drug substance and other critical materials like functional materials, manufacturing facility, equipment operating parameters, in-process and finished product controls / specifications and analytical methods, frequency of monitoring and control (Woodcock J, 2004; Yu LX 2008;).

Steps in Risk Assessment

Steps in risk management is outlined in below diagram.

1. Identification of potential sources of hazards using historical data, theoretical analysis, opinions etc.,
2. Risk analysis, exposure of risk associated with those hazards
3. Risk evaluation using quantitative or qualitative scale to determine the significance of risk
4. Risk control to reduce and or accept risk to reduce the risk to an acceptable level
5. Risk review by taking into account of new knowledge and experience.

Table 4. Critical Material Attributes assessment

Critical Material Attributes			Intermediate CQA	Remarks
Particle size distribution of drug substance	Particle size distribution of blend	Blend uniformity result	% RSD of blend uniformity	
D(90) – NMT 50 µm	D(90) – NMT 100 µm	97 to 101%	2.0%	Acceptable
D(90) – NMT 50 µm	D(90) – NMT 500 µm	93 to 110%	4.5%	No satisfactory
D(90) – NMT 50 µm	D(90) – NMT 850 µm	88 to 112%	5.5%	No satisfactory

Figure 3. Quality Risk Management Process

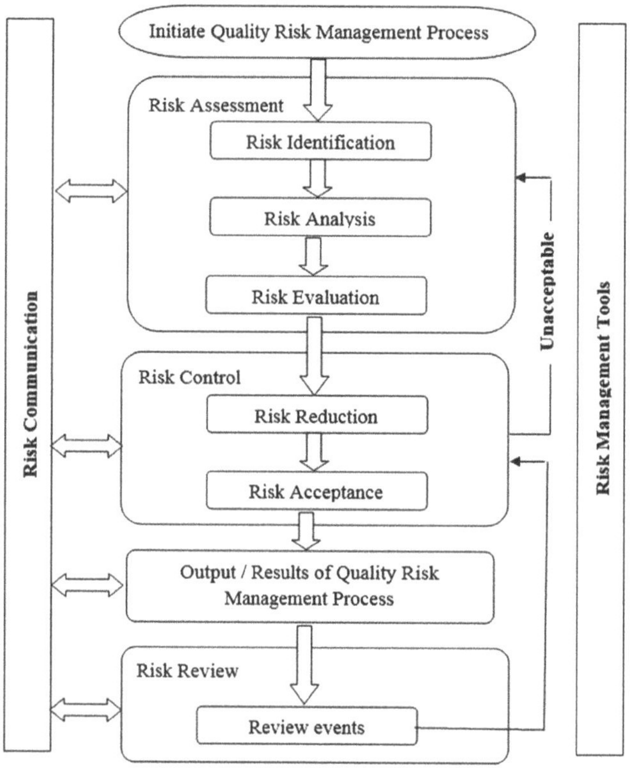

ICH Q9 provides a non-exhaustive list of 9 common risk management tools as follows: (1) Basic risk management facilitation methods (Ishikawa fishbone diagram, flowcharts, check sheets, etc.); (2) Fault tree analysis; (3) Risk ranking and filtering; (4) Preliminary hazard analysis; (5) Hazard analysis and critical control points; (6) Failure mode and effects analysis (FMEA); (7) Failure mode, effects, and criticality analysis (FMECA); (8) Hazard operability analysis; (9) Supporting statistical tools (European Medicines Agency ICH guideline Q9 on Quality risk management, Sep 2015).

Among the tools listed above, Ishikawa fishbone diagram and FMEA are widely used approaches for risk assessment, either separately or in combination.

The FMEA method can be used to perform the quantitative risk assessment, identifying the CQAs that have the greatest chance of causing product failure. The outcome of an FMEA are risk priority numbers (RPN) for each combination of failure mode severity, occurrence probability, and likelihood of detection. Where Occurrence probability (O), Severity (S), and Detectability (D) are all expressed with scale 1–10.

Alternatively, qualitative risk assessment shall be performed by categorising the risk into broad categories of low risk, medium risk and high risk with different colour codes as explained below.

As per ICH Q9 Quality Risk Management, it is not mandatory to perform formal risk management process. Internal practice of risk management process is also acceptable.

At initial stage of product development, initial Quality Risk evaluation is performed based on scientific knowledge with a rationale to ensure patient safety. Once the risk is identified, a formal risk analysis and risk evaluation performed and the risk output results are reviewed to reduce the risk level to acceptable range.

Table 5. Qualitative Risk categories system

Risk Category	Definition of Risk Category
Low (Green)	Broadly acceptable risk. No further investigation required
Medium (Yellow)	Risk is acceptable. Further investigation may be needed in order to reduce the risk
High (Red)	Risk is unacceptable. Further investigation is needed to reduce the risk

Risk Assessment and Control Strategy for Critical Material Attributes

Risk assessment to identify Critical Material Attributes is explained below by considering an example of drug product formulation.

Qualitative composition of drug product composition with the assumption that, the drug substance is of BCS class IV category with dose of 5mg in formulation. The grade and functionality details of materials are explained in below Table 6. Further risk assessment to identify the critical Material Attribute is explained in Table 7 followed by detailed of risk assessment evaluation.

Table 6. Qualitative composition of a formulation

Material Name	Grade	Functionality
Drug substance	D(90) – NMT 50 μm	Active Pharmaceutical ingredient
Microcrystalline Cellulose	Avicel PH 102	Diluent
Crospovidone	Polyplasdone XL 10	Super disintegrant
Sodium starch glycollate	Type A	Disintegrant
Colloidal silicon dioxide	Aerosil 200	Glidant
Magnesium stearate	Specific surface area of NMT 15m²/gm	Lubricant

Detailed risk assessment of Critical Material Attribute and control strategy to mitigate the risk are discussed in detail in this section.

Table 7. Risk assessment to identify Critical Material Attributes (CMA's)

Critical quality attributes	Drug substance particle size	Micro crystalline cellulose grade	Crospovidone grade	Crospovidone level	Sodium starch glycolate levels	Colloidal silicon dioxide levels	Magnesium stearate levels
Physical attributes	Low	Low	Low	Low	Low	Low	High
Stability	Low	Low	Low	Low	Low	Low	Low
Disintegration time	Low	Low	High	High	High	Low	High
Dissolution	High	Low	High	High	High	Low	High
Assay	Medium	Low	Medium	Medium	Low	High	Low
Blend uniformity	Medium	Low	Medium	Medium	Low	High	Low
Related substances	Low	Low	Low	Low	Low	Low	Low

Risk Assessment and Control Strategy for CMA: Drug Substance Particle Size Distribution (PSD)

Since, the drug substance is assumed as BCS class IV molecule with low solubility, finer particle size distribution of drug substance will have higher solubility, which in turn will have significant impact on dissolution of drug product. Hence, quality characteristic parameter of drug product – dissolution is considered as high risk and is identified as Critical Quality Attribute.

The proportion of over sized, under sized particles in drug substance will impact homogeneity of drug substance in the blend. Hence, quality characteristic of drug product like Assay and Blend uniformity are considered under medium risk.

During drug product development, different particle size distribution of drug substance will be evaluated to identify suitable particle size distribution of drug substance which will ensure desired dissolution of drug product consistently. Suitable screen size during sizing of dried granules to achieve desired particle size distribution of blend and the blending process with optimum blending time and number of revolutions will be evaluated during development to derive appropriate control. Based on these assessments, control strategy of three tier particle size distribution of drug substance as D(10), D(50) and D(90) with specification limit and blending time and number of revolutions of blender per minute for a specific blender size and occupancy of blend will be established and these parameters will be kept as control strategy.

Risk Assessment and Control Strategy for CMA: Grade, Level Disintegrants

Since, the drug substance is assumed as BCS class IV molecule with low solubility, the proportion of super disintegrant and disintegrant will impact disintegration time as well as *in-vitro* dissolution rate of drug product. The super disintegrant – crospovidone available in different grades as XL, XL10, Ultra, Ultra 10 with varying in particle size distribution and peroxide content.

By considering suitability of particle size distribution of input materials as well as by considering screen size for sizing of dried granules, suitable grade of super disintegrant and appropriate level of super disintegrant and disintegrant will be assessed during development. Suitable grade will be finalised accordingly. The CPP's, Blending time, blender speed and screen size for sizing of granules etc., will be optimised during development.

Table 8. Control strategy for CMA – Particle size distribution of drug substance

CQA	CMA	Control Strategy
Dissolution	• Particle size distribution of drug substance	• Three tier particle size distribution of drug substance with defined specification limit as D(10), D(50) and D(90) • Optimised Blending time and RPM of blender for specific size of blender and occupancy of blend. Whenever there is change in batch size or equipments these parameters will be re-assessed and optimised accordingly. • Defined screen size to size dried granules as established during development will be fixed.
Blend uniformity		
Blend Assay		

Risk Assessment and Control Strategy for CMA: Level of Glidant

The Glidant improves flowability of the blend. Inappropriate level of glidant will lead to poor flowability of blend, which might lead to poor assay, content uniformity of drug product.

During drug product development, appropriate level of Glidant will be evaluated and optimised.

Risk Assessment and Control Strategy for CMA: Level of Lubricant

Lubricants are hydrophobic in nature and imports hydrophobicity to the blend. Hence lubricant decreases the wettability of blend which retards the solubility of drug substance. This will delay the disintegration, *in-vitro* dissolution of drug product. Higher, the proportion of lubricant than that of optimum level will increase the disintegration time, delay the *in-vitro* dissolution and will lead to soft tablets.

During development, different levels of lubricant will be assessed and optimum quantity will be finalised based on comparative *in-vitro* dissolution of drug product with that of reference product.

Risk Assessment and Control Strategy for Critical Process Parameters

Risk assessment to identify Critical Process Parameters is explained below by considering an example of immediate release, uncoated, tablet formulation with 5mg dose, of BCS class IV drug substance made by High shear aqueous wet granulation process. Detailed risk assessment of Critical Process Parameter and control strategy to mitigate the risk are discussed below in detail.

Table 9. Control strategy for CMA – Grade, level of Disintegrants

CQA	CMA	Control Strategy
Disintegration time Dissolution Blend uniformity Blend Assay	• Grade of super disintegrant • Level of super dsintegrant • Level of disintegrant	• Grade of super disintegrant with specification limit for particle size distribution. • Optimised Blending time and RPM of blender for specific size of blender and occupancy of blend. Whenever there is change in batch size or equipments these parameters will be re-assessed and optimised accordingly. • Defined screen size to size granules as established during development will be fixed.

Table 10. Control strategy for CMA – level of Glidant

CQA	CMA	Control Strategy
Blend uniformity Blend Assay	• Level of Glidant	• Level of Glidant defined in quantitative composition of formulation. • Optimised Blending time and RPM of blender for specific size of blender and occupancy of blend. Whenever there is change in batch size or equipments these parameters will be re-assessed and optimised accordingly. • Defined screen size to size granules as established during development will be fixed.

Table 11. Control strategy for CMA – level of Lubricant

CQA	CMA	Control Strategy
Physical attributes Disintegration time Dissolution	• Level of lubricant	• Level of Lubricant defined in quantitative composition. • Optimised Blending time and RPM of blender for specific size of blender and occupancy of blend. Whenever there is change in batch size or equipments these parameters will be re-assessed and optimised accordingly. • Defined screen size to size granules as established during development will be fixed.

Risk Assessment and Control Strategy for CPP: Dry Mixing Process Parameters

Occupancy of dry mix materials in Rapid Mixer Granulator, Impeller Chopper speed of Rapid Mixer Granulator during dry mixing and dry mixing time are the key parameters of dry mixing process.

Based on binder quantity to be added, change in bulk density of wet mass during granulation process, in general, Pharmaceutical industries follows 30 to 75% occupancy of the Rapid Mixer granulator. Under occupancy might lead to turbulent mixing and higher occupancy might lead to poor mixing. Hence optimum occupancy to be finalised by considering bulk density of material, validated capacity range established for the equipment.

In general, Chopper is not preferred during dry mixing, until unless it is specifically required for a product.

Table 12. Process Steps of a formulation

Process Steps	Key Process Parameters	Quality characteristic of drug product
Input materials Screening	Screen size	Physical appearance of blend
Dry mixing	Dry mixing time & Speed	Blend uniformity
Binder preparation	Homogeneity of binder Binder quantity	Physical appearance of binder
Wet granulation	Binder addition time Granulation time	Physical appearance of wet mass
Drying	Drying time Drying temperature	Loss on drying of granules
Sizing	Screen size	Physical appearance of sized granules
Blending	Blend occupancy Blender speed & time	Blend uniformity
Compression	Compression force Speed of compression	Tablet Disintegration time Tablet Dissolution

Table 13. Risk assessment to identify Critical Process Parameters (CPP's)

Critical quality attributes	Dry mixing process parameters	Wet granulation process parameters	Drying process parameters	Sizing process parameters	Blending process parameters	Compression Process parameters
Physical attributes	Low	Low	High	Medium	Low	High
Stability	Low	Low	High	Low	Low	Low
Disintegration time	Low	High	High	High	Low	High
Dissolution	Low	High	High	High	Low	High
Assay	Low	Low	Medium	High	High	Low
Blend uniformity	High	Low	Medium	High	High	N/A
Uniformity of dosage units	N/A	N/A	N/A	N/A	N/A	High
Related substances	Low	Low	High	Low	Low	Low

Lower, Higher speed and time of impeller might lead to under mixing or over mixing of drug substance in the dry mix. Hence, mixing time, mixing speed, requirement of chopper etc., will be optimised during development and the optimum parameters will be defined in manufacturing process accordingly.

Based on optimisation of dry mixing process during drug product development, the critical process parameters like dry mixing time, impeller speed etc., will be finalised to achieve safe and efficient product manufactured consistently through valid manufacturing process. The control strategy will minimise the risk of non homogeneity of blend by achieving CQA – Blend uniformity.

Risk Assessment and Control Strategy for CPP: Wet Granulation Process Parameters

Quantity of Binder, Binder addition time, Impeller and chopper speed during binder addition and kneading, kneading time after binder addition are the key process parameters of wet granulation process (Defne K.T. et al., 2013).

The above mentioned wet granulation process parameters will impact strength of granules, particle size distribution of granules etc., This will affect hardness of tablets, disintegration time and dissolution etc., during compression.

Based on optimisation of wet granulation process during drug product development, the critical process parameters like binder addition time, kneading time, impeller and chopper speed during binder addition and granulation etc., will be finalised to achieve safe and efficient product manufactured consistently through valid manufacturing process. The control strategy will ensure to achieve desired CQA's disintegration time, dissolution etc.,

Risk Assessment and Control Strategy for CPP: Drying Process Parameters

Product temperature, drying time, fluidisation air flow during drying, loss on drying of granules are the key parameters of drying process.

If the drug substance is sensitive to temperature, then drying of granules at higher temperature might lead to increase in degradation product. Drying at lower temperature might lead to improper drying,

Table 14. Control strategy for CPP – Dry mixing Process Parameters

CPP	CQA	Control Strategy
• Dry mixing time • Impeller speed	• Blend uniformity	• Optimised impeller speed for dry mixing • Optimised dry mixing time

Table 15. Control strategy for CPP – Wet granulation Process Parameters

CPP	CQA	Control Strategy
• Binder quantity • Binder addition time • Impeller & chopper speed during binder addition • Kneading time • Impeller & chopper speed during kneading	• Tablet Disintegration time • Tablet dissolution	• Optimised binder quantity • Optimised impeller, chopper speed for binder addition and kneading. • Optimised binder addition time and kneading time

which will affect the quality parameters like tablet appearance (sticking, picking), increase in degradation products etc., during release / stability. Improper air flow during drying will lead to erratic fluidisation of granules, which might lead to non uniform drying or more fines generation, which will affect the appearance of tablet surface etc.,

Based on optimisation of drying process during drug product development, the critical process parameters like product temperature for drying, loss on drying of granules, drying time etc., will be finalised to achieve safe and efficient product manufactured consistently through valid manufacturing process. The control strategy will ensure to achieve the CQA's like related substances, stability, physical appearance etc.,

Risk Assessment and Control Strategy for CPP: Sizing Process Parameters

Sizing screen size, mill type, mill speed, sizing sieve size are the key parameters of sizing process.

If the dried granules were found hard, then it is preferred to use mills with knives like multi mill. If less fines are required, it is preferred to use knives forward and slow speed of mill etc., The screen size for milling to be selected to ensure that, the screened granules passes through sifting sieves. If the granules found to be more coarser, that might lead to rough surface of tablet, lower hardness, faster disintegration time and increased dissolution release rate.

Based on optimisation of sizing process during drug product development, the critical process parameters like milling screen size, mill speed, knife direction etc., will be finalised to achieve safe and efficient product manufactured consistently through valid manufacturing process. The control strategy will ensure to achieve desired CQA's - disintegration time, dissolution, assay, blend uniformity etc.,

Risk Assessment and Control Strategy for CPP: Blending Process Parameters

Blender type, Occupancy of blender, revolutions per minute of blender, blending time are the key parameters of blending process.

By considering blend characteristics and available infrastructure, the blender type will be finalised. Based on validated capacity of blender and batch size requirement of product, the blender occupancy will be finalised. The blending time and speed of blender will be optimised during development. In general, higher the capacity of blender will have low revolutions per minute. Lower the capacity of blender will have higher revolutions per minute. The blending time will be evaluated and optimised accordingly.

Lower or higher blending time and speed than that of optimum blending time and speed will lead to under mixing or over mixing of blend which will lead to non uniform blend. The same can evaluated and optimised through quality characteristic of drug product – Blend uniformity.

Table 16. Control strategy for CPP – Drying Process Parameters

CPP	CQA	Control Strategy
• Product temperature during drying. • Fluidisation airflow during drying. • Loss on drying of granules.	• Physical appearance of tablet • Stability • Related substances	• Optimised product temperature for drying • Optimised fluidisation airflow for drying • Optimised Loss on drying of granules

Table 17. Control strategy for CPP – Sizing Process Parameters

CPP	CQA	Control Strategy
• Sizing screen size • Milling speed • Knives direction during milling	• Physical appearance of tablet • Blend uniformity • Blend assay • Tablet hardness, Disintegration time, Dissolution	• Optimised screen size • Optimised mill speed • Optimised knife direction

Based on optimisation of blending process during drug product development, the critical process parameters like blending time, blender speed etc., will be finalised to achieve safe and efficient product manufactured consistently through valid manufacturing process. The control strategy will ensure to achieve desired CQA's – Blend Assay and Blend Uniformity etc.

Risk Assessment and Control Strategy for CPP: Compression Process Parameters

Compression force, Compression machine speed, force feeder speed are some of the key parameters of compression process.

Higher the compression force will lead to harder tablets which will increase disintegration time and will delay dissolution. Similarly lower compression will yield soft tablets which affects physical attributes of tablets. Force feeder speed to be optimised to synchronise to that of compression machine speed to avoid blend segregation during compression, which in turn will impact drug product CQA – Uniformity of dosage units.

Based on optimisation of compression process during drug product development, the critical process parameters like compression machine force, speed of compression machine and force feeder etc., will be finalised to achieve safe and efficient product manufactured consistently through valid manufacturing process. The control strategy will ensure to achieve desired CQA's – physical attributes, disintegration time, dissolution and uniformity of dosage units etc.,

DESIGN SPACE

Design space is a multidimensional combination and interaction of input variables (material attributes) and process parameters that have been demonstrated to provide assurance of quality. As per ICH Q8, design space is defined as "the established range of process parameters that has been demonstrated to provide assurance of quality". DOE helps to identify unclassified parameters. Efforts, experimentations are to be performed to remove non critical unclassified parameters out of design space. Critical unclassi-

Table 18. Control strategy for CPP – Blending Process Parameters

CPP	CQA	Control Strategy
• Blending time • Revolutions per minute of blender	• Blend uniformity • Blend assay	• Optimised blending time • Optimised blender speed

Table 19. Control strategy for CPP – Blending Process Parameters

CPP	CQA	Control Strategy
• Compression machine speed Vs force feeder speed • Compression force	• Physical attribute • Disintegration time • Dissolution • Uniformity of dosage units	• Optimised compression machine speed and force feeder speed • Optimum compression force.

fied parameters are identified to establish design space (Hlinak A. J., Kuriyan K., Morris K. R., Reklaitis G. W., Basu P. K. 2006; Naseem A.C., et al., 2012).

Methods for determination of design space:

1. Mechanistic approach
2. Non mechanistic – Empirical approach
3. Scale up interpretations
4. Risk analysis to determine significance of effects

CONTINUOUS IMPROVEMENT OF PRODUCT

Continuous improvement of product is implemented by trouble shooting and implementing corrective and preventive actions. Continuous improvement of product is established through input materials like CAPA, deviations, manufacturing experience, customer complains, material variabilities etc., (Lan Zhang, Shirui Mao et. al., 2017)

Validated process and approved facility helps to design and improve product quality.

Figure 4. Design space

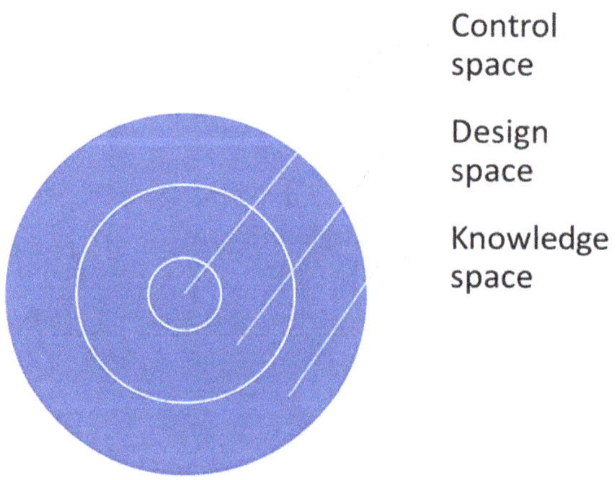

CONCLUSION

Quality by design assures quality of drug product through improved product and process design, risk assessment, monitoring, tracking of product and process, cost saving and more efficient quality of product. Assessment of tools like Quality Target Product Profile (QTPP), Critical Quality Attributes (CQA's), Critical Material Attributes (CMA's), Critical Process Parameters (CPP's), establishing design space etc., helps to develop a quality product. Continuous improvement of product helps to further improve quality of drug product.

REFERENCES

Asma Siddiqua, S. (2013). QBD- A Challenge to the Pharma Industry. International Journal of Innovative Pharmaceutical Sciences and Research, 23, 47-54.

Defne, K. T. (2013). Quality by Design for Wet Granulation in Pharmaceutical processing: Assessing Models for a Priori Design and Scaling. Powder Technology, 240, 7-8.

Delasko, J.M., Cocchetto, D.M., & Burke, L.B. (2005). *Target Product Profile: Beginning Drug Development with the End in Mind*. Academic Press.

European Medicines Agency ICH guideline Q10 on Pharmaceutical quality system, Sep 2015

European Medicines Agency ICH guideline Q8(R2) on Pharmaceutical development, Jun 2017

European Medicines Agency ICH guideline Q9 on Quality risk management, Sep 2015

FDA. (n.d.). *EMA Announce Pilot for Parallel Assessment of Quality by Design Applications*. Retrieved from https://www.qualitydigest.com/inside/fda-compliance-news/fda-ema-announce-pilot-parallel-assessment-quality-design-applications.ht

Food and Drug Administration CDER. (2007). *Draft Guidance for Industry and Review Staff: Target Product Profile- A Strategic Development Tool*. Author.

Glodek, M., Liebowitz, S., & McCarthy, R. (2006). Process robustness: A PQRI white paper. *Pharmaceutical Engineering*, 1-11.

Hlinak, A. J., Kuriyan, K., Morris, K. R., Reklaitis, G. W., & Basu, P. K. (2006). Understanding critical material properties for solid dosage form design. Journal of Pharmaceutical Innovation, 1, 12-17. doi:10.1007/BF02784876

ICH endorsed guide for ICH Q8/Q9/Q10 implementation. Dec 2011.

Implementation of Quality by Design (QbD): status, challenges and next steps. (n.d.). FDA advisory committee for pharmaceutical sciences. Retrieved from http://slideplayer.com/slide/4127998/

Khatri, Saini, Gangawat, & Gurubalaji. (2014). Pharmaceutical QbD: Concepts for Drug Product Development. *Int. J. Pharm. Sci., 13*, 84-91.

Kumar & Gupta. (2015). A review of quality by design approach (QbD) for Pharmaceuticals. International of Drug Development and Research, 7(1), 52-60.

Lawrence, X. Y. (2008). Pharmaceutical Quality by Design: Product and Process Development, Understanding, and Control. Pharmaceutical Research, 25(4).

Lawrence, X. Yu., Amidon, G., Khan, M. A., Hoag, S. W., Polli, J., Raju, G. K., & Woodcock, J. (2014). Understanding Pharmaceutical Quality by Design. The AAPS Journal, 16(4).

Leuenberger, H., Puchkov, M., Krausbauer, E., & Betz, G. (2009). Manufacturing pharmaceutical granules, Is the granulation end-point a myth. Powder Technology, 189, 141–148.

Lionberger, Lee, Lee, Raw, & Yu. (2008). Quality by design: concepts for ANDAs. The AAPS Journal, 10, 268-276.

Moreton. (2009). Functionality and Performance of Excipients in Quality-by-Design World Part V: Changes in the Sourcing and Supply of Pharmaceutical Excipients. *American Pharmaceutical Review.* Retrieved from https://www.americanpharmaceuticalreview.com/Featured-Articles/118926-Functionality-and-Performance-of-Excipients-in-Quality-by-Design-World-Part-V-Changes-in-the-Sourcing-and-Supply-of-Pharmaceutical-Excipients/

Narke, R. M., & Singh, R. P. (2014). Qverview of QbD: A challenge to the Pharmaceuticval industry. Asian Journal of Pharmaceutical Research and Development, 2, 42-53.

Naseem, A. C. (2012). A Case Study of Dispersible Tablets. *Quality by Design Approach for Formulation Development*, *423*, 167–178.

Nosal, R. (2006). Industry perspective of risk-based CMC assessment under QbD. *AAPS Annual Meeting*.

PAT - A Framework for Innovative Pharmaceutical Development, Manufacturing, and Quality Assurance. (2004). U.S. Department of Health and Human Services Food and Drug Administration Guidance.

Rockville, M. D. (2011). Good manufacturing practice for bulk pharmaceutical excipients. *USP*, *2011*, 1415–1420.

Rockville, M. D. (2011). USP and NF Excipients, Listed by Category. *USP*, *2011*, 583–595.

Shah. (2009). Quality by Design in Pharmaceutical Manufacturing. American Association of Pharmaceutical Scientist.

Siddiqua, Kumar, & Kumar. (2013). QBD – A challenge to the Pharma industry. *International Journal of Innovative Pharmaceutical Sciences and Research, 1*, 1-21.

U. S. Food and Drug Administration. Guidance for industry. (2014). *CMC post approval manufacturing changes to be documented in annual reports*. Author.

U. S. Food and Drug Administration. (2012). *Quality by design for ANDs: an example for immediate-release dosage forms*. Author.

U. S. Food and Drug Administration. (2011). *Quality by design for ANDs: an example for modified-release dosage forms*. Author.

U. S. Food and Drug Administration. (1997). *Guidance for industry: modified release solid oral dosage forms scale-up and post approval changes: chemistry, manufacturing, and controls, in vitro dissolution testing, and in vivo bioequivalence documentation*. Author.

U. S. Food and Drug Administration. (1995). *Guidance for industry: immediate release solid oral dosage forms scale-up and post approval changes: chemistry, manufacturing, and controls, in vitro dissolution testing, and in vivo bioequivalence documentation*. Author.

U.S. Food and Drug Administration CDER. (2004). *Guidance for industry: PAT—a framework for innovative pharmaceutical development, manufacturing, and quality assurance*. Author.

Van Arnum. (2007). A FDA Perspective on Quality by Design. Advancing Development & Manufacturing Pharmaceutical Technology, 3(12).

Woodcock, J. (2004). The concept of pharmaceutical quality. *American Pharmaceutical Review*, 1–3.

Wu, Tawakkul, White, & Khan. (2009). Quality-by-design (QbD): and integrated multivariate approach for the component quantification of powder blends. *International Journal of Pharmaceutics, 372*(1-2).

Wu, H., & Khan, M. A. (2009). Quality-by-design (QbD): An integrated approach for evaluation of powder blending process kinetics and determination of powder blending end-point. *Journal of Pharmaceutical Sciences*, *98*(8), 2784–2798. doi:10.1002/jps.21646 PMID:19116952

Yu, L. X. (2008). Pharmaceutical quality by design: product and process development, understanding, and control. Pharmaceutical Research, 25, 781-791.

Zhang, L., & Mao, S. (2017). Application of quality by design in the current drug development. Asian Journal of Pharmaceutical Sciences, 12, 1-8.

Chapter 11
The Next Generation Sequencing Techniques and Application in Drug Discovery and Development

Afzal Hussain
Maulana Azad National Institute of Technology, India

ABSTRACT

Next-generation sequencing or massively parallel sequencing describe DNA sequencing, RNA sequencing, or methylation sequencing, which shows its great impact on the life sciences. The recent advances of these parallel sequencing for the generation of huge amounts of data in a very short period of time as well as reducing the computing cost for the same. It plays a major role in the gene expression profiling, chromosome counting, finding out the epigenetic changes, and enabling the future of personalized medicine. Here the authors describe the NGS technologies and its application as well as applying different tools such as TopHat, Bowtie, Cufflinks, Cuffmerge, Cuffdiff for analyzing the high throughput RNA sequencing (RNA-Seq) data.

INTRODUCTION

The human genome contains too much complexity and diversity and shows its effects on health and diseases. The journey started with the discovery of the structure of DNA. A large number of innovations in reagents and the development in the instrumentation supported the Human Genome Project initiative (Mardis, 2013; Watson & Crick, 1953). The Human genome project completion shown a need for more advanced technologies for giving the answer of complex biological questions because of the high cost and limited throughput barriers. First high-throughput sequencing platform released in the mid-2000s and dropped the cost of human genome sequencing since the human genome project and lead to the next generation sequencing. Over the past decade, next generation sequencing continued to evolve. It showed advances in the read length and reducing the cost of sequencing. The next generation sequencing

DOI: 10.4018/978-1-5225-7326-5.ch011

technologies are more advanced than the previous technologies such as DNA microarray, NanoString, qPCR and Optical mapping. The DNA microarrays are used to identify common polymorphisms related to diseases, including cancer, cardiovascular disease and genome-wide association study (DeRisi *et al.*, 1996; Jia *et al.*, 2010; Keating *et al.*, 2008; Rhodes *et al.*, 2004; Welter *et al.*, 2013).

Different Types of NGS Technologies

There are different Next generation sequencing are available, some of the main sequencing technologies were explained below such as

1. Illumina sequencing
2. Roche 454 sequencing
3. Ion PGM from Ion Torrent sequencing

Illumina Sequecning

Solexa released the Genome analyzer in 2006 and later in 2007, it was purchased by Illumina. It adopts the technology of, sequencing by synthesis (Mardis, 2008).

It has a few steps for the sequencing

- The input samples cleaved into short sections. The length of the sections depends on the sequencing machinery used.
- In Illumina sequencing 100 to 150bp reads are used for the sequencing. Fragments are ligated with generic adaptors and annealed to a slide using the adaptors.
- The PCR is used to amplify each read and creating a spot with so many copies of the same read and then separated into single strands to be sequenced.
- The Sequencing slide is filled with nucleotides and DNA polymerase. These all the nucleotides are fluorescently labelled and also have a terminator for adding one base at a time.
- An image is taken of the slide, At each read site, there will be a fluorescent signal which indicates the base that has been added.
- The slide goes for the next cycle, the process is repeated, at a time only one nucleotide added and imaging in between.
- Computers detect the base at each site in each image and construct a sequence.
- The overall Illumina sequencing technique was shown in Figure 1.

Roche 454 Sequencing

Roche 454 was the first successful next generation system which was commercially used. It uses a pyrosequencing technology (Goodwin *et al.*, 2016; Liu *et al.*, 2012b; Margulies *et al.*, 2005).

Few steps of the sequencing

- DNA or RNA is fragmented up to 1kb.
- The library DNAs with generic adaptors are added to the ends and annealed to beads.

Figure 1. Illumina sequencing technology

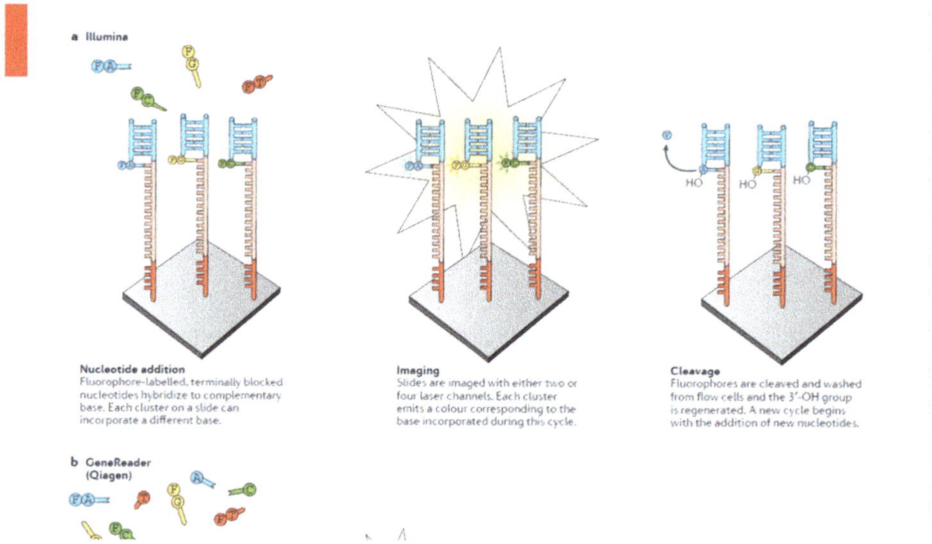

- The fragments were amplified by emulsion PCR using adaptor specific primers.
- The single well of the slide contains each bead, covered in many PCR copies of a single sequence. The well is also being full of DNA polymers as well as sequencing buffers.
- The slide is filled with one of the NTP species among four species. If the single base repeats, after that more will be added.
- Every time addition of each nucleotide generates visible light.
- Each cycle the different number of bases will be added and the sequencing determined computationally.
- The overall Roche 454 sequencing technique was shown in Figure 2.

Ion PGM From Ion Torrent Sequencing

Ion Torrent released Ion PGM at the end of 2010. It uses semiconductor sequencing technology (Flusberg *et al.*, 2010).

Few steps of the sequencing

- The input DNA or RNA is fragmented.
- Adaptors are added, molecules are amplified on the bead by emulsion PCR.
- Addition of a DNTP to DNA polymer releases an H+ ion.
- The changes in PH are detected, PH change is used to determine the number of bases were added with each cycle.
- The overall Ion Torrent sequencing technique was shown in Figure 3.

Figure 2. Roche 454 sequencing technology

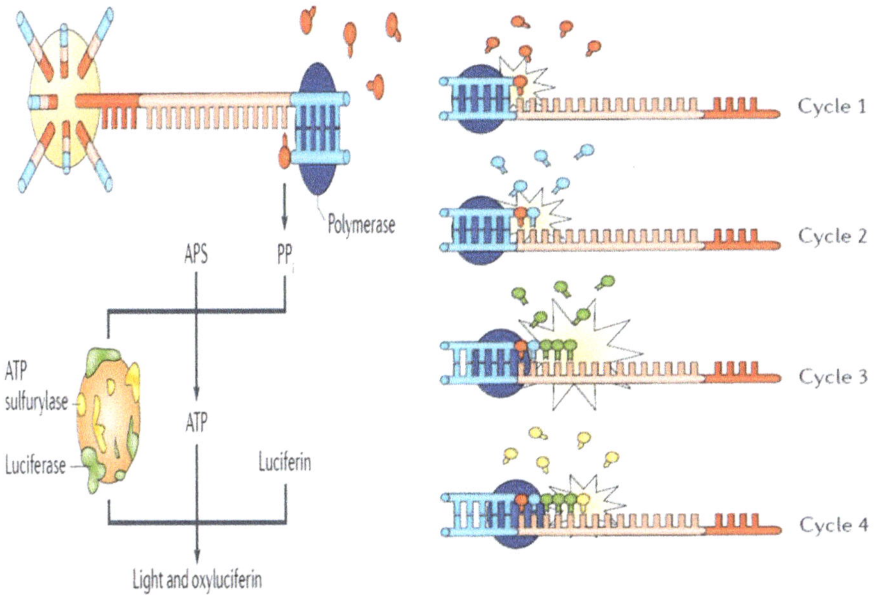

Figure 3. Ion Torrent sequencing technology

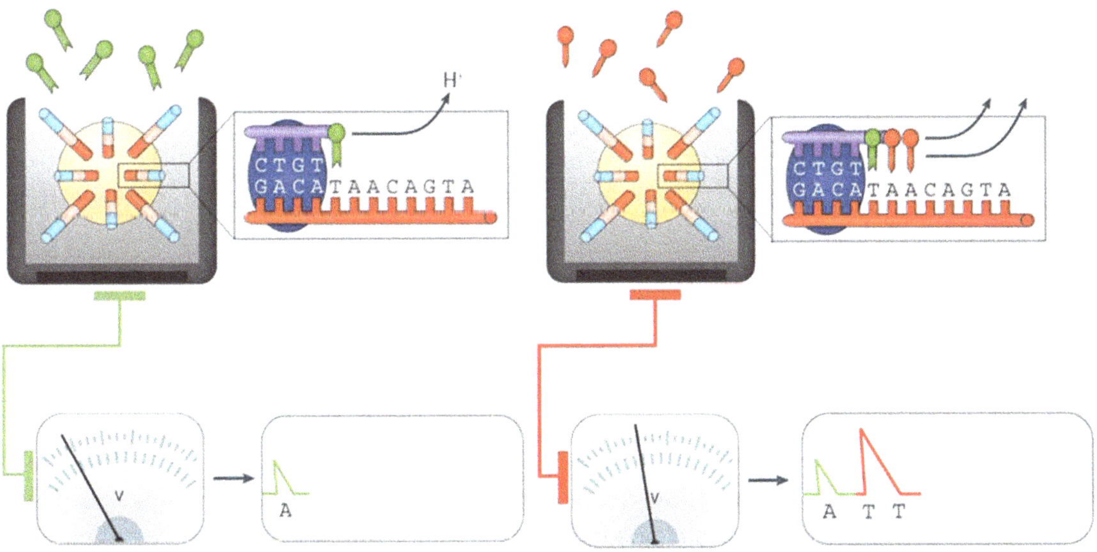

NEXT GENERATION SEQUENCING DATA ANALYSIS (TOOLS AND TECHNIQUES)

RNA-Seq has become the most accepted technique of the next generation sequencing, used for gene expression analysis, which can estimate the nature and the quantity of expressing mRNAs by sequencing a complete transcriptome. RNA-Seq detect as well as quantify the expression profile for a large number of genes in specific pathological and physiological condition for understanding the biological process and its regulation (Conesa *et al.*, 2016; Kukurba & Montgomery, 2015; Lea *et al.*, 2011).

Several pipelines and tools were investigated for RNA-Seq data analysis.

1. NGSQC toolkit
2. Bowtie
3. TopHat
4. Cufflinks
5. Cuffmerge
6. Cuffdiff
7. R language

NGSQC Toolkit

Next generation sequencing generates a large amount of data so there is need an efficient and fast processing tool for quality control for meaningful downstream analysis of sequencing data. NGSQC toolkit is a standalone and open source application for quality check and filtering of high quality data. It is freely available and very user friendly application. A variety of additional tools has been incorporated in this toolkit such as QC (sequence format converter and trimming tools) and analysis (statistical tools) for Roche 454 and Illumina platforms generated data. This tool allows to filter out Low quality data and increase the overall quality of the dataset (Patel & Jain, 2012).

NGSQC Toolkit Applications

- Quality control: IllQC (Illumina data), 454QC (Roche 454 data).
- Trimming: Trimming Reads, HomoPloymer Trimming.
- Format Conversion: Fatsq to 454, Fastq to Fasta, SangerFastq to Illu Fastq, Solexa Fastq to IlluFastq.
- Statistics: Average Quality, N50Stat.

Bowtie

After checking the quality of the NGS submitted data, there is another step to detect the novel splicing events. So a spliced aligner is needed to map reads to the genome, across the introns. Bowtie package enables memory efficient and an ultrafast alignment of large sets of sequencing reads to a reference sequence. The Bowtie packages contain tools for building reference genome indexes for aligning short reads using an index. It uses FM index to align reads at a rate of tens of millions per CPU hour (Langmead, 2010).

TopHat

TopHat is a fast splice junction mapper for RNA-Seq reads. It aligns RNA-Seq reads to reference genome using the Ultra high-throughput short read aligner Bowtie and analyzes the mapping results to identify splice junctions between exons (Trapnell *et al.*, 2009).

Cufflinks

Cufflinks assembles individual transcripts from RNA-Seq reads that have been aligned to the reference genome. After this assembly phase, Cufflinks quantifies the expression level of each tranfrag in the sample which filtered out the background or artificial tranfrags (Ghosh & Chan, 2016).

Cuffmerge

Cuffmerge is a meta-assembler. It treats the assembled transfrags the way cufflinks treats reads, merging them together parsimoniously. It can integrate the reference transcript into the merged assembly and produce a single annotation file for use in downstream differential analysis (Trapnell *et al.*, 2012).

Cuffdiff

Cuffdiff calculates an expression in two or more samples and tests the statistical significance of each observed change in expression between them (Trapnell *et al.*, 2012).

R Language

R is a language for statistical computing and graphs. It provides a wide number of statistics such as linear and nonlinear modelling, time-series analysis, classical statistical tests, classification, clustering and graphical techniques. It is a free software ("R Language,").

RNA-SEQ ANALYSIS WORKFLOW

The next generation sequencing (RNA-Seq) data is very huge and for analyzing the sequencing data, different algorithms and computational tools were developed for read mapping, transcript reconstruction and expression quantification (Garber *et al.*, 2011; Mortazavi *et al.*, 2008). The RNA-Seq data analysis pipeline was shown in Figure 4. The different software and tools were used for analyzing the gene expression data. TopHat is a software tool which uses the Bowtie tool for aligning the reads to the reference genome for finding out the transcript splice sites. The Tophat and the Bowtie is freely available tools (Trapnell *et al.*, 2009). After using the TopHat and bowtie the further analysis has been done using Cufflinks software suit. In which the mapped reads counting was performed using cufflinks, cuffmerge was used to merge the separate assembled transcript into cohesive set and in the last step, the Cuffdiff was used to find out the differential expressed transcript. R language and CuumeRbund are statistical analysis tools utilized for the heat map generation of the differential expression data (Trapnell *et al.*, 2012; Trapnell *et al.*, 2010).

Therefore Next generation sequencing is very vital techniques for differential gene expression analysis. In this chapter, we describe that these techniques are very crucial for finding out the Up-regulated, Down-regulated genes of the kidney tumor and the gene enrichment analysis was also being done for the same. The RNA-Seq data analysis workflow was illustrated in Figure 4.

Figure 4. RNA-Seq data analysis workflow

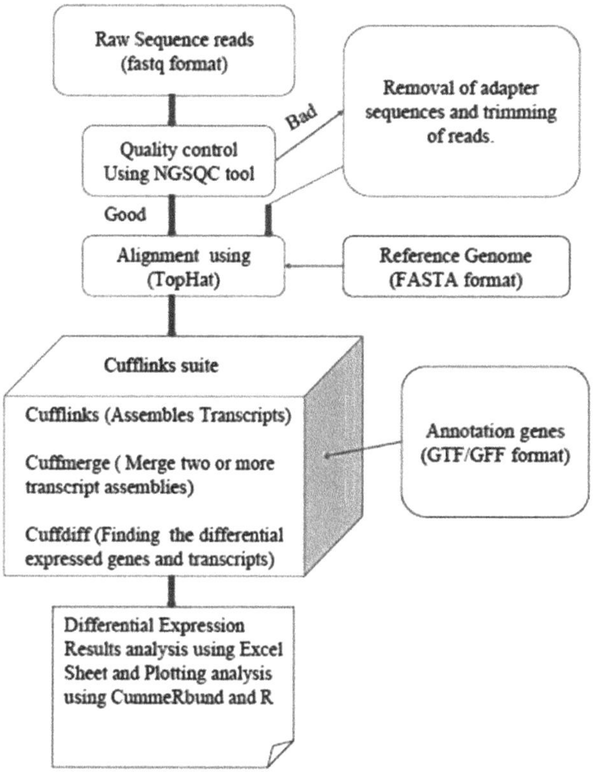

BACKGROUND AND MAIN FOCUS

We planned a step by step pipeline for searching out the up-regulated and down-regulated gene for further analysis and the further analysis goes for gene enrichment.

RNA-Seq Data Retrieval

The RNA-Seq raw data were retrieved from the SRA (Sequence Read Archive) which is under the NCBI (National Center for Biotechnology Information) http://www.ncbi.nlm.nih.gov/sra.

We have retrieved four sample runs

Normal 1 SRR2064424
Normal 2 SRR2064425
Tumor 1 SRR2064426
Tumor 2 SRR2064427

The Fastq file of the samples were downloaded using the accession number which were entered in the ebi site http://www.ebi.ac.uk/ena/data/view/ and clicked on the Fastq file. After clicking it download the Fastq file from the FTP site.

Normal 1 SRX1059892
Normal 2 SRX1059893
Normal 3 SRX1059894
Normal 4 SRX1059895

Normal 1 Sample

ftp://ftp.sra.ebi.ac.uk/vol1/fastq/SRR206/004/SRR2064424/SRR2064424.fastq.gz

Normal 2 Sample

ftp://ftp.sra.ebi.ac.uk/vol1/fastq/SRR206/005/SRR2064425/SRR2064425.fastq.gz

Tumor 1 Sample

ftp://ftp.sra.ebi.ac.uk/vol1/fastq/SRR206/006/SRR2064426/SRR2064426.fastq.gz

Tumor 2 Sample

ftp://ftp.sra.ebi.ac.uk/vol1/fastq/SRR206/007/SRR2064427/SRR2064427.fastq.gz

Raw Sample Quality Analysis/ Adapter Trimming/ Quality Trimming

The generated huge amount of data using the next generation technology contain numerous sequence artifact, contain read error, primer and poor quality reads as well as adapter contaminations. Therefore, checking the quality of the raw data, adapter trimming and the quality trimming is needed for extracting the meaningful information. For this purpose NGSQC toolkit was used which is an open source and standalone application available at http://www.nipgr.res.in/ngsqctoolkit.html. It contains different tools such as QC tools, trimming tools, format converter tools and the statistical tools for performing next generation sequencing data analysis.

NGSQC toolkit was used for quality checking and filtering the raw sequencing data which has been generated using Illumina technology (Patel & Jain, 2012).

Retrieval of the Reference Genome, Preparing Genome File and Mapping the Reads

The reference genome was downloaded form UCSC genome browser like first of all open the UCSC genome browser, then go to the download link, then genome data, human, The full data set and then click on the link

The link presented here for the human genome

(hg38.fa.gz)

(http://hgdownload.soe.ucsc.edu/goldenPath/hg38/bigZips/)

Like that .GTF file was also downloaded using the UCSC site.

The read mapping was done using Bowtie and TopHat, Tophat was used for aligning the processed sequence reads to the reference human genome, with this purpose it uses Bowtie for the indexing (Langmead & Salzberg, 2012; Li *et al.*, 2009; Trapnell *et al.*, 2009).

Bowtie perform the indexing and prepare the genome.fa file for the TopHat program for performing the alignment process.

Source of the Bowtie Program: http://bowtie-bio.sourceforge.net/index.shtml
Source of the TopHat Program: http://ccb.jhu.edu/software/tophat/index.shtml

Cufflinks/Cuffmerge/Cuffdiff Read Counting

The cufflink program was used for counting of the mapped reads and Cuffmerge program was used for merging the separate assembled transcript into a organized set and finally the differentially expressed transcript were identified using Cuffdiff program (Trapnell *et al.*, 2012).

The Source of the Cufflink Program: http://cole-trapnell-lab.github.io/cufflinks/

Heat Map Generating Using the R Language and CummeRbund

The R language was used to generate the Heat map of the differentially expressed genes.

EXPERIMENTAL RESULT AND DISCUSSION

Quality Analysis of the Raw Data and Filtering

The kidney tumor raw data samples Normal 1, Normal 2, Tumor 1 and Tumor 2 were retrieved from NCBI SRA search and further downloaded form ebi site http://www.ebi.ac.uk/ena/data/view/

The NGSQC toolkit was used for checking the quality of the raw data, adapter trimming as well as quality trimming. The Perl script was used for running the NGSQC program through command prompt. The final quality checked and trimmed data with statistical analysis was found. The overall quality of the samples were presented in Figure 5.

The statistics for quality check and filtered data were generated in the text files and graphs. It represents the quality score at each base position as well as average quality distribution, base composition, GC content, input and filtered reads and showed the quality control analysis summary in the form of a pie chart. The overall analysis result was illustrated in Figure 5.

Normal vs. Tumor Sample: Differential Gene Expression Analysis

After performing all the quality checking and trimming, filtering, merging using Bowtie, Tophat, cufflink, cuffmerge and cuffdiff.

The final Cuffdiff result file was opened into the excel sheet and the p-value has been kept <0.05 for finding out the significant genes and fold change is kept > 0.8 for upregulated genes and < -0.8 for down regulated genes.

Figure 5. Quality analysis of the raw sequencing data of RNA-Seq using the NGSQC toolkit. Showing the average quality score at each base position, base position, average quality distribution and the summary of quality control analysis of the sample (a) Normal 1, (b) Normal 2, (c) Tumor 1, (d) Tumor 2

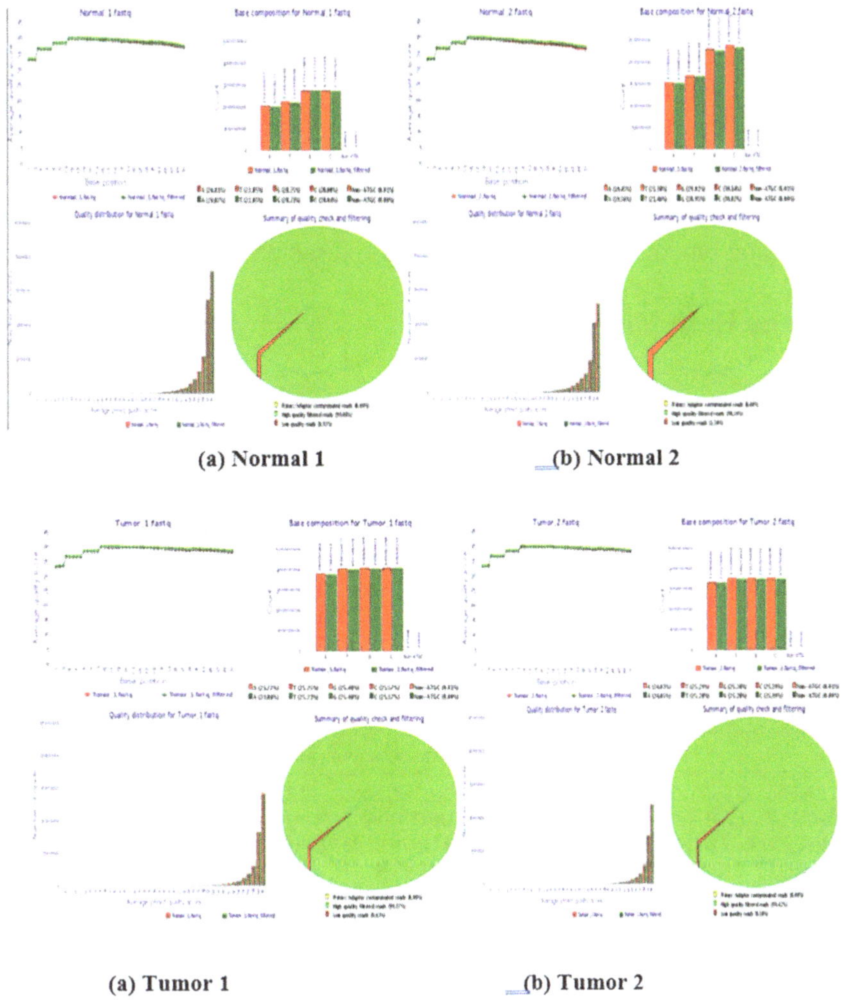

Gene Ontology and Gene Enrichment Analysis

Gene set enrichment analysis is a method to identify the classes of protein and genes that are over-represented in a huge set of genes or proteins and also may have the relation with disease phenotypes. After getting the result the cutoff was decided and further analysis was performed using DAVID (The database for annotation, visualization and integrated discovery) database and other source database. We have found the total number of genes are 26, 840 then further filtering was done and got 1,692 unique genes. The up-regulated genes were 742 and the down regulated genes were 764 has been recognized with full annotations. The gene enrichment analysis better describes the gene's association with biological process, cellular components and the molecular function. Talking about the Tumor 1 vs. Normal up-regulated genes, the enrichment analysis shows that the lots of genes involve in regulation of transcription, the cellular components are intrinsic to membrane and the molecular functions of the huge number of genes are ATP binding as well as Tumor 1 vs. Normal down-regulated genes, the enrichment analysis shows that a lot of genes involve in the regulation of transcription, The cellular components are intracellular non-membrane bounded organelle and the molecular function is related to ion-binding. The similar enrichment analysis was also being done for the Tumor 2 vs. Normal up-regulated genes, the enrichment analysis shows a huge number of genes involved in regulation of transcription, the cellular components are intrinsic to membrane and the molecular function is ion binding likewise the Tumor 2 vs. Normal down-regulated gene enrichment suggest that the huge number of genes involved in regulation of transcription, the cellular component is an intracellular non-membrane-bounded organelle and the molecular functions are ion-binding. The overall Results are presented in Table 1 and Figures 6, 7, 8 and 9.

Cluster Analysis by Heat Map

The differential expressed genes cluster was plotted by using R statistical language. The R code was run on the fold change value, the differential expressed genes plot of Tumor 1 vs. Normal and Tumor 2 vs. Normal is almost showing the similar expression patterns. The highly expressed genes were shown in red color, Average expressed genes were shown in yellow color and the green color presented the lower expressed genes respectively. The Heat map has been presented in Figure 10.

Table 1. Few genes are presented which involve in the regulation of the Transcription Process in the up-regulated and Down-regulated

S. No.	Samples	Some of the gene names among all	Biological Process
1.	Tumor 1 Vs Normal up-regulated	ZNF664, VPS25, PTHLH, MCM3, RHOA, ZNF395, XRN2, ENO1, NR3C1, TGFB1, LBH, RAN, CALR, PRKAR1A, CSDE1, BACH1, UBC, EPAS1, SORBS3, NOTCH3, DNAJB6, PPP2R1A, YWHAB, SAP18, CIAO1, MEF2A, RUVBL1, LITAF, RPS3, CHMP1A, HMOX1, CREM, PUF60, ZHX2, CARHSP1, CTNNB1, TCEAL8, TP53, UBA52, CREG1, AEBP1	Regulation of the Transcription
2.	Tumor 1 Vs Normal Down-regulated	MLXIPL, DDIT3, SUPT5H, SUPT6H, NFX1, SRCAP, THRAP3, KDM6B, ERC1, KDM4C, HNF1B, KAT5, MTA1, ZNF274, HOXC6, ZGPAT, HOXB3, SF1, EWSR1, PNN, DNM2, AFF4, EP300, TSC22D2, CCAR1, TSPYL2, STAT6, ZNF133, FUBP1, TAF1, SPEN, ARHGEF10L, MZF1, CALCOCO1, SMAD3, FUBP3, SREBF2, PHF1, NFKBIZ	Regulation of the Transcription
3.	Tumor 2 Vs Normal up-regulated	PFDN5, HSBP1, MCM3, NOTCH3, CHMP1A, HNRNPAB, MAGED1, RPS3, CRK, ZNF395, CREG1, YWHAB, DNAJB6, TGIF2, CREM, XRN2, UBA52, HMOX1, BACH1, EPAS1, MED13L, S1PR1, TP53, UBB, CNOT1, MEF2A, PUF60, CARHSP1, PTHLH, VPS25, NDUFA13, YWHAH, EID1, TGFB1, LITAF, UBC, ENO1, ZNF664, CALR, DPF2, APP,LBH, VEGFA, SORBS3, XRCC6, RPL6, NR3C1, PRKAR1A, INSR, AEBP1, PKIG, ZHX2, CIAO1, CTNNB1, CREB3L2, ATP6AP1, RAN, RHOA, PPP2R1A, SAP18, NCOA4, NFE2L1, RUVBL1, MAF1, TCEAL8, CSDE1	Regulation of the Transcription
4.	Tumor 2 Vs Normal Down-regulated	SMARCA2, RSC1A1, BCL6, SF1, MOV10, SMARCA4, HDAC7, EHMT1, POLR2A, SRCAP, PNN, ELF3, CHD3, MZF1, KDM2B, AFF4, CXXC1, MTA1, GABPB2, NCOA1, ATN1, ARHGEF10L, EWSR1, SOX13, ZNF462, MED15, CHD2, HSF1, HIF1A, NRF1, ZBTB16, ZBTB37, DNM2, HOXC5, TAF1, MAFK, NRG1, PER3, PER1, KDM6B, AFF1, TCF25, SPEN, BRD8, ZGPAT, MBD1, PHF1, TSC22D2, MLLT6, NCOR1, SUPT6H, THRAP3, SALL1, RING1, DDIT3, EGR1, SMAD3, CCNL1, EYA3, DMTF1, RCOR3, KAT5, SLTM, LRCH4, SMARCC2, HNF4A, SAFB2, CRY2, PTOV1, FOS, EP300, SETDB1, ZNF274, NR2C1, CNOT3, SREBF2, CSRNP1, CALCOCO1, TRIB1, BDP1, CCNL2, BTAF1, SUPT5H, CCAR1, FUBP3, ATF3, TGIF1, NFKBIZ, SIN3B, ZNF224, NFKB2	Regulation of the Transcription

Figure 6. Tumor 1 vs. Normal Up-regulated genes-enrichment analysis has been shown using Pie chart

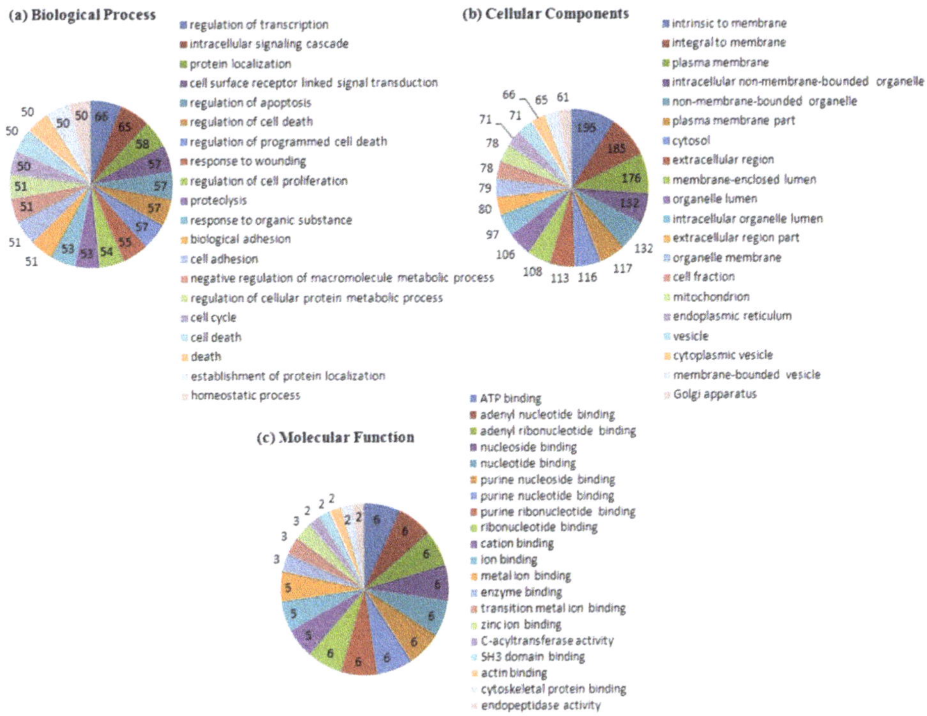

Figure 7. Tumor 1 vs. Normal down-regulated genes-enrichment analysis has been shown using Pie chart

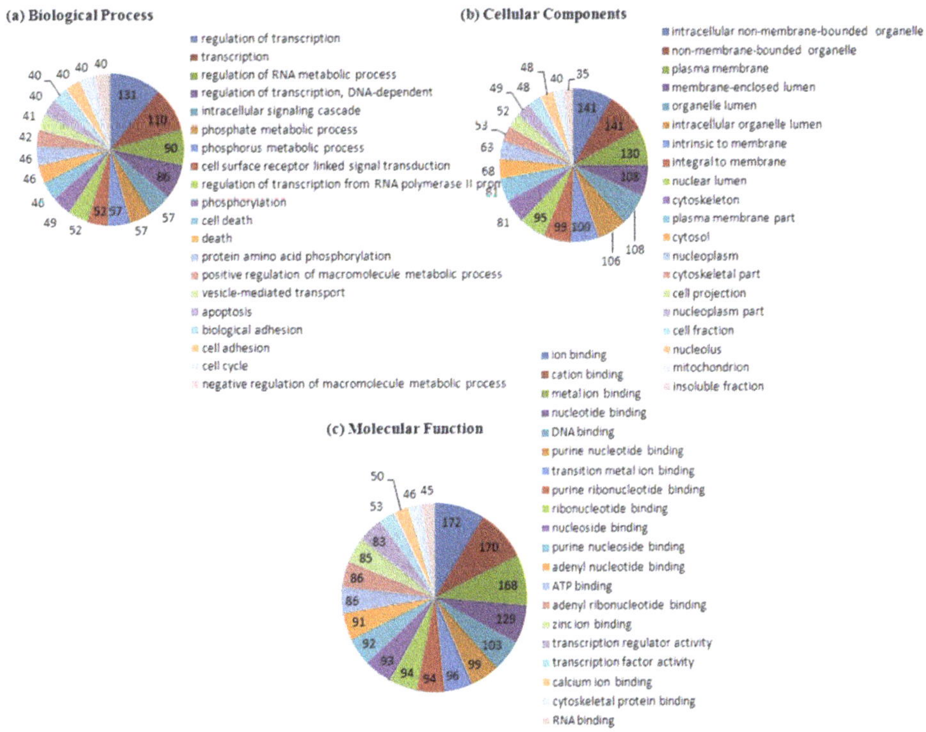

Figure 8. Tumor 2 vs. Normal Up-regulated genes-enrichment analysis has been shown using Pie chart

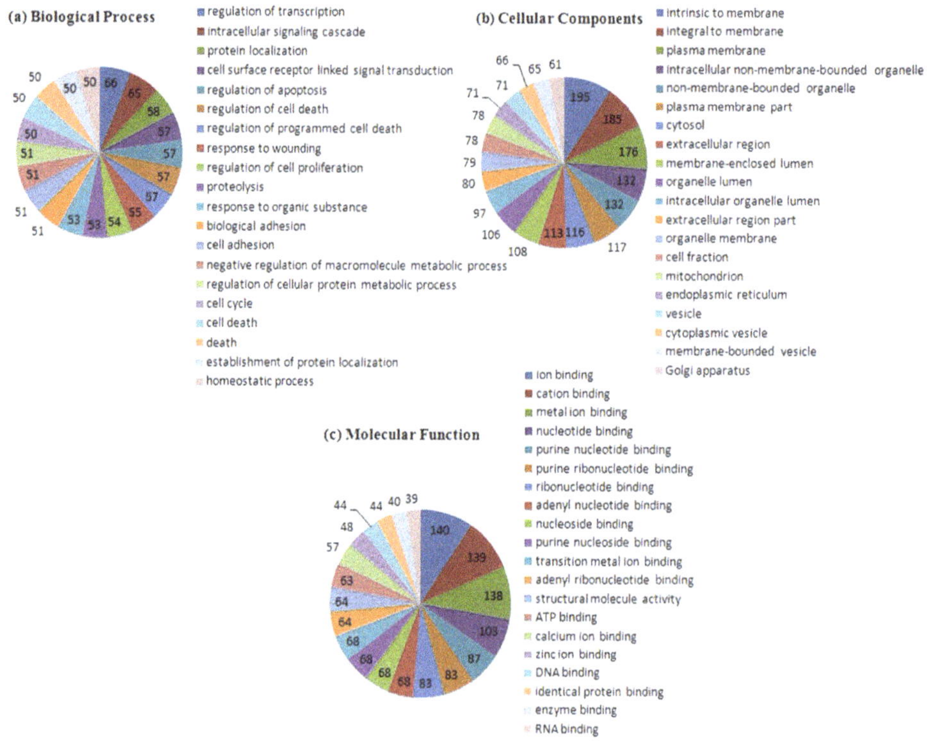

Figure 9. Tumor 2 vs. Normal down-regulated genes-enrichment analysis has been shown using Pie chart

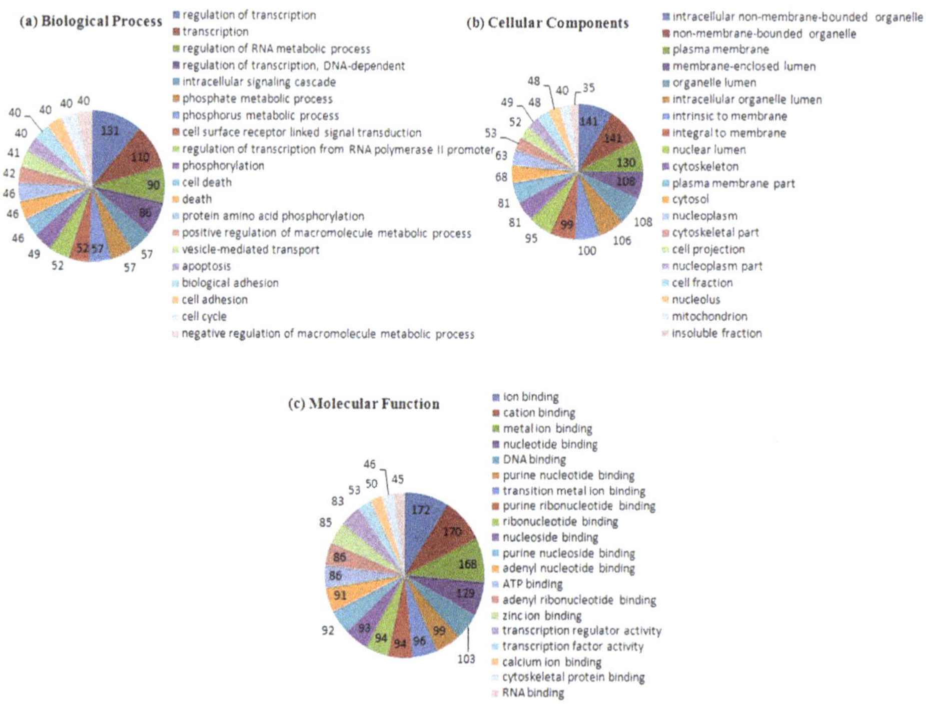

Figure 10. Differential expressed genes identified by using Heat Map, generated by using R

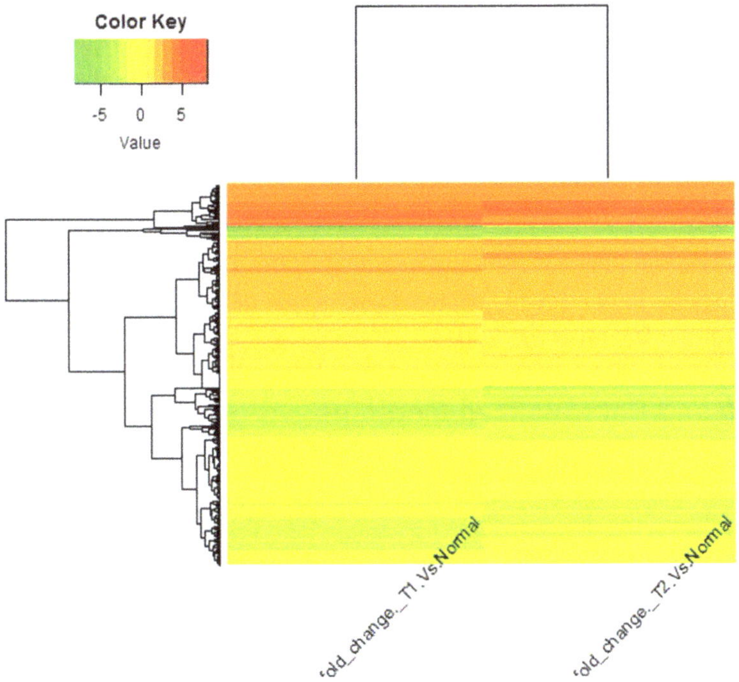

APPLICATION OF SEQUENCING TECHNOLOGIES

Next generation sequencing technologies shows reduction in costs and increased accuracy as well. Because of the less time sequencing more and more organism being sequenced and due to showing the progress in the genomics studies such as exomics, metagenomics, epigenomics as well as transcriptomics. It is also very crucial as therapeutic aspects for cancer and other complex diseases (Liu *et al.*, 2012a).

Gene Expression Analysis

Earlier the Microarray technologies were used for the gene expression analysis but because of some drawback such as detection of low expressed genes was limited by background noise. Nowadays The Next generation sequencing is widely used in gene expression profiling. It has also been used to study miRNA expression, Transcriptome analysis, Ribosome profiling etc. (Andersson *et al.*, 2014; Berezikov *et al.*, 2006; Klerk *et al.*, 2012; Ingolia *et al.*, 2009; Lappalainen *et al.*, 2013; Nolte-'t Hoen *et al.*, 2012; Valen *et al.*, 2009).

ChIP-Sequencing

ChIP-sequencing is also known as CHIP-seq, it is the another application of NGS technology. This method is used to analyze the protein binding sites in genomic DNA specially for transcription factor binding sites based on Chromatin Immunoprecipitation (Blat & Kleckner, 1999).

De Novo Genome Sequencing

De novo sequencing is the main application of NGS technology. In this sequencing the complete characterization of the entire genome of a particular organism were performed such as yeast, Drosophila, mouse, Arabidopsis etc. (Lie *et al.*, 2010., Reich *et al.*, 2010; Rohland *et al.*, 2010).

Metagenomics

Next generation sequencing play a significant role in Metagenomics. Metagenomics is the analysis of DNA from microbial communities in environmental samples, does not need prior culturing of the organism (Ercolini *et al.*, 2012; Venter *et al.*, 2004).

Human Disease and Personalized Medicine

Next generation sequencing is very crucial for investigating the genetic variations in human and their roles in health and causing the disease. Therefore the personalized medicine provides the possibility to treat diseases which is based on the genetic makeup of the patient (Rabbani *et al.*, 2016).

ALL THE COMMAND USED IN THIS CHAPTER FOR NGS (RNA-SEQ) DATA ANALYSIS

Command for Quality Analysis

```
        system("perl NGSQCToolkit_v2.3.3/QC/IlluQC.pl -se Normal_1.fastq N A
-o Normal_1
        -t 2 -l 70 -s 20");
        system("perl NGSQCToolkit_v2.3.3/QC/IlluQC.pl -se Normal_2.fastq N A
-o Normal_2
        -t 2 -l 70 -s 20");
        system("perl NGSQCToolkit_v2.3.3/QC/IlluQC.pl -se Tumor_1.fastq N A -o
Tumor_1 -t
        2 -l 70 -s 20");
        system("perl NGSQCToolkit_v2.3.3/QC/IlluQC.pl -se Tumor_2.fastq N A -o
Tumor_2 -t
        2 -l 70 -s 20");
```

Command: Bowtie

```
system("bowtie2-build genome.fa genome");
```

Command: TopHat

```
system("tophat2 -p 4 -o Tophat_Normal_1 -G genome.gtf genome Normal_1.fastq_
filtered");
system("tophat2 -p 4 -o Tophat_Normal_2 -G genome.gtf genome Normal_2.fastq_
filtered");
system("tophat2 -p 4 -o Tophat_Tumor_1 -G genome.gtf genome Tumor_1.fastq_fil-
tered");
system("tophat2 -p 4 -o Tophat_Tumor_2 -G genome.gtf genome Tumor_2.fastq_fil-
tered");
```

Command: Cufflinks

```
$ cufflinks -o  cufflinks_Normal_1 -G genome.gtf /Tophat_Normal_1/accepted_
hits.bam
$ cufflinks -o  cufflinks_Normal_2 -G genome.gtf /Tophat_Normal_2/accepted_
hits.bam
$ cufflinks -o  cufflinks_Tumor_1 -G genome.gtf /Tophat_Tumor_1/accepted_hits.
bam
$ cufflinks -o  cufflinks_Tumor_2 -G genome.gtf /Tophat_Tumor_2/accepted_hits.
bam
```

Command: Cuffmerge

```
$ cuffmerge -o cuffmerge_result -g genome.gtf -s genome.fa assembly.txt
        assembly.txt file
        (
         cufflinks_Normal_1/Transcripts.gtf
        cufflinks_Normal_2/Transcripts.gtf
         cufflinks_Tumor_1/Transcripts.gtf
         cufflinks_Tumor_2/Transcripts.gtf
        )
```

Command: Cuffdiff

```
$cuffdiff -o -cuffdiff_Normal_vs_Tumor_1 -u /cuffmerge_result /merged.gtf  /
Tophat_Normal_1/accepted_hits.bam, /Tophat_Normal_2/accepted_hits.bam Tophat_
Tumor_1/accepted_hits.bam
$cuffdiff -o -cuffdiff_Normal_vs_Tumor_2 -u /cuffmerge_result /merged.gtf /
Tophat_Normal_1/accepted_hits.bam, /Tophat_Normal_2/accepted_hits.bam
/Tophat_Tumor_2/accepted_hits.bam
```

Command: Heat Map Generation

```
Library("gdata")
library("gplots")
setwd("C:/rna_seq/Heatmap")
Normdata<-read.xls("DEG_significant.xlsx",sheet=1)
drawimage = function(Normdata,file,colplot,colpval,cexcol,pval)
{
   ind=which(Normdata[,colpval] <pval)
 Normdata=as.matrix(Normdata[ind,colplot])
   heatmap.2(Normdata,Colv=T,trace="none",offsetRow=0,labRow="",density.info="
none",srtCol=45,key=T,cexCol=cexcol,cexRow=cexcol,adjCol=c (0.5,3),col=colorRa
mpPalette(c("green", "yellow", "red")));
   dev.print(jpeg,width = 550,height = 480,file)
}
drawimage(Normdata,"Normalized_HeatMap.jpeg",2:3,4,1,0.05)
```

CONCLUSION

Nowadays the high-throughput sequencing technologies is very important to address increasing different biological problems. In this chapter, differential gene expression analysis was done on the kidney tumor vs. normal sample using next generation sequencing data analysis. The gene enrichment analysis showed the genes involved in the cancer. The Up-regulated and the down-regulated genes were found which are showing their expressions in the cancer cells and these differential expressions are very essential for finding out the novel drug against the target protein. Future research work is very significant for designing a drug against the death leading diseases. The NGS data analysis gives a better way for the development of personalized medicine.

REFERENCES

Andersson, R., Gebhard, C., Miguel-Escalada, I., Hoof, I., Bornholdt, J., Boyd, M., ... Sandelin, A. (2014). An atlas of active enhancers across human cell types and tissues. *Nature*, *507*(7493), 455–461. doi:10.1038/nature12787 PMID:24670763

Berezikov, E., Thuemmler, F., van Laake, L. W., Kondova, I., Bontrop, R., Cuppen, E., & Plasterk, R. H. A. (2006). Diversity of microRNAs in human and chimpanzee brain. *Nature Genetics*, *38*(12), 1375–1377. doi:10.1038/ng1914 PMID:17072315

Blat, Y., & Kleckner, N. (1999). Cohesins bind to preferential sites along yeast chromosome III, with differential regulation along arms versus the centric region. *Cell*, *98*(2), 249–259. doi:10.1016/S0092-8674(00)81019-3 PMID:10428036

Conesa, A., Madrigal, P., Tarazona, S., Gomez-Cabrero, D., Cervera, A., McPherson, A., ... Mortazavi, A. (2016). A survey of best practices for RNA-seq data analysis. *Genome Biology*, *17*(1), 13. doi:10.118613059-016-0881-8 PMID:26813401

de Klerk, E., Venema, A., Anvar, S. Y., Goeman, J. J., Hu, O., Trollet, C., ... 't Hoen, P. A. C. (2012). Poly (A) binding protein nuclear 1 levels affect alternative polyadenylation. *Nucleic Acids Research*, *40*(18), 9089–9101. doi:10.1093/nar/gks655 PMID:22772983

DeRisi, J., Penland, L., Bittner, M., Meltzer, P., Ray, M., Chen, Y., & .... (1996). Use of a cDNA microarray to analyse gene expression. *Nature Genetics*, *14*(4), 457–460. doi:10.1038/ng1296-457 PMID:8944026

Ercolini, D., De Filippis, F., La Storia, A., & Iacono, M. (2012). "Remake" by high-throughput sequencing of the microbiota involved in the production of water buffalo mozzarella cheese. *Applied and Environmental Microbiology*, *78*(22), 8142–8145. doi:10.1128/AEM.02218-12 PMID:22941080

Flusberg, B. A., Webster, D. R., Lee, J. H., Travers, K. J., Olivares, E. C., Clark, T. A., ... Turner, S. W. (2010). Direct detection of DNA methylation during single-molecule, real-time sequencing. *Nature Methods*, *7*(6), 461–465. doi:10.1038/nmeth.1459 PMID:20453866

Garber, M., Grabherr, M. G., Guttman, M., & Trapnell, C. (2011). Computational methods for transcriptome annotation and quantification using RNA-seq. *Nature Methods*, *8*(6), 469–477. doi:10.1038/nmeth.1613 PMID:21623353

Ghosh, S., & Chan, C.-K. K. (2016). Analysis of RNA-Seq data using TopHat and Cufflinks. In Plant Bioinformatics (pp. 339-361). Academic Press.

Goodwin, S., McPherson, J. D., & McCombie, W. R. (2016). Coming of age: Ten years of next-generation sequencing technologies. *Nature Reviews. Genetics*, *17*(6), 333–351. doi:10.1038/nrg.2016.49 PMID:27184599

Ingolia, N. T., Ghaemmaghami, S., Newman, J. R., & Weissman, J. S. (2009). Genome-wide analysis in vivo of translation with nucleotide resolution using ribosome profiling. *Science*, *324*(5924), 218-223.

Jia, P., Wang, L., Meltzer, H. Y., & Zhao, Z. (2010). Common variants conferring risk of schizophrenia: A pathway analysis of GWAS data. *Schizophrenia Research*, *122*(1), 38–42. doi:10.1016/j.schres.2010.07.001 PMID:20659789

Keating, B. J., Tischfield, S., Murray, S. S., Bhangale, T., Price, T. S., Glessner, J. T., ... FitzGerald, G. A. (2008). Concept, design and implementation of a cardiovascular gene-centric 50 k SNP array for large-scale genomic association studies. *PLoS One*, *3*(10), e3583. doi:10.1371/journal.pone.0003583 PMID:18974833

Kukurba, K. R., & Montgomery, S. B. (2015). RNA sequencing and analysis. *Cold Spring Harbor Protocols*, *2015*(11).

Langmead, B. (2010). Aligning short sequencing reads with Bowtie. *Current Protocols in Bioinformatics*.

Langmead, B., & Salzberg, S. L. (2012). Fast gapped-read alignment with Bowtie 2. *Nature Methods*, *9*(4), 357–359. doi:10.1038/nmeth.1923 PMID:22388286

Lappalainen, T., Sammeth, M., Friedländer, M. R., & C't Hoen, A. (2013). Transcriptome and genome sequencing uncovers functional variation in humans. *Nature*, *501*(7468), 506–511. doi:10.1038/nature12531 PMID:24037378

Lea, K., Qu, L., Whitley, P., Schageman, J., Gu, J., & Bramlett, K. (2011). Transcriptome Analysis Using Next-Generation Sequencing Technology. *Journal of Biomolecular Techniques: JBT*, *22*(Suppl), S44.

Li, H., Handsaker, B., Wysoker, A., Fennell, T., Ruan, J., Homer, N., ... Durbin, R. (2009). The sequence alignment/map format and SAMtools. *Bioinformatics (Oxford, England)*, *25*(16), 2078–2079. doi:10.1093/bioinformatics/btp352 PMID:19505943

Li, R., Fan, W., Tian, G., Zhu, H., He, L., Cai, J., ... Wang, J. (2010). The sequence and de novo assembly of the giant panda genome. *Nature*, *463*(7279), 311–317. doi:10.1038/nature08696 PMID:20010809

Liu, L., Li, Y., Li, S., Hu, N., He, Y., & Pong, R. (2012a). Comparison of Next-Generation Sequencing Systems. *Journal of Biomedicine & Biotechnology*, *11*. doi:10.1155/2012/251364 PMID:22829749

Liu, L., Li, Y., Li, S., Hu, N., He, Y., & Pong, R. (2012b). Comparison of next-generation sequencing systems. *BioMed Research International*. PMID:22829749

Mardis, E. R. (2008). The impact of next-generation sequencing technology on genetics. *Trends in Genetics*, *24*(3), 133–141. doi:10.1016/j.tig.2007.12.007 PMID:18262675

Mardis, E. R. (2013). Next-generation sequencing platforms. *Annual Review of Analytical Chemistry (Palo Alto, Calif.)*, *6*(1), 287–303. doi:10.1146/annurev-anchem-062012-092628 PMID:23560931

Margulies, M., Egholm, M., Altman, W. E., Attiya, S., Bader, J. S., Bemben, L. A., ... Rothberg, J. M. (2005). Genome sequencing in microfabricated high-density picolitre reactors. *Nature*, *437*(7057), 376–380. doi:10.1038/nature03959 PMID:16056220

Mortazavi, A., Williams, B. A., McCue, K., Schaeffer, L., & Wold, B. (2008). Mapping and quantifying mammalian transcriptomes by RNA-Seq. *Nature Methods*, *5*(7), 621–628. doi:10.1038/nmeth.1226 PMID:18516045

Nolte-'t Hoen, E. N., Buermans, H. P., Waasdorp, M., Stoorvogel, W., Wauben, M. H., & 't Hoen, P. A. (2012). Deep sequencing of RNA from immune cell-derived vesicles uncovers the selective incorporation of small non-coding RNA biotypes with potential regulatory functions. *Nucleic Acids Research*, *40*(18), 9272–9285. doi:10.1093/nar/gks658 PMID:22821563

Patel, R. K., & Jain, M. (2012). NGS QC Toolkit: A toolkit for quality control of next generation sequencing data. *PLoS One*, *7*(2), e30619. doi:10.1371/journal.pone.0030619 PMID:22312429

Rabbani, B., Nakaoka, H., Akhondzadeh, S., Tekin, M., & Mahdieh, N. (2016). Next generation sequencing: Implications in personalized medicine and pharmacogenomics. *Molecular BioSystems*, *12*(6), 1818–1830. doi:10.1039/C6MB00115G PMID:27066891

Reich, D., Green, R. E., Kircher, M., Krause, J., Patterson, N., Durand, E. Y., ... Pääbo, S. (2010). Genetic history of an archaic hominin group from Denisova Cave in Siberia. *Nature*, *468*(7327), 1053–1060. doi:10.1038/nature09710 PMID:21179161

Rhodes, D. R., Yu, J., Shanker, K., Deshpande, N., Varambally, R., Ghosh, D., ... Chinnaiyan, A. M. (2004). Large-scale meta-analysis of cancer microarray data identifies common transcriptional profiles of neoplastic transformation and progression. *Proceedings of the National Academy of Sciences of the United States of America*, *101*(25), 9309–9314. doi:10.1073/pnas.0401994101 PMID:15184677

Rohland, N., Reich, D., Mallick, S., Meyer, M., Green, R. E., Georgiadis, N. J., ... Hofreiter, M. (2010). Genomic DNA sequences from mastodon and woolly mammoth reveal deep speciation of forest and savanna elephants. *PLoS Biology*, *8*(12), e1000564. doi:10.1371/journal.pbio.1000564 PMID:21203580

Trapnell, C., Pachter, L., & Salzberg, S. L. (2009). TopHat: Discovering splice junctions with RNA-Seq. *Bioinformatics (Oxford, England)*, *25*(9), 1105–1111. doi:10.1093/bioinformatics/btp120 PMID:19289445

Trapnell, C., Roberts, A., Goff, L., Pertea, G., Kim, D., Kelley, D. R., ... Pachter, L. (2012). Differential gene and transcript expression analysis of RNA-seq experiments with TopHat and Cufflinks. *Nature Protocols*, *7*(3), 562–578. doi:10.1038/nprot.2012.016 PMID:22383036

Trapnell, C., Williams, B. A., Pertea, G., Mortazavi, A., Kwan, G., van Baren, M. J., ... Pachter, L. (2010). Transcript assembly and quantification by RNA-Seq reveals unannotated transcripts and isoform switching during cell differentiation. *Nature Biotechnology*, *28*(5), 511–515. doi:10.1038/nbt.1621 PMID:20436464

Valen, E., Pascarella, G., Chalk, A., Maeda, N., Kojima, M., Kawazu, C., ... Carninci, P. (2009). Genome-wide detection and analysis of hippocampus core promoters using DeepCAGE. *Genome Research*, *19*(2), 255–265. doi:10.1101/gr.084541.108 PMID:19074369

Venter, J. C., Remington, K., Heidelberg, J. F., Halpern, A. L., Rusch, D., Eisen, J. A. *et al.*, (2004). Environmental genome shotgun sequencing of the Sargasso Sea. *Science*, *304*(5667), 66-74.

Watson, J. D., & Crick, F. H. (1953). *The structure of DNA*. Paper presented at the Cold Spring Harbor symposia on quantitative biology. 10.1101/SQB.1953.018.01.020

Welter, D., MacArthur, J., Morales, J., Burdett, T., Hall, P., Junkins, H., ... Parkinson, H. (2013). The NHGRI GWAS Catalog, a curated resource of SNP-trait associations. *Nucleic Acids Research*, *42*(D1), D1001–D1006. doi:10.1093/nar/gkt1229 PMID:24316577

Chapter 12
Semantic Technologies for Medical Knowledge Representation

Shridevi S.
VIT Chennai, India

Saleena B.
VIT Chennai, India

Viswanathan V.
VIT Chennai, India

ABSTRACT

The ongoing rapid growth of diversity of data and their wide use to solve different complex tasks resulted in a significant number of semantic reference systems enriched with vocabularies, thesauri, terminologies, and ontologies. The extensive use of ontologies stemmed a new approach to build modern intelligent systems in reusing and sharing pieces of declarative knowledge. A lot of effort has been made to produce standard ontologies for medical knowledge representation. This chapter brings an overview of semantic knowledge representation frameworks such as RDF and OWL for developing ontology-based medical systems. The chapter presents the state of the art in ontology resources/systems so that it could be useful for learners and researchers involved in interdisciplinary research areas that include medicine and information technology. Also, a clinical use case is illustrated highlighting the role of ontology in the medical domain.

INTRODUCTION

Knowledge representation plays a vital role in reasoning which is a part of the Decision Support Systems (DSS). Medical ontology can be a model of the information from a clinical domain that will contain all the relevant ideas related to the patient information, treatment, their medicine and clinical procedures. Ontology allows knowledge inference and reasoning. The benefits of applying ontology for information illustration are: information sharing, standardization of medical terms and support for automatic semantic

DOI: 10.4018/978-1-5225-7326-5.ch012

reasoning (Wang et al, 2004). In this manner, ontologies integrate descriptive, actionable and factual information and they can be populated using the PIKES approach. (Francesco et al, 2016)

In this chapter, our aim is to discuss different knowledge representation frameworks, manipulation of data and metadata and their storage (Petar, 2016). Representation and Inference must be the core of any knowledge representation systems. So here, we have two Ontology representation mechanisms – namely RDF *and* OWL Frameworks. Rules and query languages for handling such metadata repositories are discussed in the below sections.

RDF Metadata Framework

RDF is a W3C standard (RDF Working group, 2004) for describing metadata and modeling the resources in the Web. It is written in XML format. Any kind of knowledge available in RDF can be decomposed into triples. Semantics and rules can be applied to relate the knowledge based on their meanings (Chakkarwar et al, 2016) and with their timestamps (Barbieri et al, 2010). RDF triples are a combination of three variables- Subject, Predicate and the Object. The objects are always literals and the subjects and predicates are resources. Resources are identified by Uniform Resource Identifiers (URI) when the data is from a Web repository and a set of statements when the data is from text or relational databases. For instance, <http://en.wikipedia.org/wiki/Dopamine#, http://en.wikipedia.org/wiki/Functions#, http://en.wikipedia.org/wiki/Neurotransmitter#> is a triple communicating that the subject Dopamine functions as a Neurotransmitter which is an object. URL (Uniform Resource Locator) has been utilized to find a Web page we need to get to. RDF uses two unique sorts of URI to recognize a given resource, in particular slash URI and hash URI. URI using slash is basically an ordinary URI that we all know and URI using hash is used as below:

Ordinary URI + # + fragment identifier

URI using hash and slash to recognize a Sick person on the Web can be used as mentioned below.

http://www.clinic.org/Sickpersons/Sickperson1

http://www.clinic.org/Sickpersons#Sickperson1

The ordinary URI for hash URI is given by http://www.clinic.org/Sickpersons/ Sickperson1and its fragment identity is given by # Sickperson1. An RDF file must have the below format.

The RDF root element is <rdf:RDF> which defines that an RDF document is referenced with a namespace xmlns. <rdf:Description> gives description about the resources to be stored in the RDF file.

```
<rdf:RDF
xmlns:rdf="http://www.w3.org/1999/02/22-rdf-syntax-ns#">
<rdf:Description
  ...Description of resources
</rdf:Description>
</rdf:RDF>
```

Example 1: A simple set of statements describing the hill station Kodaikanal is considered. The area of Kodaikanal is 21.45 sq-km. Its altitude is 2133 metres. The food crops in Kodaikanal are plums, peaches and pears. The locations (place of interest) of Kodaikanal are stored in URI http://www.hill-stations-india.com/kodaikanal/. Converting this statement into triples (Subject –Object –Predicate) will take the form as in Table 1.

The below statements gives the RDF representation for the above Example.

```
<rdf:RDF
 xmlns:rdf='http://www.w3.org/1999/02/22-rdf-syntax-ns#'
 xmlns:NS="http://tamilnadutourism.org/HillStation/HillStationMain.aspx" >
<rdf:Description  rdf:about ='Kodaikanal'>
<NS:Area> Area 21.45-sq-km </NS:Area>
<NS:Altitude> Altitude 2,133 metres  </NS:Altitude>
<NS:Foodcrop> peaches, plums, pears </NS:Foodcrop>
<NS:Location rdf:resource="http://tamilnadutourism.org/HillStation/TNHillSta-
tions/HS_Kodaikkanal.aspx?catid=030101P01 "/>
</rdf:Description>
</rdf:RDF>
```

Representing the information in the Web using RDF in the above format will help the user group the information based on the subjects and predicates. BM25F ranking function for RDF data, can also be used in RDF searching and organizing data.(Blanco et al, 2011) To ensure that the RDF statements are valid, they can be validated through the W3C RDF validator. The results are shown in Figure 1.

RDF Container Classes

RDF Properties can occur as single or a group of elements. The group of elements can be represented using anyone of the following RDF containers

Bag – Which contain an unordered list of items, which can also have duplicates.
Sequence – Which contain the sequence of elements
Alternative – Provides alternative value for the group

BAG: BAG defines a set of unordered resources or literals. Bags convey that a property can have numerous values and no importance is considered for the order of given values. The below RDF example lists all the available physicians in a hospital.

Table 1. RDF triples

Subject	Predicate	Object
Kodaikanal	Area	"Area 21.45-sq-km"
Kodaikanal	Altitude	"Altitude 2,133 metres"
Kodaikanal	Foodcrop	"peaches, plums, pears "
Kodaikanal	Location	"http://tamilnadutourism.org/HillStation/TNHillStations/HS_Kodaikkanal.aspx?catid=030101P01"

Figure 1. Validated RDF file

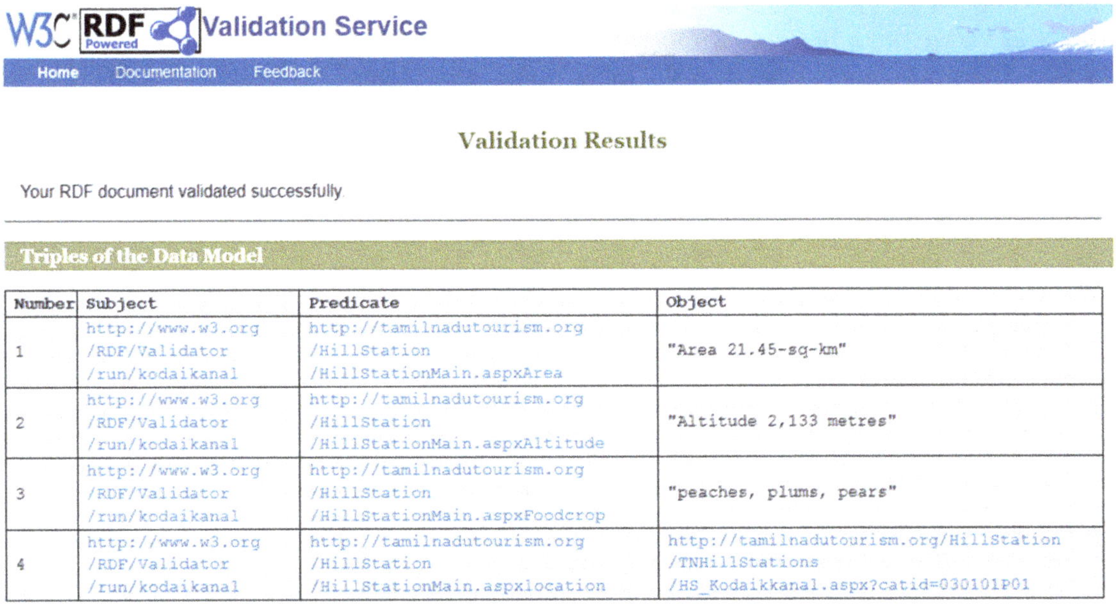
W3C RDF Powered Validation Service

Home Documentation Feedback

Validation Results

Your RDF document validated successfully

Triples of the Data Model

Number	Subject	Predicate	Object
1	http://www.w3.org /RDF/Validator /run/kodaikanal	http://tamilnadutourism.org /HillStation /HillStationMain.aspxArea	"Area 21.45-sq-km"
2	http://www.w3.org /RDF/Validator /run/kodaikanal	http://tamilnadutourism.org /HillStation /HillStationMain.aspxAltitude	"Altitude 2,133 metres"
3	http://www.w3.org /RDF/Validator /run/kodaikanal	http://tamilnadutourism.org /HillStation /HillStationMain.aspxFoodcrop	"peaches, plums, pears"
4	http://www.w3.org /RDF/Validator /run/kodaikanal	http://tamilnadutourism.org /HillStation /HillStationMain.aspxlocation	http://tamilnadutourism.org/HillStation /TNHillStations /HS_Kodaikkanal.aspx?catid=030101P01

```
<?xml version="1.0"?>
<rdf:RDFxmlns:rdf=http://www.w3.org/1999/02/22-rdf-syntax-ns#>
<xmlns:d="http://www.hospital.org/doctors#">
<rdf:Description
rdf:about="http://www.hospital.org/doctors/general">
  <d:physicians>
    <rdf:Bag>
      <rdf:li>Dr.John</rdf:li>
      <rdf:li>Dr.Paul</rdf:li>
      <rdf:li>Dr.George</rdf:li>
      <rdf:li>Dr.Ringo</rdf:li>
    </rdf:Bag>
  </d:physicians>
</rdf:Description>
</rdf:RDF>
```

Sequence: An unordered set of resources or literals. Sequence conveys that a property can have numerous values and values order is important. For instance, to demonstrate the pattern of temperature values of a patient based on time, sequence can be applied and here also duplicates are allowed.

Alternative: Property values can be chosen from a list of choices of resources or literals.

Figure 2. Mapping of RDF to RDF Schema

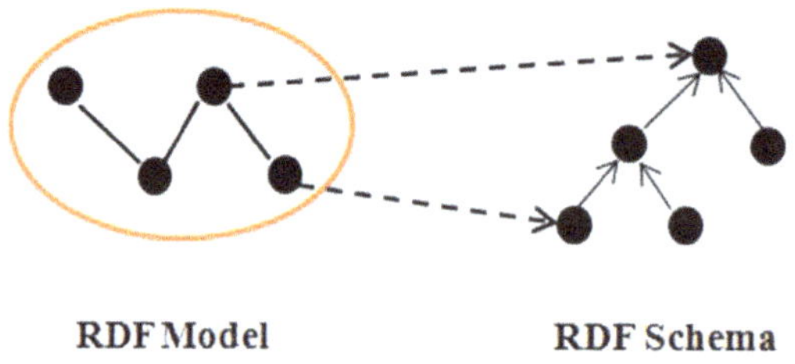

RDF Schema

RDF has the most basic syntaxes. RDF Schema has few additional features to enhance the definition of the schema as shown in Figure 2 and the class hierarchy is depicted Figure 3. The vocabulary helps us to define classes, properties and relationship between them.

Given below is a simple example using the constructs of RDF schema.

```
<?xml version ="1.0"?>
<rdf: RDF
xmlns:rdf='http://www.w3.org/1999/02/22-rdf-syntax-ns#'
xml:base:"http://hospital.org">
              <rdfs:Class rdf:about="#WardBoy">
        <rdfs:subClassOf rdf:resource="#Staff"/>
</rdfs:Class>
<rdf:Property rdf:ID="MobileNumber">
                 <rdfs:domain rdf:resource="#Staff"/>
                 <rdfs:range rdf:resource="#Literal"/>
</rdf:Property>
 <rdf:RDF>
```

Figure 3. RDFS Class Hierarchy

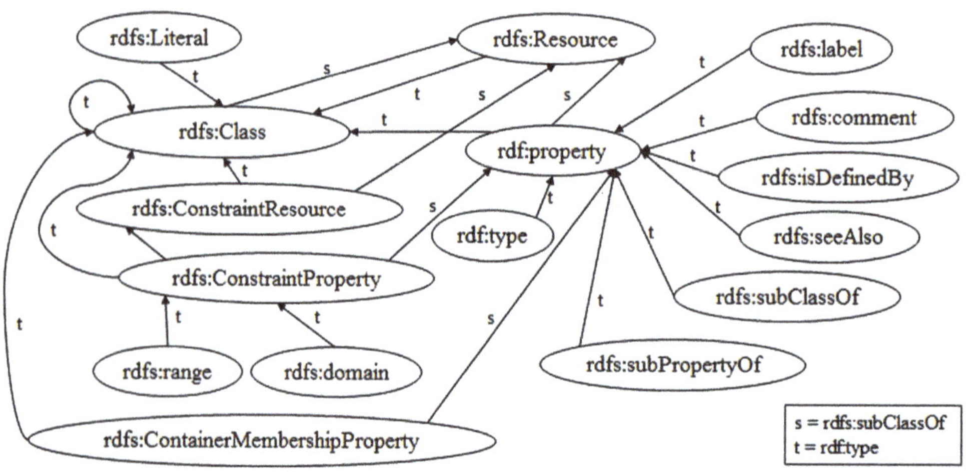

RDF Serialization

RDF has several serialization formats. The encoding of resources varies from format to format. RDF/XML is the first standard and official serialization format for RDF data.

Few of the common serialization formats are listed below

- **Turtle:** It is a very human-friendly and compact model
- **N-Triples:** It is a very simple line based format and east to parse
- **JSON-LD:** It is a java based serialization.
- **N-Quads:** It is a superset of N-Triples, for serializing multiple RDF graphs.
- **N3 or Notation3:**This format is very similar to Turtle, with but with extended features to define inference rules.

An example of RDF/XML format and its serialized version in turtle is given below.

```
RDF/XML Format:
<?xml version="1.0"?>
<rdf:RDF xmlns:rdf="http://www.w3.org/1999/02/22-rdf-syntax-ns#"
 xmlns:ex="http://hospital.org/">
 <rdf:Description rdf:about="http://hospital.org/Alice">
<ex:age>19</ex:age>
 </rdf:Description>
 </rdf:RDF>
Turtle Format:
@prefix rdf: <http://www.w3.org/1999/02/22-rdf-syntax-ns#>.
@prefix ex: <http://hospital.org/">.
<http://hospital.org/Alice> ex:age "19"
```

SPARQL

Without a query language, the data representation model cannot be utilized in an efficient manner. This section gives an overview of the query pattern involved in retrieving data from the linked data sets. The Simple Protocol and RDF Query Language (SPARQL) is a standard query language for RDF. A SPARQL query is defined as a set of triples (subject, predicate and object) which consist of variables. Solutions to the query is identified by matching the triples of SPARQL query with the existing RDF triples . SPARQL 1.0 only allows limited operations on matching results or solutions such as filter or duplicate elimination, ordering, projection and triple construction. We need to provide more flexible operations such as aggregates, grouping, and assignment and select expressions. SPARQL 1.1 provides all these features. In SPARQL, SELECT statement is used to give the subset of the selected data, WHERE clause defines the graph patterns through one of more triples to find a match in the query data set.

SPARQL General Form

PREFIX (Namespace Prefixes)
e.g. PREFIX iot: < http://purl.org/IoT/iot#>
SELECT (Result Set)
e.g. SELECT ?sensorname
WHERE (Query Triple Pattern)
e.g. WHERE iot:?sensorname iot:location iot:?room1
ORDER BY(modifier)
e.g. ORDER BY ?sensorname

For example, consider the below query that lists the hospitals within 40 km of distance where cardiologists are available.

```
SELECT  ?clinic ?doctor
WHERE { ?clinic rdf:value ?distance.
                  ?doctor category ?cardiologist.
              FILTER (?distance<=40). }
```

OWL-BASED METADATA FRAMEWORK

OWL is an extension of RDF which adds a rich semantic layer (Bechhofer, 2016).

Web Ontology Language is a description of knowledge and ontologies of a given domain such as

- Axioms/constraints capture knowledge about a given domain, e.g.,
    - ***class(Patient), class(Person)***
    - ***Patient*** $\subseteq$ ***Person***
- Axioms/constraints are imposed on underlying RDF Graph instances
- ***URIs (URLs)*** are used as identifiers for: Resources, Properties, Values, Namespaces and Ontological Elements
- ***Namespaces*** contain:
    - Tags for RDF and OWL languages
    - Ontological elements (classes, properties) that are instantiated by these RDF Graphs
    - Ontological elements or XML Schema data types that are dimensions of identifiers such as ***LSIDs***

Figure 4 gives an overview of RDF and OWL vocabulary constructs.

Using these constructs, the Ontology developed can be defined as a collective vocabulary, a common appreciative for re-use of domain knowledge. And is an obvious explanation of a domain using concepts (classes, subclasses and super classes), properties and attributes of concepts, constraints on properties and attributes and Individuals.

Figure 4. RDF and OWL vocabulary

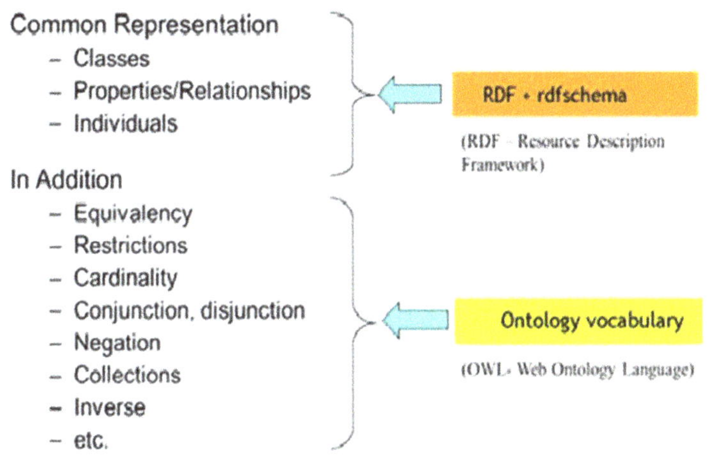

SWRL

This section explains the need for rules in inferring knowledge from the data representation models discussed in the previous sections. Rule languages are commonly used in most of the business applications. The main goal of the Semantic Web is to achieve the Interoperability. Expressing all relations using OWL 2 language is very difficult. By adding SWRL rules (Horrocks et al, 2004 and Edmond et al, 2017) to ontology, the expressivity of OWL can be improved. SWRL is similar to rules in DATALOG or Prolog languages. SWRL allows users to write rules expressed in terms of OWL concepts to reason about OWL individuals (Lehmann, 2009). Figure 5 illustrates rules for a simple scenario.

Important and Relevant Biomedical Resources/Ontologies

As ontologies attract a significant amount of attention in different research communities, this section provides an overview of terminologies and ontologies in medicine. The content highlights the most attractive resources/systems for industry and academia in medical and biological terminologies, ontologies, resources/systems and tools. The section intends to give an informative and instructive overview of resources/systems that could be useful for newcomers in the multidisciplinary fields that include biology, medicine and information technology.

FMA

In the field of biomedical informatics, Foundational Model of Anatomy Ontology (**FMA**) is used as a computer-based knowledgebase. To represent phenotypic structure of the human body in a user understandable form classes and relationships are used. It is also traversable, parse-able and interpretable by machine-based systems. Structural Informatics Group at University of Washington is developed and maintaining the FMA ontology.

Figure 5. RDFS rules

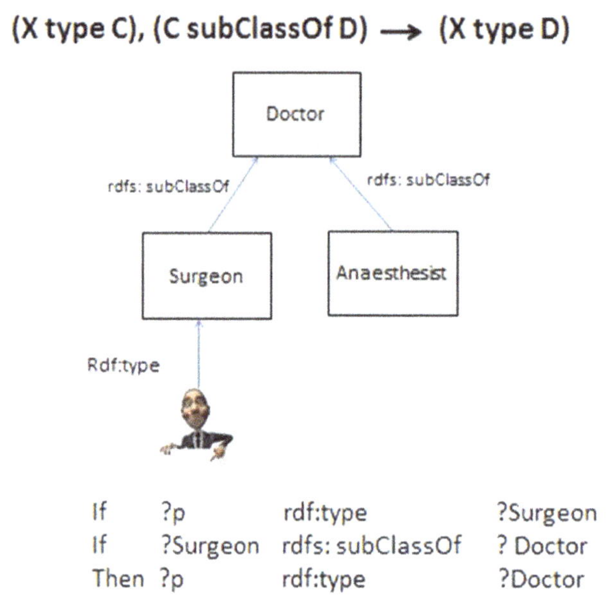

ICD-10

International Statistical Classification of Diseases and Related Health Problems (ICD) is a medical classification list and it is revised as ICD-10 by the World Health Organization (WHO, 2017). Unique codes are assigned for diseases, symptoms, signs, complaints, abnormal findings, social circumstances and external causes of injury or diseases. ICD-10 encompasses a set of codes that permits the tracking of symptoms through new diagnoses. These codes can be expanded by using optional sub-classifications.

RadLex

RadLex has more than 68000 terms to satisfy the needs of the software developers, radiology users and system vendors to fill the critical gaps in existing terminologies by adopting new terms from the best features of the variety of terminologies and standards in its existing terminology systems (RadLex, 2015). To organize and retrieve the imaging report, the radiologists need a unified language with single lexicon that serves all of their requirements.

MFOEM

To describe affective phenomena influencing human behaviour an emotional ontology is being developed by the Swiss Centre for Affective Sciences, in collaboration with the University at Buffalo. Emotion ontology encompasses all important aspects of affective phenomena which includes the different types of emotions, moods etc. including their bearers. It also includes the degrees of variations in different parts of human body, human facial and vocal expressions that explains the role of emotions and affective phenomena influencing the human behaviour.

UMLS

US National Library of Medicine is developed a repository of biomedical vocabularies called Unified Medical Language System (UMLS) with 2.5 million names for 900,551 concepts from more than 60 families of biomedical vocabularies and 12 million relations among these concepts. Ontologies integrated in the UMLS meta-thesaurus include the Medical Subject Headings (MeSH), the NCBI taxonomy, Gene Ontology (GO), Online Mendelian Inheritance in Man(OMIM), University of Washington Digital Anatomist symbolic knowledge base (UWDA) and Systematized Nomenclature of Medicine—Clinical Terms(SNOMED CT). Some of UMLS ontologies listed in the Table 2.

How It Supports Decision Making?

Reasoning of ontologies supports decision making which can be applied to any domain of interest. Personalized ontologies can be developed to store the fitness record of a sick person that can aid domain professionals to arrive at a decision and also to analyse and detect lack of accuracy in finding the physical condition of the patient (Linda et al, 2015). These lacks of precisions may severely impact the care and worth of the action that the patient is supposed to receive. In order to help minimize such irregularities, a decision support system can be integrated with the ontologies that enable the doctors to detect incorrect analyses, ignored comorbidities, partial descriptions of the patient illness, related sicknesses and avoidance.

Clinical Scenario

For a better understanding of the use of ontologies in health care domain, we have discussed a case study in this section. Here, a smart application is discussed which is developed to help patients for getting possible suggestions for their medical requirements, be it medicine or any other aid in the form of medical devices, or physicians, or specialists they need for their treatment. The high level architecture of the semantic health care application is depicted in Figure 6.

Table 2. UMLS Ontologies

Name	Creator	Description	Application
National Center for Biotechnology Information (NCBI)Taxonomy	National Library of Medicine	All of the **organisms** in public sequence database	Identify organisms
University of Washington Digital Anatomist Source Information (UWDA1	University of Washington Structural Informatics Group	Symbolic models of the structures and relationships that constitute the human body.	Identify terms in anatomy
Gene Ontologv(G01	Gene Ontology Consortium	Gene **product** characteristics and gene product annotation data	Gene product annotation
Medical Subject Headings (MeS1-11	National Library of Medicine	Vocabulary thesaurus used for indexing articles for pubmed	Convert terms in biomedical literature
Online Mendelian Inheritance in Man(OMIM1	cMc Kusick-Nathans Institute of Genetic Medicine Johns Hopkins University	human genes and genetic phenotypes	Annotate human genes
Systematized Nomenclature of Medicine--Clinical Terms (SNOMED CT)	College of American Pathologists	Comprehensive, multi lingual clinical **healthcare terminology** in the world	Identify clinical terms

Table 3. Biomedical ontologies

Web link	Description
http://bioportal.bioontology.org/	The most comprehensive repository of biomedical ontologies
http://www.obofoundry.org/	Open Biomedical Ontologies is an umbrella web address for well-structured controlled vocabularies for shared use across different biological domains.
http://mged.sourceforge.net/ontologies/ MGEDontology.php	An ontology for microarray experiments in support of Micro Array Gene Expression Data (MGED) version 1.0
http://www.biopax.org/	Biological Pathway Exchange (BioPAX) is a standard language that aims to enable integration, exchange, visualization and analysis of biological pathway data.
https://www.nlm.nih.gov/research/umls/knowledge_ sources/metathesaurus/release/index.html	Unified Medical Language System ontology by National Library of Medicine's (US)
http://goat.man.ac.uk/	Gene Ontology Annotation Tool (GOAT). It helps the users in biomedical researchers, in the annotation of gene products with terms from the Gene Ontology.
http://www.cs.man.ac.uk/~stevensr/rash/	Reconcile and Share (RASH) aims to address the problem of semantic heterogeneity in bioinformatics resources.
http://www.hybrow.org/	HyBrow Computer aided hypothesis evaluation

Figure 6. Design of semantic application

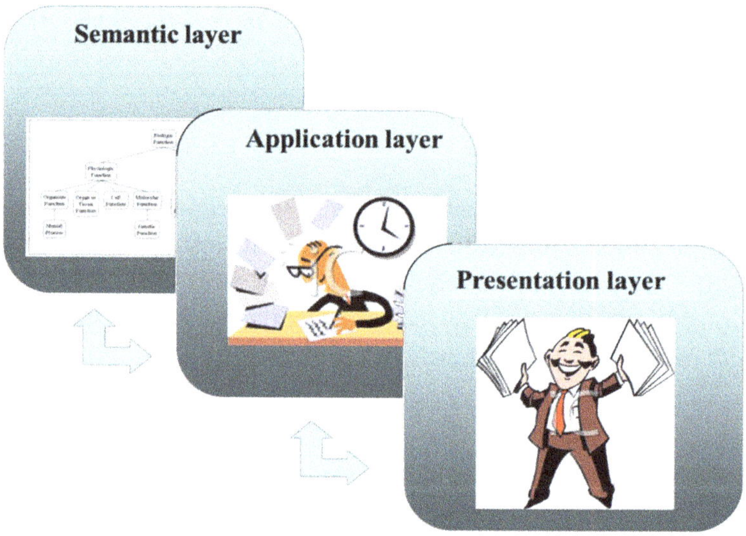

The health care ontology for semantic layer of the application would be as in Figure 7. The class and subclass hierarchy is depicted as below:

- Health_care
    - Competences
        - Care competences
        - Cure competences
        - Prevention competences
        - Suppliers competences

Figure 7. Health care ontology

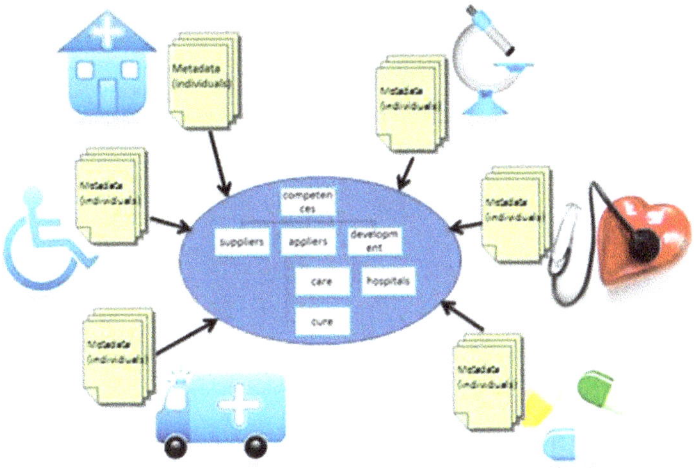

  - Wellness competences

- Prevention
- Suppliers
- Wellness
- Competences development
- Competences warehouse
- Diseases
  - Symptom

Using protégé tool, the ontology can be developed as in Figure 8.

As illustrated above, a smart healthcare application can be developed using the ontology in the semantic layer with inference capability using a reasoner that makes use of the defined rules and the application can be queried to get expected possible outcomes to help the patients. Consider the below example where the differently abled persons requirements are considered as inputs and their aids details are the expected output as depicted in Figure 9.

Input: help apparatus need for elderly or restricted persons

- Assistance for poor-vision or sightless persons
- Assistance for movement disabilities
- Hearing impaired persons
- Prolonged diseases
- Emergency service

Output:

Links of the apparatus with its description.

Figure 8. Ontology development using protégé

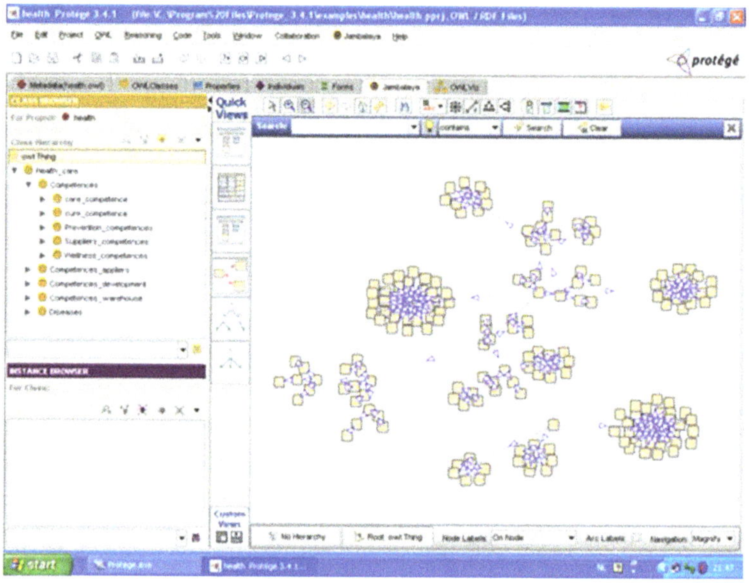

Figure 9. Semantic applications that help differently abled people to find their device

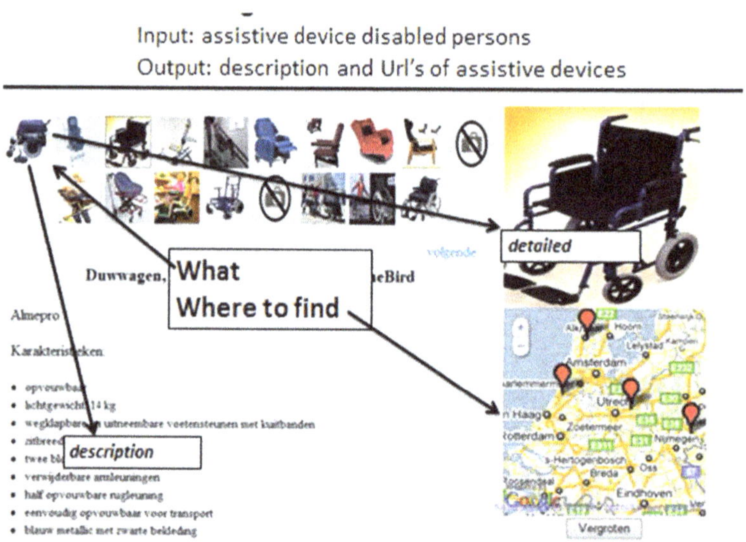

Benefits of Ontology-based applications:

- Healthcare applications can be designed more interoperable and powerful by enabling ontologies as their knowledge representation model.
- Patient data sharing, re-usage and transmission can be well supported by the inclusion of ontology based systems.
- Different statistical aggregations for various purposes can be provided by Ontologies.

- The support for indispensable incorporation of knowledge and info is possibly the most important advantage that ontologies may bring to healthcare systems.
  On the negative side:
- The upkeep of real-world healthcare information systems based on semantic technologies has got a skeptical impact about the design of domain ontologies.

SUMMARY

It is evident that the use of ontologies in medical domain and the tools and practices for semantic interoperability can improve a healthcare system in the following ways: to improve accuracy of diagnoses, to construct more authoritative and more interoperable info systems in healthcare, to upkeep process to transmit, reuse and share patient data, to deliver semantic-based standards to offer different statistical combinations, and to support the necessary assimilation of knowledge and data. Having this in mind, they recommend the following necessary key points, a healthcare organization have to think through with Ontologies and Semantic Interoperability: Establishing a workgroup to identify requirements and/or uses of medical ontologies, Detailed literature search and obtaining lessons learned from medical ontologies and semantic interoperability projects, Identifying potential organizations to collaborate with, Investigating changes in clinical and IT practices and concentrating on utilizing medical ontologies and semantic interoperability systems. Given the diversity and rapid, continuous development of biomedical ontologies, resources and tools, we tried in this chapter to present the current situation in this field. Our primary motivation was to highlight the relevant research efforts in medical and biological terminologies, ontologies, resources/systems and tools. We wanted to give an informative and instructive overview of resources/systems that could be useful for newcomers in the multidisciplinary fields that include biology, medicine, and information technology.

REFERENCES

Allemang, D., & Hendler, J. (2008). *Semantic Web for the Working Ontologist: Effective Modelling in RDFS and OWL*. Morgan Kaufmann Publishers.

Allemang, D., & Hendler, J. (2011). *Semantic Web for the Working Ontologist* (2nd ed.). Morgan Kaufmann Publishers.

Antoniou, G., & Harmelen, F. V. (2008). *A Semantic Web Primer* (2nd ed.). The MIT Press.

Baader, F., Calvanese, D., Mcguinness, D. L., Patel-Schneider, P., & Nardi, D. (2003). *The Description Logic Handbook: Theory, Implementation and Applications*. Cambridge University Press.

Barbieri, D. F., Braga, D., Ceri, S., Valle, E. D., & Grossniklaus, M. (2010). C-Sparql: A Continuous Query Language for RDF Data Streams. *International Journal of Semantic Computing*, *4*(1), 3–25. doi:10.1142/S1793351X10000936

Bechhofer, S. (2016). *Owl Web Ontology Reference*. Available: Https://Www.W3.Org/Tr/2004/Rec-Owl-Ref-20040210/

Berners-Lee, T., Hendler, J., & Lassila, O. (2001). The Semantic Web. A New Form of Web Content That Is Meaningful to Computers Will Unleash a Revolution of New Possibilities. *Scientific American, 284*, 1–5.

Bizer, C., Heath, T., & Berners-Lee, T. (2009). Linked Data, The Story so far. *International Journal on Semantic Web and Information Systems, 5*(3), 1–22. doi:10.4018/jswis.2009081901

Bizer, C., Heath, T., & Berners-Lee, T. (2009). Linked Data, The Story so far. *International Journal on Semantic Web and Information Systems, 5*(3), 1–22. doi:10.4018/jswis.2009081901

Blanco, R., Mika, P., & Vigna, S. (2011, October). Effective and Efficient Entity Search in RDF Data. *Proceedings of the 10th International Conference on the Semantic Web (Iswc'11).* 10.1007/978-3-642-25073-6_6

Brickley, D., & Guha, R. V. (2004). *RDF Vocabulary Description Language 1.0: Schema.* W3c Recommendation.

Brickley, D., & Miller, L. (2005). FOAF Vocabulary Specification. *Namespace Document.* Retrieved from Http://Xmlns.Com/Foaf/0.1

Carroll, J. J., & Klyne, G. (2004). *Resource Description Framework (RDF): Concepts And Abstract Syntax.* W3c Recommendation.

Castaneda, C., Nalley, K., Mannion, C., Bhattacharyya, P., Blake, P., Pecora, A., ... Suh, K. S. (2015). Clinical Decision Support Systems for Improving Diagnostic Accuracy and Achieving Precision Medicine. *Journal of Clinical Bioinformatics, 5*(4), 1–16. PMID:25834725

Chakkarwar, V. A., & Joshi, A. A. (2016). Semantic Web Mining Using Rdf Data. *International Journal of Computers and Applications, 133*(10), 14–19. doi:10.5120/ijca2016908022

Corcoglioniti, F., Rospocher, M., & Aprosio, A. P. (2016). Frame-Based Ontology Population with Pikes. *IEEE Transactions on Knowledge and Data Engineering, 28*(12), 3261–3275. doi:10.1109/TKDE.2016.2602206

Ducharme & Bob. (2011). *Learning Sparql.* O'Reilly Media, Inc.

Garg, A. X., Adhikari, N. K., McDonald, H., Rosas-Arellano, M. P., Devereaux, P. J., Beyene, J., ... Haynes, R. B. (2005). Effects of Computerized Clinical Decision Support Systems on Practitioner Performance and Patient Outcomes: A systematic Review. *Journal of the American Medical Association, 293*(10), 1223–1238. doi:10.1001/jama.293.10.1223 PMID:15755945

Hitzler, P., Krötzsch, M., & Rudolph, S. (2009). *Foundations of Semantic Web Technologies.* CRC Press.

Jajaga, E., & Ahmedi, L. (2017). C-SWRL: SWRL for Reasoning Over Stream Data. *11th International Conference on Semantic Computing (ICSC).* 10.1109/ICSC.2017.64

Jaspers, M. W., Smeulers, M., Vermeulen, H., & Peute, L. W. (2011). Effects of Clinical Decision-Support Systems on Practitioner Performance and Patient Outcomes: A Synthesis of High-Quality Systematic Review Finding. *Journal of the American Medical Informatics Association, 18*(3), 327–334. doi:10.1136/amiajnl-2011-000094 PMID:21422100

Keet, C. M. (2011). The Use of Foundational Ontologies in Ontology Development: An Empirical Assessment. *8th Extended Semantic Web Conference.*

Lehmann, J. (2009). DL-Learner: Learning Concepts in Description Logics. *Journal of Machine Learning Research, 10*, 2639–2642.

Mhadhb, L., Akaichi, J., Karray, M. H., & Archimde, B. (2015, April). Ontologies for Location Based Services Quality Enhancement: The Case of Emergency Services. *Second International Conference on Edemocracy & Egovernment (Icedeg).* 10.1109/ICEDEG.2015.7114469

Passin, T. B. (2004). *Explorer's Guide to the Semantic Web.* Manning Publication.

Patel-Schneider, P. F., Hayes, P., & Horrocks, I. (2004). *OWL Web Ontology Language Semantics and Abstract Syntax.* W3c Recommendation.

Pollock, J. T. (2009). *Semantic Web for Dummies.* Wiley.

Riañoa, D., Reala, F., López-Vallverdúa, J. A., Campanab, F., Ercolanic, S., Mecoccic, P., ... Caltagironed, C. (2012). An Ontology-Based Personalization of Health-Care Knowledge to Support Clinical Decisions for Chronically Ill Patients. *Journal of Biomedical Informatics, 45*(3), 429–446. doi:10.1016/j.jbi.2011.12.008 PMID:22269224

Ristoski, P., & Paulheim, H. (2016). Semantic Web in Data Mining and Knowledge Discovery: A Comprehensive Survey. *Journal of Web Semantics, 36*, 1–22. doi:10.1016/j.websem.2016.01.001

Sikos, L. F. (2015). *Mastering Structured Data On The Semantic Web.* A Press.

Sim, G., Gorman, P., Greenes, R. A., Haynes, R. B., Kaplan, B., Lehmann, H., & Tang, P. C. (2001). Clinical Decision Support Systems for the Practice of Evidence-Based Medicine. *Journal of the American Medical Informatics Association, 8*(6), 527–534. doi:10.1136/jamia.2001.0080527 PMID:11687560

Wang, H., Zhou, T., Tian, L., Qian, Y., & Li, J. (2014). Creating Hospital-Specific Customized Clinical Pathways By Applying Semantic Reasoning To Clinical Data. *Journal of Biomedical Informatics, 52*, 354–363. doi:10.1016/j.jbi.2014.07.017 PMID:25109270

Yu, L. (2014). *A Developer's Guide to the Semantic Web* (2nd ed.). Springer.

Zenuni, X., Raufi, B., Ismaili, F., & Ajdari, J. (2015). State Of The Art of Semantic Web For Healthcare. *Procedia: Social and Behavioral Sciences, 195*, 1990–1998. doi:10.1016/j.sbspro.2015.06.213

Compilation of References

23. Subbaramaiah, K., Hart, J. C., Norton, L., & Dannenberg, A. J. (2000). Microtubule-interfering Agents Stimulate the Transcription of Cyclooxygenase-2. *The Journal of Biological Chemistry*, *275*(20), 14838–14845. doi:10.1074/jbc.275.20.14838 PMID:10809726

Aarthi, G., Jennifer, P. M., Duncan, I. J., & Owen, J. S. (2015). GEMMs as preclinical models for testing pancreatic cancer therapies. *Disease Models & Mechanisms*, *8*(10), 1185–1200. doi:10.1242/dmm.021055 PMID:26438692

Accelrys. TOPKAT (TOxicity Prediction by Komputer Assisted Technology). (2015). Available at: http://accelrys.com/products/discovery-studio/admet.html

Adams, S. E. (2010). *Molecular Similarity and Xenobiotic Metabolism* (Ph.D. thesis). University of Cambridge.

Adams, C. P., & Brantner, V. V. (2006). Estimating the cost of new drug development: Is it really 802 million dollars? *Health Affairs*, *25*(2), 420–428. doi:10.1377/hlthaff.25.2.420 PMID:16522582

Adl, A., Zein, M., & Hassanien, A. E. (2016). PQSAR. Expert System with application. *International Journal (Toronto, Ont.)*, *54*, 219–227.

Agapito, G., Guzzi, P., & Cannataro, M. (2013). Visualization of protein interaction networks: Problems and solutions. *BMC Bioinformatics*, *14*(Suppl 1). doi:10.1186/1471-2105-14-S1-S1 PMID:23368786

Agrafiotis, D. K., Gibbs, A. C., Zhu, F., Izrailev, S., & Martin, E. (2007). Conformational sampling of bioactive molecules: A comparative study. *Journal of Chemical Information and Modeling*, *47*(3), 1067–1086. doi:10.1021/ci6005454 PMID:17411028

Agyres, N., & Silverman, B. (2004). R&D, Organizational Structure, and the Development of Corporate Technological Knowledge. *Strategic Management Journal*, *25*(8–9), 929–958. doi:10.1002mj.387

Ahmad, Fazal, & Abbasi. (2012). Biological role of piper nigrum L. (Black pepper): A review. *Asian Pacific Journal Tropical Biomedicine,* 1945-1953.

Ahmetaj-Shala, B., Kirkby, N. S., Knowles, R., Al'Yamani, M., Mazi, S., Wang, S. Z., ... Mitchell, J. A. (2015). Evidence That Links Loss of Cyclooxygenase-2 With Increased Asymmetric Dimethylarginine. *Circulation*, *131*(7), 633–642. doi:10.1161/CIRCULATIONAHA.114.011591 PMID:25492024

Ajay, A., & Murcko, M. A. (1995). Computational methods to predict binding free energy in ligand-receptor complexes. *Journal of Medicinal Chemistry*, *38*(26), 4953–4967. doi:10.1021/jm00026a001 PMID:8544170

Alexander, S., Oliver, G., & Markus, H. (2016). Changing R&D models in research-based pharmaceutical companies. *Journal of Translational Medicine*, *14*(1), 105. doi:10.118612967-016-0838-4 PMID:27118048

Al-Hourani, B. J., Sharma, S. K., Mane, J. Y., Tuszynski, J., Baracos, V., Kniess, T., ... Wuest, F. (2011). Synthesis and evaluation of 1,5-diaryl-substituted tetrazoles as novel selective cyclooxygenase-2 (COX-2) inhibitors. *Bioorganic & Medicinal Chemistry Letters*, *21*(6), 1823–1826. doi:10.1016/j.bmcl.2011.01.057 PMID:21316237

Al-Hussaini, M., & DiPersio, J. F. (2014). Small Molecule Inhibitors in Acute Myeloid Leukemia: From the Bench to the Clinic. *Expert Review of Hematology*, *7*(4), 439–464. doi:10.1586/17474086.2014.932687 PMID:25025370

Allemang, D., & Hendler, J. (2008). *Semantic Web for the Working Ontologist: Effective Modelling in RDFS and OWL*. Morgan Kaufmann Publishers.

Allemang, D., & Hendler, J. (2011). *Semantic Web for the Working Ontologist* (2nd ed.). Morgan Kaufmann Publishers.

Allen, T. J., & Fusfeld, A. (1975). Research laboratory architecture and the structuring of communications. *R & D Management*, *5*(2), 153–163. doi:10.1111/j.1467-9310.1975.tb01230.x

Alper, P. B., Hendrix, M., Sears, P., & Wong, C. (1998). Probing the Specificity of Aminoglycoside–Ribosomal RNA Interactions with Designed Synthetic Analogs. *Journal of the American Chemical Society*, *120*(9), 1965–1978. doi:10.1021/ja972599h

Amadasi, A., Spyrakis, F., Cozzini, P., Abraham, D. J., Kellogg, G. E., & Mozzarelli, A. (2006). Mapping the energetics of water-protein and water-ligand interactions with the "natural" HINT forcefield: Predictive tools for characterizing the roles of water in biomolecules. *Journal of Molecular Biology*, *358*(1), 289–309. doi:10.1016/j.jmb.2006.01.053 PMID:16497327

Amadasi, A., Surface, J. A., Spyrakis, F., Cozzini, P., Mozzarelli, A., & Kellogg, G. E. (2008). Robust classification of "relevant" water molecules in putative protein binding sites. *Journal of Medicinal Chemistry*, *51*(4), 1063–1067. doi:10.1021/jm701023h PMID:18232647

Andersen, M. R., Almen, M. S., & Schioth, H. B. (2011). Trends in the exploitation of novel drug targets. *Nature Reviews. Drug Discovery*, *10*(8), 579–590. doi:10.1038/nrd3478 PMID:21804595

Anderson, C. G., & Yuji, T. (1992). Calculation of molecular surface area with numerical factors. *Computers & Chemistry*, *16*(4), 277–284. doi:10.1016/0097-8485(92)80047-4

Anderson, V. R., & Perry, C. M. (2007). Fludarabine: A review of its use in non-Hodgkin's lymphoma. *Drugs*, *67*(11), 1633–1655. doi:10.2165/00003495-200767110-00008 PMID:17661532

Andersson, R., Gebhard, C., Miguel-Escalada, I., Hoof, I., Bornholdt, J., Boyd, M., ... Sandelin, A. (2014). An atlas of active enhancers across human cell types and tissues. *Nature*, *507*(7493), 455–461. doi:10.1038/nature12787 PMID:24670763

Andersson, S., Armstrong, A., Bjore, A., Bowker, S., Chapman, S., Davies, R., ... Whittamore, P. (2009). Making medicinal chemistry more effective – application of lean sigma to improve processes, speed and quality. *Drug Discovery Today*, *14*(11-12), 598–604. doi:10.1016/j.drudis.2009.03.005 PMID:19508922

Andrea, T. A., & Kalayeh, H. (1991). Applications of neural networks in quantitative structure-activity-relationships of dihydrofolate-reductase inhibitors. *Journal of Medicinal Chemistry*, *34*(9), 2824–2836. doi:10.1021/jm00113a022 PMID:1895302

Andrew, L. H., & Colin, R. G. (2002). The druggable genome. *Nature Reviews. Drug Discovery*, *1*(9), 727–730. doi:10.1038/nrd892 PMID:12209152

Andrew, R. L. (2001). *Molecular Modelling Principles and Applications*. Pearson Education Limited.

Andrews, C. W., Bennett, L., & Yu, L. X. (2000). Predicting human oral bioavailability of a compound: Development of a novel quantitative structure-bioavailability relationship. *Pharmaceutical Research*, *17*(6), 639–644. doi:10.1023/A:1007556711109 PMID:10955834

Antoniou, G., & Harmelen, F. V. (2008). *A Semantic Web Primer* (2nd ed.). The MIT Press.

Araz, Jac., & Bayly. (2002). Fast, Efficient Generation of High-Quality Atomic Charges. AM1-BCC Model: II. Parameterization and Validation. *Journal of Computational Chemistry*, *23*(16), 1623–41.

Arkin, M. R., & Wells, J. A. (2004). Small-molecule inhibitors of protein-protein interactions: Progressing towards the dream. *Nature Reviews. Drug Discovery*, *3*(4), 301–317. doi:10.1038/nrd1343 PMID:15060526

Arono, V. A. M. (2005). Predictive *in silico* modeling for hERG channel blockers. *Drug Discovery Today*, *10*(2), 149–155. doi:10.1016/S1359-6446(04)03278-7 PMID:15718164

Arrowsmith, J. (2011). Phase II failures: 2008–2010. *Nature Reviews. Drug Discovery*, *10*(5), 328–329. doi:10.1038/nrd3439 PMID:21532551

Arrowsmith, J., & Miller, P. (2013). Trial Watch: Phase II and Phase III attrition rates 2011–2012. *Nature Reviews. Drug Discovery*, *12*(8), 569. doi:10.1038/nrd4090 PMID:23903212

Ashraf, M. I., Ong, S. K., Mujawar, S., Pawar, S., More, P., Paul, S., & Lahiri, C. (2018). A side-effect free method for identifying cancer drug targets. *Scientific Reports*, 8. PMID:29703908

Asma Siddiqua, S. (2013). QBD- A Challenge to the Pharma Industry. International Journal of Innovative Pharmaceutical Sciences and Research, 23, 47-54.

Ayrton, A., & Morgan, P. (2001). The role of transport proteins in drug absorption, distribution and excretion. *Xenobiotica*, *31*(8-9), 469–497. doi:10.1080/00498250110060969 PMID:11569523

Baader, F., Calvanese, D., Mcguinness, D. L., Patel-Schneider, P., & Nardi, D. (2003). *The Description Logic Handbook: Theory, Implementation and Applications*. Cambridge University Press.

Bader, G. D., Betel, D., & Hogue, C. W. V. (2003). BIND: The Biomolecular Interaction Network Database. *Nucleic Acids Research*, *31*(1), 248–250. doi:10.1093/nar/gkg056 PMID:12519993

Bains, W., Gilbert, R., Sviridenko, L., Gascon, J. M., Scoffin, R., & Birchall, K. (2002). Evolutionary computational methods to predict oral bioavailability QSPRs. *Current Opinion in Drug Discovery & Development*, *5*, 44–51. PMID:11865672

Bajorath, J. (2002). Integration of virtual and high-throughput screening. *Nature Reviews. Drug Discovery*, *1*(11), 882–894. doi:10.1038/nrd941 PMID:12415248

Bakheet, T. M., & Doig, A. J. (2009). Properties and identification of human protein drug targets. *Bioinformatics (Oxford, England)*, *25*(4), 451–457. doi:10.1093/bioinformatics/btp002 PMID:19164304

Balasubramanian, S., Ramos, J., Luo, W., Sirisawad, M., Verner, E., & Buggy, J. J. (2008). A novel histone deacetylase 8 (HDAC8)-specific inhibitor PCI-34051 induces apoptosis in T-cell lymphomas. *Leukemia*, *22*(5), 1026–1034. doi:10.1038/leu.2008.9 PMID:18256683

Baldwin, E. L., & Osheroff, N. (2005). Etoposide, topoisomerase II and cancer. *Current Medicinal Chemistry. Anti-Cancer Agents*, *5*(4), 363–372. doi:10.2174/1568011054222364 PMID:16101488

Bali, A., Ohri, R., & Deb, P. K. (2012). Synthesis, evaluation and docking studies on 3-alkoxy-4-methanesulfonamido acetophenone derivatives as non-ulcerogenic anti-inflammatory agents. *European Journal of Medicinal Chemistry*, *49*, 397–405. doi:10.1016/j.ejmech.2012.01.018 PMID:22318166

Barabasi, A. L., Gulbahce, N., & Loscalzo, J. (2011). Network medicine: A network-based approach to human disease. *Nature Reviews. Genetics*, *12*(1), 56–68. doi:10.1038/nrg2918 PMID:21164525

Barbieri, D. F., Braga, D., Ceri, S., Valle, E. D., & Grossniklaus, M. (2010). C-Sparql: A Continuous Query Language for RDF Data Streams. *International Journal of Semantic Computing*, *4*(1), 3–25. doi:10.1142/S1793351X10000936

Barnash, K. D., James, L. I., & Frye, S. V. (2017). Target class drug discovery. *Nature Chemical Biology*, *13*(10), 1053–1056. doi:10.1038/nchembio.2473 PMID:28926557

Baxter, A., Bennion, C., Bent, J., Boden, K., Brough, S., Cooper, A., ... Unitt, J. (2003). Hit-to-lead studies: The discovery of potent, orally bioavailable triazolethiol CXCR2 receptor antagonists. *Bioorganic & Medicinal Chemistry Letters*, *13*(16), 2625–2628. doi:10.1016/S0960-894X(03)00561-4 PMID:12873480

Bechhofer, S. (2016). *Owl Web Ontology Reference*. Available: Https://Www.W3.Org/Tr/2004/Rec-Owl-Ref-20040210/

Beeler, A.B., Porco, J.A., Ingham, O.J. & Bradner, J.E. (2014). *Selective histone deacetylase 8 inhibitors*. PCT/US2014/012968.

Begley, D. J. (1996). The blood-brain barrier: Principles for targeting peptide and drugs to the central nervous system. *The Journal of Pharmacy and Pharmacology*, *48*(2), 136–140. doi:10.1111/j.2042-7158.1996.tb07112.x PMID:8935161

Bemporad, D., Luttmann, C., & Essex, J. W. (2005). Behaviour of small solutes and large drugs in a lipid bilayer from computer simulations. *Biochimica et Biophysica Acta Biomembranes*, *1718*(1-2), 1–21. doi:10.1016/j.bbamem.2005.07.009 PMID:16321606

Benfenati, E., Benigni, R., Demarini, D. M., Helma, C., Kirkland, D., Martin, T., ... Yang, C. (2009). Predictive models for carcinogenicity and mutagenicity: Frameworks, state-of-the-art, and perspectives. *Journal of Environmental Science and Health. Part C, Environmental Carcinogenesis & Ecotoxicology Reviews*, *27*(2), 57–90. doi:10.1080/10590500902885593 PMID:19412856

Benigni, R., Cotta-Ramusino, M., Giorgi, F. & Gallo, G. (1995). Molecular similarity matrices and quantitative structure-activity relationships: a case study with methodological implications. *Journal of Medicinal Chemistry*, *38*(4), 629-635.

Benigni, R., Battistelli, C. L., Bossa, C., Colafranceschi, M., & Tcheremenskaia, O. (2013). Mutagenicity, carcinogenicity, and other end points. In B. Reisfeld & A. N. Mayeno (Eds.), *Computational Toxicology* (Vol. 930, pp. 67–98). New York: Humana Press. doi:10.1007/978-1-62703-059-5_4

Bento, A. P., Gaulton, A., Hersey, A., Bellis, L. J., Chambers, J., Davies, M., ... Overington, J. P. (2014). The ChEMBL bioactivity database: An update. *Nucleic Acids Research*, *42*(Database issue), D1083–D1090. doi:10.1093/nar/gkt1031 PMID:24214965

Berezikov, E., Thuemmler, F., van Laake, L. W., Kondova, I., Bontrop, R., Cuppen, E., & Plasterk, R. H. A. (2006). Diversity of microRNAs in human and chimpanzee brain. *Nature Genetics*, *38*(12), 1375–1377. doi:10.1038/ng1914 PMID:17072315

Berners-Lee, T., Hendler, J., & Lassila, O. (2001). The Semantic Web. A New Form of Web Content That Is Meaningful to Computers Will Unleash a Revolution of New Possibilities. *Scientific American*, *284*, 1–5.

Betz, U. A., Farquhar, R., & Ziegelbauer, K. (2005). Genomics: Success or failure to deliver drug targets? *Current Opinion in Chemical Biology*, 9, 387–391. PMID:15990354

Bieliauskas, A. V., & Pflum, M. K. H. (2008). Isoform-selective histone deacetylase inhibitors. *Chemical Society Reviews*, *37*(7), 1402–1413. doi:10.1039/b703830p PMID:18568166

Birnbaumer, L., Abramowitz, J., & Brown, A. M. (1990). Receptor-effector coupling by G proteins. *Biochimica et Biophysica Acta Biomembranes*, *1031*(2), 163–224. doi:10.1016/0304-4157(90)90007-Y PMID:2160274

Bizer, C., Heath, T., & Berners-Lee, T. (2009). Linked Data, The Story so far. *International Journal on Semantic Web and Information Systems*, *5*(3), 1–22. doi:10.4018/jswis.2009081901

Blanco, R., Mika, P., & Vigna, S. (2011, October). Effective and Efficient Entity Search in RDF Data. *Proceedings of the 10th International Conference on the Semantic Web (Iswc'11)*. 10.1007/978-3-642-25073-6_6

Blat, Y., & Kleckner, N. (1999). Cohesins bind to preferential sites along yeast chromosome III, with differential regulation along arms versus the centric region. *Cell*, *98*(2), 249–259. doi:10.1016/S0092-8674(00)81019-3 PMID:10428036

Bleckmann, A., & Meiler, J. (2003). Quantitative structure activity relations studied by support vector machines and artificial neural networks. *QSAR & Combinatorial Science*, *22*(7), 722–728. doi:10.1002/qsar.200330837

Bleicher, K. H., Bohm, H. J., Muller, K., & Alanine, A. I. (2003). Hit and lead generation: Beyond high-throughput screening. *Nature Reviews. Drug Discovery*, *2*(5), 369–378. doi:10.1038/nrd1086 PMID:12750740

Boehm, H. J., Boehringer, M., Bur, D., Gmuender, H., Huber, W., Klaus, W., ... Mueller, F. (2000). Novel inhibitors of DNA gyrase: 3-D structure based biased needle screening, hit validation by biophysical methods, and 3-D guided optimization A promising alternative to random screening. *Journal of Medicinal Chemistry*, *43*(14), 2664–2674. doi:10.1021/jm000017s PMID:10893304

Bohacek, R. S., & McMartin, C. (1994). Multiple highly diverse structures complementary to enzyme binding sites: Results of extensive application of a *de novo* design method incorporating combinatorial growth. *Journal of the American Chemical Society*, *116*(13), 5560–5571. doi:10.1021/ja00092a006

Bohm, H. (1994). The development of a simple empirical scoring function to estimate the binding constant for a protein-ligand complex of known three-dimensional structure. *Journal of Computer-Aided Molecular Design*, *8*, 243–256. doi:10.1007/BF00126743 PMID:7964925

Bolden, J. E., Peart, M. J., & Johnstone, R. W. (2006). Anticancer activities of histone deacetylase inhibitors. *Nature Reviews. Drug Discovery*, *5*(9), 769–784. doi:10.1038/nrd2133 PMID:16955068

Bolis, G., Dipace, L., & Fabrocini, F. (1991). A machine learning approach to computer-aided molecular design. *Journal of Computational Methods in Molecular Design*, *5*(6), 617–628. doi:10.1007/BF00135318 PMID:1818094

Bologa, C. G., Revankar, C. M., Young, S. M., Edwards, B. S., Arterburn, J. B., Kiselyov, A. S., ... Prossnitz, E. R. (2006). Virtual and biomolecular screening converge on a selective agonist for GPR30. *Nature Chemical Biology*, *2*(4), 207–212. doi:10.1038/nchembio775 PMID:16520733

Boobis, A., Gundert-Remy, U., Kremers, P., Macheras, P., & Pelkonen, O. (2002). *In silico* prediction of ADME and pharmacokinetics. Report of an expert meeting organised by COST B15. *European Journal of Pharmaceutical Sciences*, *17*(4-5), 183–193. doi:10.1016/S0928-0987(02)00185-9 PMID:12453607

Borrotti, M., De March, D., Slanzi, D., & Poli, I. (2013). Designing Lead Optimization of MMP-12 Inhibitors. Computational and Mathematical Methods in Medicine. *Article ID*, *258627*. doi:10.1155/2014/258627

Bourne, P. E., & Weissig, H. (2005). *Structural Bioinformatics*. Hoboken, NJ: John Wiley & Sons, Inc.

Brenk, R., Naerum, L., Grädler, U., Gerber, H. D., Garcia, G. A., Reuter, K., ... Klebe, G. (2003). Virtual screening for sub micromolar leads of tRNA-guanine transglycosylase based on new unexpected binding model detected by crystal structure analysis. *Journal of Medicinal Chemistry*, *46*(7), 1133–1143. doi:10.1021/jm0209937 PMID:12646024

Brickley, D., & Guha, R. V. (2004). *RDF Vocabulary Description Language 1.0: Schema.* W3c Recommendation.

Brickley, D., & Miller, L. (2005). FOAF Vocabulary Specification. *Namespace Document.* Retrieved from Http://Xmlns.Com/Foaf/0.1

Brooks, B. R., Bruccoleri, R. E., Olafson, B. D., States, D. J., Swaminathan, S., & Karplus, M. (1983). CHARMM: A program for macromolecular energy, minimization and dynamics calculations. *Journal of Computational Chemistry*, *4*(2), 187–217. doi:10.1002/jcc.540040211

Brooks, W. H., Guida, W. C., & Daniel, K. G. (2011). The significance of chirality in drug design and development. *Current Topics in Medicinal Chemistry*, *11*(7), 760–770. doi:10.2174/156802611795165098 PMID:21291399

Buchan, N. S., Rajpal, D. K., Webster, Y., Alatorre, C., Gudivada, R. C., Sanseau, P., & .... (2011). The role of translational bioinformatics in drug discovery. *Drug Discovery Today*, *16*(9-10), 426–434. doi:10.1016/j.drudis.2011.03.002 PMID:21402166

Buchwald, P., & Bodor, N. (2002). Computer aided drug design: The role of quantitative structure-property, structure-activity and structure-metabolism relationships (QSPR, QSAR, QSMR). *Drugs of the Future*, *15*(6), 577–588. doi:10.1358/dof.2002.027.06.856934

Buckingham, J., Glen, R. C., Hill, A. P., Hyde, R. M., Martin, G. R., Robertson, A. D., ... Woollard, P. M. (1995). Computer-Aided Design and Synthesis of 5-Substituted Tryptamines and Their Pharmacology at the 5-HT1D Receptor: Discovery of Compounds with Potential Anti-Migraine Properties. *Journal of Medicinal Chemistry*, *38*(18), 3566–3580. doi:10.1021/jm00018a016 PMID:7658443

Buggy, J. J., Sideris, M. L., Mak, P., Lorimer, D. D., McIntosh, B., & Clark, J. M. (2000). Cloning and characterization of a novel human histone deacetylase, HDAC8. *The Biochemical Journal*, *350*(1), 199–205. doi:10.1042/bj3500199 PMID:10926844

Burgess, A., Ruefli, A., Beamish, H., Warrener, R., Saunders, N., Johnstone, R., & Gabrielli, B. (2004). Histone deacetylase inhibitors specifically kill nonproliferating tumour cells. *Oncogene*, *23*(40), 6693–6701. doi:10.1038j.onc.1207893 PMID:15235588

Butcher, E. C. (2005). Can cell systems biology rescue drug discovery? *Nature Reviews. Drug Discovery*, *4*(6), 461–467. doi:10.1038/nrd1754 PMID:15915152

Camenisch, G., Folkers, G., & van de Waterbeemd, H. (1996). Review of theoretical passive drug absorption models: Historical background, recent developments and limitations. *Pharmaceutica Acta Helvetiae*, *71*(5), 309–327. doi:10.1016/S0031-6865(96)00031-3 PMID:8973162

Carroll, J. J., & Klyne, G. (2004). *Resource Description Framework (RDF): Concepts And Abstract Syntax.* W3c Recommendation.

Castaneda, C., Nalley, K., Mannion, C., Bhattacharyya, P., Blake, P., Pecora, A., ... Suh, K. S. (2015). Clinical Decision Support Systems for Improving Diagnostic Accuracy and Achieving Precision Medicine. *Journal of Clinical Bioinformatics*, *5*(4), 1–16. PMID:25834725

Cavasotto, C. N., & Phatak, S. S. (2009). Homology modeling in drug discovery: Current trends and applications. *Drug Discovery Today*, *14*(13-14), 676–683. doi:10.1016/j.drudis.2009.04.006 PMID:19422931

Centerwatch. (2007). *Drugs approved by the FDA*. Retrieved from http://www.centerwatch.com/patient/drugs/druglist.html

Chakkarwar, V. A., & Joshi, A. A. (2016). Semantic Web Mining Using Rdf Data. *International Journal of Computers and Applications*, *133*(10), 14–19. doi:10.5120/ijca2016908022

Chan, C. C., Boyce, S., Brideau, C., Charleson, S., Cromlish, W., Ethier, D., ... Riendeau, D. (1999). Rofecoxib(Vioxx, MK-0966; 4-(4′-methylsulfonylphenyl)-3-phenyl-2(5H)-furanone): A potent and orally active cyclooxygenase-2 inhibitor. Pharmacological and biochemical profiles. *The Journal of Pharmacology and Experimental Therapeutics*, *290*, 551–560. PMID:10411562

Chandramohan Reddy, T., Aparoy, P., Kishore Babu, N., Anil Kumar, K., Kumar Kalangi, S., & Reddanna, P. (2010). Kinetics and docking studies of a COX-2 inhibitor isolated form terminalia bellerica fruits. *Protein and Peptide Letters*, *17*(10), 1251–1257. doi:10.2174/092986610792231537 PMID:20441561

Changxiao, L., Panayiotis, P. C., & Yazhuo, L. (2014). Research and development in drug innovation: Reflections from the 2013 bioeconomy conference in China, lessons learned and future perspectives. *Acta Pharmaceutica Sinica. B*, *4*(2), 112–119. doi:10.1016/j.apsb.2014.01.002 PMID:26579372

Charifson, P. S., Corkerey, J. J., Murcko, M. A., & Walters, W. P. (1999). Consensus scoring: A method for obtaining improved hit rates from docking databases of three-dimensional structures into proteins. *Journal of Medicinal Chemistry*, *42*(25), 5100–5109. doi:10.1021/jm990352k PMID:10602695

Chatonnet, A., Krejci, E., Duval, N., Vincens, P., & Massoulie, J. (1991). Cholinesterase-like domains in enzymes and structural proteins: Functional and evolutionary relationships and identification of a catalytically essential aspartic acid. *Proceedings of the National Academy of Sciences of the United States of America*, *88*(15), 6647–6651. doi:10.1073/pnas.88.15.6647 PMID:1862088

Chatr-aryamontri, A., Ceol, A., Palazzi, L. M., Nardelli, G., Schneider, M. V., Castagnoli, L., & Cesareni, G. (2007). MINT: The Molecular INTeraction database. *Nucleic Acids Research*, *35*(Database), D572–D574. doi:10.1093/nar/gkl950 PMID:17135203

Chaturvedi, P. R., Decker, C. J., & Odinecs, A. (2001). Prediction of pharmacokinetic properties using experimental approaches during early drug discovery. *Current Opinion in Chemical Biology*, *5*(4), 452–463. doi:10.1016/S1367-5931(00)00228-3 PMID:11470610

Chaudhary, P., Sharma, P. K., Sharma, A., & Varshney, J. (2010). Recent AdvancesIn Pharmacological Activity Of Benzothiazole Derivatives. *International Journal of Current Pharmaceutical Research*, *4*, 5–11.

ChEMBL. (n.d.a). Retrieved February 10, 2018, from https://www.ebi.ac.uk/chembl/

ChEMBL. (n.d.b). Retrieved February 15, 2018, from ftp://ftp.ebi.ac.uk/pub/databases/chembl/ChEMBLdb/releases/chembl_23/chembl_23_release_notes.txt

Chem-X version 96. (2001). Oxford Molecular Group, Inc.

Chen, Duan, Zhang, & Zhang. (2016). Survivin and tumorigenesis: molecular mechanism and therapeutic strategies. *Journal of Cancer, 7*(3), 314-323.

Cheng, A., & Dixon, S. L. (2003). In silico models for the prediction of dose-dependent human hepatotoxicity. *Journal of Computer-Aided Molecular Design*, *17*(12), 811–823. doi:10.1023/B:JCAM.0000021834.50768.c6 PMID:15124930

Cheng, A., & Merz, K. (2003). Prediction of aqueous solubility of a diverse set of compounds using quantitative structure-property relationships. *Journal of Medicinal Chemistry*, *46*(17), 3572–3580. doi:10.1021/jm020266b PMID:12904062

Chen, L. S., Nowak, B. J., Ayres, M. L., Krett, N. L., Rosen, S. T., Zhang, S., & Gandhi, V. (2009). Inhibition of ATP synthase by chlorinated adenosine analogue. *Biochemical Pharmacology*, *78*(6), 583–591. doi:10.1016/j.bcp.2009.05.019 PMID:19477165

Chen, Z., Li, H. L., Zhang, Q. J., Bao, X. G., Yu, K. Q., Luo, X. M., ... Jiang, H. (2009). Pharmacophore-based virtual screening versus docking-based virtual screening: A benchmark comparison against eight targets. *Acta Pharmacologica Sinica*, *30*(12), 1694–1708. doi:10.1038/aps.2009.159 PMID:19935678

Choi, S. E., & Pflum, M. K. H. (2012). The structural requirements of histone deacetylase inhibitors: Suberoyl anilide hydroxamic acid analogs modified at the C6 position. *Bioorganic & Medicinal Chemistry Letters*, *22*(23), 7084–7086. doi:10.1016/j.bmcl.2012.09.093 PMID:23089527

Choi, S. E., Weerasinghe, S. V. W., & Pflum, M. K. H. (2011). The structural requirements of histone deacetylase inhibitors: Suberoyl anilide hydroxamic acid analogues modified at the C3 position display isoform selectivity. *Bioorganic & Medicinal Chemistry Letters*, *21*(20), 6139–6142. doi:10.1016/j.bmcl.2011.08.027 PMID:21889343

Chopra, M., Beswick, H., Clapperton, M., Dargie, H. J., Smith, W. E., & McMurray, J. (1992). Antioxidant effects of angiotensin-converting enzyme (ACE) inhibitors: Free radical and oxidant scavenging are sulfhydrl dependent, but lipid peroxidation is inhibited by both sulfhydryl-and non sulfhydryl-containing ACE inhibitors. *Journal of Cardiovascular Pharmacology*, *19*(3), 330–340. doi:10.1097/00005344-199203000-00005 PMID:1378110

Christen, M., Hunenberger, P. H., Bakowies, D., Baron, R., Burgi, R., Geerke, D. P., ... van Gunsteren, W. F. (2005). The GROMOS software for biomolecular simulation: GROMOS05. *Journal of Computational Chemistry*, *26*(16), 1719–1751. doi:10.1002/jcc.20303 PMID:16211540

Christopher, S. (1999). The role of cyclooxygenases in inflammation, cancer, and development. *Oncogene*, *18*(55), 7908–7916. doi:10.1038j.onc.1203286 PMID:10630643

Citeline Pharma R&D annual review. (2014). Retrieved from http://maxicool5.free.fr/Bourse/Valo%20Pharma/Annual-Review-2014b.pdf

Clark, D. E. (2003). *In silico* prediction of blood-brain barrier permeation. *Drug Discovery Today*, *8*(20), 927–933. doi:10.1016/S1359-6446(03)02827-7 PMID:14554156

Clark, D. E., Frenkel, D., Levy, S. A., Li, J., Murray, C. W., & Robson, B. (1995). PRO_LIGAND: An approach to *de novo* Drug Design. *Journal of Computer-Aided Molecular Design*, *9*, 13–32. doi:10.1007/BF00117275 PMID:7751867

Clark, R. D., Strizhev, A., Leonard, J. M., Blake, J. F., & Matthew, J. B. (2002). Consensus scoring for ligand/protein interactions. *Journal of Molecular Graphics & Modelling*, *20*(4), 281–295. doi:10.1016/S1093-3263(01)00125-5 PMID:11858637

Claussen, H., Buning, C., Rarey, M., & Lengauer, T. (2001). FlexE: Efficient molecular docking considering protein structure variations. *Journal of Molecular Biology*, *308*(2), 377–395. doi:10.1006/jmbi.2001.4551 PMID:11327774

Cole, C. J., & Pfund, W. P. (2000). Permeability Assays. *Modern Drug Discovery*, *3*, 73–76.

Comes, K. M., & Schurdak, M. E. (2004). Affinity-based screening techniques for enhancing lead discovery. *Current Opinion in Drug Discovery & Development*, *7*, 411–416. PMID:15338950

Conesa, A., Madrigal, P., Tarazona, S., Gomez-Cabrero, D., Cervera, A., McPherson, A., ... Mortazavi, A. (2016). A survey of best practices for RNA-seq data analysis. *Genome Biology*, *17*(1), 13. doi:10.118613059-016-0881-8 PMID:26813401

Congressional Budget Office (CBO) study. (2016). *Research and Development in the Pharmaceutical Industry*. Retrieved from https://www.cbo.gov/sites/default/files/109th-congress-2005-2006/reports/10-02-drugr-d.pdf

Congressional Budget Office (CBO) study. (n.d.). *Research and Development in the Pharmaceutical Industry*. Retrieved from https://www.cbo.gov/sites/default/files/109th-congress-2005-2006/reports/10-02-drugr-d.pdf

Congreve, M. S. (2003). Detection of ligands from a dynamic combinatorial library by X-ray crystallography. Angewandate Chemie (International Ed. in English), 42, 4479–4482.

Cooper, T., & Cramer, K. A. (n.d.). Designed chemical libraries for hit/lead optimization. *Innovations in Pharmaceutical Technology*, 46-53. Retrieved from http://www.iptonline.com/articles/public/iptfive46np.pdf

Copeland, R. A. (2013). Why Enzymes as Drug Targets? In *Evaluation of Enzyme Inhibitors in Drug Discovery: A Guide for Medicinal Chemists and Pharmacologists* (2nd ed.). Hoboken, NJ: John Wiley & Sons, Inc.; doi:10.1002/9781118540398.ch1

Copeland, R. A., Pompliano, D. L., & Meek, T. D. (2006). Drug–target residence time and its implications for lead optimization. *Perspectives*, *5*, 730–740. PMID:16888652

Corcoglioniti, F., Rospocher, M., & Aprosio, A. P. (2016). Frame-Based Ontology Population with Pikes. *IEEE Transactions on Knowledge and Data Engineering*, *28*(12), 3261–3275. doi:10.1109/TKDE.2016.2602206

Cornell, W. D., Cieplak, P., Bayly, C. I., Gould, I. R., Merz, K. M., Ferguson, D. M., ... Kollman, P. A. (1995). A second generation force field for the simulation of proteins, nucleic acids, and organic molecules. *Journal of the American Chemical Society*, *117*(19), 5179–5197. doi:10.1021/ja00124a002

Cruciani, G., Crivori, P., Carrupt, P. A., & Testa, B. (2000). Molecular fields in quantitative structure-permeation relationships: The VolSurf approach. *Theochem*, *53*(1-2), 17–30. doi:10.1016/S0166-1280(99)00360-7

da Silva, C., da Silva, E. C., & Nascimento, M. A. C. (1999). Ab Initio Calculations of Absolute pKa Values in Aqueous Solution I. Carboxylic Acids. *The Journal of Physical Chemistry A*, *103*(50), 11194–11199. doi:10.1021/jp9836473

Dai, Y., Guo, Y., Curtin, M. L., Li, J., Pease, L. J., Guo, J., ... Michaelides, M. R. (2003). A novel series of histone deacetylase inhibitors incorporating hetero aromatic ring systems as connection units. *Bioorganic & Medicinal Chemistry Letters*, *13*(21), 3817–3820. doi:10.1016/j.bmcl.2003.07.012 PMID:14552787

Damanhouri & Ahmad. (2014). A review on therapeutic potential of *Piper nigrum* L. (Black Pepper): The king of spices. *Medicinal & Aromatic Plants*, *3*(3), 1–6.

David, C. Y. (2009). *Computational Drug Design*. Hoboken, NJ: John Wiley & Sons.

David, E. G. (2008). Gerber Targeted Therapies: A New Generation of Cancer Treatments. *American Family Physician*, *77*(3), 311–319. PMID:18297955

David, E., Tramontin, T., & Zemmel, R. (2009). Pharmaceutical R&D: The road to positive returns. *Nature Reviews. Drug Discovery*, *8*(8), 609–610. doi:10.1038/nrd2948 PMID:19644471

Davidson, B. L., & McCray, P. B. Jr. (2011). Current prospects for RNA interference based therapies. *Nature Reviews. Genetics*, *12*(5), 329–340. doi:10.1038/nrg2968 PMID:21499294

Davies, M. N., Secker, A., Freitas, A. A., Mendao, M., Timmis, J., & Flower, D. R. (2007). On the hierarchical classification of G protein-coupled receptors. *Bioinformatics (Oxford, England)*, *23*(23), 3113–3118. doi:10.1093/bioinformatics/btm506 PMID:17956878

de Klerk, E., Venema, A., Anvar, S. Y., Goeman, J. J., Hu, O., Trollet, C., ... 't Hoen, P. A. C. (2012). Poly (A) binding protein nuclear 1 levels affect alternative polyadenylation. *Nucleic Acids Research*, *40*(18), 9089–9101. doi:10.1093/nar/gks655 PMID:22772983

Debouck, C., & Metcalf, B. (2000). The impact of genomics on drug discovery. *Annual Review of Pharmacology and Toxicology*, *40*(1), 193–207. doi:10.1146/annurev.pharmtox.40.1.193 PMID:10836133

Deepali, G., Gauri, S., & Ashish, M. (2016). Re-thinking drug discovery: *In silico* method. *Journal of Chemical and Pharmaceutical Research*, *8*(8), 1092–1099.

Defne, K. T. (2013). Quality by Design for Wet Granulation in Pharmaceutical processing: Assessing Models for a Priori Design and Scaling. Powder Technology, 240, 7-8.

Delasko, J.M., Cocchetto, D.M., & Burke, L.B. (2005). *Target Product Profile: Beginning Drug Development with the End in Mind*. Academic Press.

Delcuve, G. P., Khan, D. H., & Davie, J. R. (2013). Targeting class I histone deacetylases in cancer therapy. *Expert Opinion on Therapeutic Targets*, *17*(1), 29–41. doi:10.1517/14728222.2013.729042 PMID:23062071

Deprez, B., & Deprez-Poulain, R. (2006). Trends in hit-to-lead:an update. *Frontiers in Medicinal Chemistry*, *3*, 653–673.

DeRisi, J., Penland, L., Bittner, M., Meltzer, P., Ray, M., Chen, Y., & … . (1996). Use of a cDNA microarray to analyse gene expression. *Nature Genetics*, *14*(4), 457–460. doi:10.1038/ng1296-457 PMID:8944026

Devillers, J. (2013). Methods for building QSARs. In B. Reisfeld & A. N. Mayeno (Eds.), *Computational Toxicology* (pp. 3–27). New York: Humana Press.

DeWitt, R. & SMOG. (1997). *de novo* design method based on simple, fast, and accurate free energy estimates 2 case studies in molecular design. *J Am Chem Soc, 119*, 4608-17.

Dhivyan, M. A. J. E., & Anoop, M. N. (n.d.). *Virtual screening and lead optimization to identify novel inhibitors for HDAC-8*. Retrieved from https://arxiv.org/abs/1209.2793

Dickson, M., & Gagnon, J. P. (2004). Key factors in the rising cost of new drug discovery and development. *Nature Reviews. Drug Discovery*, *3*(5), 417–429. doi:10.1038/nrd1382 PMID:15136789

Dijkhorst-Oei, L. T., Stroes, E. S., Koomans, H. A., & Rabenlink, T. J. (1999). Acute simultaneous stimulation of nitric oxide and oxygen radicals by angiotensin II in humans invivo. *Journal of Cardiovascular Pharmacology*, *33*(3), 420–424. doi:10.1097/00005344-199903000-00012 PMID:10069678

DiMasi, J. A. (2002). The value of improving the productivity of the drug development process. *PharmacoEconomics*, *20*(S3), 1–10.

DiMasi, J. A. (2001). Risks in new drug development: Approval success rates for investigational drugs. *Clinical Pharmacology and Therapeutics*, *69*(5), 297–307. doi:10.1067/mcp.2001.115446 PMID:11371997

DiMasi, J. A., Feldman, L., Seckler, A., & Wilson, A. (2010). Trends in risks associated with new drug development: Success rates for investigational drugs. *Clinical Pharmacology and Therapeutics*, *87*(3), 272–277. doi:10.1038/clpt.2009.295 PMID:20130567

DiMasi, J. A., Hansen, R. W., Grabowski, H. G., & Lasagna, L. (1991). Cost of innovation in the pharmaceutical industry. *Journal of Health Economics*, *10*(2), 107–142. doi:10.1016/0167-6296(91)90001-4 PMID:10113009

DiMasi, J., Hansen, R., & Grabowski, H. (2003). The price of innovation: New estimates of drug development costs. *Journal of Health Economics*, *22*(2), 151–185. doi:10.1016/S0167-6296(02)00126-1 PMID:12606142

Doman, T. N., McGovern, S. L., Witherbee, B. J., Kasten, T. P., Kurumbail, R., Stallings, W. C., ... Shoichet, B. K. (2002). Molecular docking and high-throughput screening for novel inhibitors of protein tyrosine phosphatase-1B. *Journal of Medicinal Chemistry*, *45*(11), 2213–2221. doi:10.1021/jm010548w PMID:12014959

Domenico, F. (2015). Hypothesis for changing models: Current pharmaceutical paradigms, trends and approaches in drug discovery. *PeerJ PrePrints, 813*(1).

Doniger, S., Hofmann, T., & Yeh, J. (2002). Predicting CNS permeability of drug molecules: Comparison of neural network and support vector machine algorithms. *Journal of Computational Biology, 9*(6), 849–864. doi:10.1089/10665270260518317 PMID:12614551

Douguet, D., Thoreau, E., & Grassy, G. A. (2000). Genetic algorithm for the automated generation of small organic molecules: Drug Design using an evolutionary algorithm. *Journal of Computer-Aided Molecular Design, 14*(5), 449–466. doi:10.1023/A:1008108423895 PMID:10896317

Dowling, D. P., Gantt, S. L., Gattis, S. G., Fierke, C. A., & Christianson, D. W. (2008). Structural studies of human histone deacetylase 8 and its site-specific variants complexed with substrate and inhibitors. *Biochemistry, 47*(51), 13554–13563. doi:10.1021/bi801610c PMID:19053282

Drews, J. (2000). Drug discovery: A historical perspective. *Science, 287*(5460), 1960–1964. doi:10.1126cience.287.5460.1960 PMID:10720314

Dror, O., Shulman-Peleg, A., Nussinov, R., & Wolfson, H. J. (2004). Predicting molecular interactions in silico: I. A guide to pharmacophore identification and its applications to drug design. *Current Medicinal Chemistry, 11*(1), 71–90. doi:10.2174/0929867043456287 PMID:14754427

Drug Discovery and Development. (n.d.). Retrieved from http://www.slideshare.net/anisha88shah/rd-brochure

DRUGBANK. (n.d.). Retrieved from https://www.drugbank.ca/

Dubois, R. N., & Abramson, S. B. (1998). Cyclooxygenase in biology and disease. *The FASEB Journal, 12*(12), 1063–1073. doi:10.1096/fasebj.12.12.1063 PMID:9737710

Ducharme & Bob. (2011). *Learning Sparql.* O'Reilly Media, Inc.

Du-Cuny, L., Son, Z., Moses, S., Powis, G., Mas, E. A., Meuillet, E. J., & Zhang, S. (2009). Computational MODELLING of novel inhibitors targeting the Aktpleckstrin homology domain. *Bioorganic & Medicinal Chemistry, 17*(19), 6983–6992. doi:10.1016/j.bmc.2009.08.022 PMID:19734051

Dudek, A. Z., Arodz, T., & Galvez, J. (2006). Computational methods in developing quantitative structure–activity relationships (QSAR): A review. *Combinatorial Chemistry & High Throughput Screening, 9*(3), 213–228. doi:10.2174/138620706776055539 PMID:16533155

Duncia, J. V., Chiu, A. T., Carini, D. J., Gregory, G. B., Johnson, A. L., Price, W. A., ... Timmermans, P. B. M. W. M. (1990). The discovery of potent nonpeptide angiotensin II receptor antagonists: A new class of potent antihypertensives. *Journal of Medicinal Chemistry, 33*(5), 1312–1329. doi:10.1021/jm00167a007 PMID:2329553

Dunne, A., Jowett, M., & Rees, S. (2009). Use of primary cells in high throughput screens. *Methods in Molecular Biology (Clifton, N.J.), 565*, 239–257. doi:10.1007/978-1-60327-258-2_12 PMID:19551366

Durham, S. K., & Pearl, G. M. (2001). Computational methods to predict drug safety liabilities. *Drug Disc Dev, 4*, 110–115. PMID:11727316

Durrant, J. D., & McCammon, J. A. (2011). Molecular dynamics simulations and drug discovery. *BMC Biology, 9*(1), 71. doi:10.1186/1741-7007-9-71 PMID:22035460

Durst, K. L., Lutterbach, B., Kummalue, T., Friedman, A. D., & Hiebert, S. W. (2003). The inv (16) fusion protein associates with corepressors via a smooth muscle myosin heavy-chain domain. *Molecular and Cellular Biology*, *23*(2), 607–619. doi:10.1128/MCB.23.2.607-619.2003 PMID:12509458

Duvic, M., Talpur, R., Ni, X., Zhang, C., Hazarika, P., Kelly, C., ... Frankel, S. R. (2007). Phase 2 trial of oral vorinostat (suberoylanilide hydroxamic acid, SAHA) for refractory cutaneous T-cell lymphoma (CTCL). *Blood*, *109*(1), 31–39. doi:10.1182/blood-2006-06-025999 PMID:16960145

Ecker, D. J., & Griffey, R. H. (1999). RNA as a small-molecule drug target: Doubling the value of genomics. *Drug Discovery Today*, *4*(9), 420–429. doi:10.1016/S1359-6446(99)01389-6 PMID:10461152

Egan, W. J., & Lauri, G. (2002). Prediction of intestinal permeability. *Advanced Drug Delivery Reviews*, *54*(3), 273–289. doi:10.1016/S0169-409X(02)00004-2 PMID:11922948

Egan, W. J., Merz, K. M., & Baldwin, J. J. (2000). Prediction of Drug Absorption Using Multivariate Statistics. *Journal of Medicinal Chemistry*, *43*(21), 3867–3877. doi:10.1021/jm000292e PMID:11052792

Ehrhardt, P. W. (1999). *Drug Metabolism Databases and High–Throughput Testing During Drug Design and Development. Blackwell Science.*

Eisen, M. B., Wiley, D. C., Karplus, M., & Hubbard, R. E. (1994). HOOK: A program for finding novel molecular architectures that satisfy the chemical and steric requirements of a macromolecule binding site. *Proteins*, *19*(3), 199–221. doi:10.1002/prot.340190305 PMID:7937734

Ekins, S., Bravi, G., Binkley, S., Gillespie, J. S., Ring, B. J., & Wikel, J. H. (2000). Three- and four-dimensional quantitative structure-activity relationship (3D/4D-QSAR) analyses of CYP2C9 inhibitors. *Drug Metabolism and Disposition: the Biological Fate of Chemicals*, *28*, 994–1002. PMID:10901712

Ekins, S., De Groot, M., & Jones, J. P. (2001). Pharmacophore and three-dimensional quantitative structure-activity relationship methods for modeling cytochrome P450 active sites. *Drug Metabolism and Disposition: the Biological Fate of Chemicals*, *29*, 936–944. PMID:11408357

Ekins, S., Kim, R. B., Leake, B. F., Dantzig, A. H., Schuetz, E. G., Lan, L. B., & .... (2002). Three-dimensional quantitative structure-activity relationships of inhibitors of P-glycoprotein. *Molecular Pharmacology*, *61*(5), 964–973. doi:10.1124/mol.61.5.964 PMID:11961113

Ekins, S., Mestres, J., & Testa, B. (2007). *In silico* pharmacology for drug discovery: Methods for virtual ligand screening and profiling. *British Journal of Pharmacology*, *152*(1), 9–20. doi:10.1038j.bjp.0707305 PMID:17549047

Ekins, S., Ring, B. J., Grace, J., McRobie-Belle, D. J., & Wrighton, S. A. (2000). Present and further *in vitro* approaches for drug metabolism. *Journal of Pharmacological and Toxicological Methods*, *44*(1), 313–324. doi:10.1016/S1056-8719(00)00110-6 PMID:11274898

Ekins, S., & Wang, B. (2006). *Computer Applications in Pharmaceutical Research and Development*. Wiley-Interscience. doi:10.1002/0470037237

Eldridge, M. D., Murray, C. W., Auton, T. R., Paolini, G. V., & Mee, R. P. (1997). Empirical scoring functions: I. The development of a fast empirical scoring function to estimate the binding affinity of ligands in receptor complexes. *Journal of Computer-Aided Molecular Design*, *11*(5), 425–445. doi:10.1023/A:1007996124545 PMID:9385547

eMolecule. (n.d.a). Retrieved February 25, 2018, from https://www.emolecules.com/

eMolecule. (n.d.b). Retrieved February 25, 2018, from https://www.emolecules.com/info/support-intro-to-searching.html

eMolecule. (n.d.c). Retrieved February 25, 2018, from https://www.emolecules.com/info/products-data-downloads.html

Englebienne, P., & Moitessier, N. (2009). Docking ligands into flexible and solvated macromolecules. 5. Force-field-based prediction of binding affinities of ligands to proteins. *Journal of Chemical Information and Modeling*, *49*(11), 2564–2571. doi:10.1021/ci900251k PMID:19928836

Enslein, K., Gombar, V. K., & Blake, B. W. (1994). Internation commission for protection against environmental mutagens and carcinogens. Use of SAR in computer-assisted prediction of carcinogenicity and mutagenicity of chemicals by the TOPKAT program. *Mutation Research*, *305*, 47–61. doi:10.1016/0027-5107(94)90125-2 PMID:7508547

Enyedy, I. J., Sakamuri, S., Zaman, W. A., Johnson, K. M., & Wang, S. M. (2003). Pharmacophore-based discovery of substituted pyridines as novel dopamine transporter inhibitors. *Bioorganic & Medicinal Chemistry Letters*, *11*, 1123–1135. PMID:12565962

Enyedy, I. J., Zaman, W. A., Sakamuri, S., Kozikowski, A. P., Johnson, K. M., & Wang, S. M. (2001). Pharmacophore-based discovery of 3, 4-disubstituted pyrrolidines as a novel class of monoamine transporter inhibitors. *Bioorganic & Medicinal Chemistry Letters*, *11*(9), 1113–1118. doi:10.1016/S0960-894X(01)00132-9 PMID:11354356

Ercolini, D., De Filippis, F., La Storia, A., & Iacono, M. (2012). "Remake" by high-throughput sequencing of the microbiota involved in the production of water buffalo mozzarella cheese. *Applied and Environmental Microbiology*, *78*(22), 8142–8145. doi:10.1128/AEM.02218-12 PMID:22941080

Ernst, & Young, L.L.P. (2001). *Pharmaceutical Industry R&D Costs: Key Findings about the Public Citizen Report.* Retrieved from http://www.cptech.org/ip/health/econ/phrmaresponse.pdf

Esser, R., Berry, C., Du, Z., Dawson, J., Fox, A., Fujimoto, R. A., ... Marshall, P. J. (2005). Preclinical pharmacology of lumiracoxib: A novel selective inhibitor of cyclooxygenase-2. *British Journal of Pharmacology, 144*, 538−550. Marnett, L. J. (2009). The COXIB experience: A look in the rear-view mirror. *Annual Review of Pharmacology and Toxicology*, *49*, 265–290.

Estiu, G., West, N., Mazitschek, R., Greenberg, E., Bradner, J. E., & Wiest, O. (2010). On the inhibition of histone deacetylase 8. *Bioorganic & Medicinal Chemistry*, *18*(11), 4103–4110. doi:10.1016/j.bmc.2010.03.080 PMID:20472442

Eswar, N., Webb, B., Marti-Renom, M. A., Madhusudhan, M. S., Eramian, D., Shen, M. Y., & ... . (2006). Comparative Protein Structure Modeling Using Modeller. *Current Protocols in Bioinformatics*, *5*(5-6). doi:10.1002/0471250953.bi0506s15 PMID:18428767

European Medicines Agency ICH guideline Q10 on Pharmaceutical quality system, Sep 2015

European Medicines Agency ICH guideline Q8(R2) on Pharmaceutical development, Jun 2017

European Medicines Agency ICH guideline Q9 on Quality risk management, Sep 2015

Evaluate Pharma orphan drug report. (2017). Retrieved from http://info.evaluategroup.com/rs/607-YGS-364/images/wp15.pdf

Ewing, T. J., Makino, S., Skillman, A. G., & Kuntz, I. D. (2001). DOCK 4.0: Search strategies for automated molecular docking of flexible molecule databases. *Journal of Computer-Aided Molecular Design*, *15*(5), 411–428. doi:10.1023/A:1011115820450 PMID:11394736

Fabio, P., Laura, M., & Massimo, R. (2011). The productivity crisis in pharmaceutical R&D. *Nature Reviews. Drug Discovery*, *10*(6), 428–438. doi:10.1038/nrd3405 PMID:21629293

Falkenberg, K. J., & Johnstone, R. W. (2014). Histone deacetylases and their inhibitors in cancer, neurological diseases and immune disorders. *Nature Reviews. Drug Discovery*, *13*(9), 673–691. doi:10.1038/nrd4360 PMID:25131830

Fang, Wu, Yang, Gao, Li, Wang, … Du. (2014). Inhibition of acetylcholinesterase by two geinstein derivatives: Kinetic analysis, molecular docking and molecular dynamics simulation. *Acta Pharmaceutica (Zagreb, Croatia)*, *4*(6), 430–437.

FDA. (n.d.). *EMA Announce Pilot for Parallel Assessment of Quality by Design Applications*. Retrieved from https://www.qualitydigest.com/inside/fda-compliance-news/fda-ema-announce-pilot-parallel-assessment-quality-design-applications.ht

Ferreira, S. H., Moncada, S., & Vane, J. R. (1971). Indomethacin and aspirin abolish prostaglandin release from the spleen. *Nature: New Biology*, *231*(25), 237–239. doi:10.1038/newbio231237a0 PMID:5284362

Flusberg, B. A., Webster, D. R., Lee, J. H., Travers, K. J., Olivares, E. C., Clark, T. A., ... Turner, S. W. (2010). Direct detection of DNA methylation during single-molecule, real-time sequencing. *Nature Methods*, *7*(6), 461–465. doi:10.1038/nmeth.1459 PMID:20453866

Folkers, G., Chretien, J. R., & Raevsky, O. A. (1998). Estimation of blood-brain barrier crossing of drugs using molecular size and shape, and H-bonding descriptors. *Journal of Drug Targeting*, *6*(2), 151–165. doi:10.3109/10611869808997889 PMID:9886238

Foloppe, N., & Hubbard, R. (2006). Towards predictive ligand design with free-energy based computational methods? *Current Medicinal Chemistry*, *13*(29), 3583–3608. doi:10.2174/092986706779026165 PMID:17168725

Food and Drug Administration CDER. (2007). *Draft Guidance for Industry and Review Staff: Target Product Profile- A Strategic Development Tool*. Author.

Fox, T., & Haaksma, E. E. J. (2000). Computer based screening of compound database: 1 preselection of benzamidine-based thrombin inhibitor. *Journal of Computer-Aided Molecular Design*, *14*(5), 411–425. doi:10.1023/A:1008167012101 PMID:10896314

Franz, F. H. (2008). Requirements for a lead compound to become a clinical candidate. *BMC Neuroscience*, *9*(3), S7. PMID:19091004

Fu, J. Y., Masferrer, J. L., Seibert, K., Raz, A., & Needleman, P. (1990). The induction and suppression of prostaglandin H2 synthase (cyclooxygenase) in human monocytes. *The Journal of Biological Chemistry*, *265*(28), 16737–16740. PMID:2120205

Fulcher, M. L., Gabriel, S. E., Olsen, J. C., Tatreau, J. R., Gentzsch, M., Livanos, E., ... Randell, S. H. (2009). Novel human bronchial epithelial cell lines for cystic fibrosis research. *American Journal of Physiology. Lung Cellular and Molecular Physiology*, *296*(1), L82–L91. doi:10.1152/ajplung.90314.2008 PMID:18978040

Galletti, P., Quintavalla, A., Ventrici, C., Giannini, G., Cabri, W., Penco, S., ... Giacomini, D. (2009). Azetidinones as zinc-binding groups to design selective HDAC8 inhibitors. *ChemMedChem*, *4*(12), 1991–2001. doi:10.1002/cmdc.200900309 PMID:19821480

Galperin, M. Y., & Koonin, E. V. (1999). Searching for drug targets in microbial genomes. *Current Opinion in Biotechnology*, *10*(6), 571–578. doi:10.1016/S0958-1669(99)00035-X PMID:10600691

Gangwal, R. P., Damre, M. V., Das, N. R., Dhoke, G. V., Bhadauriya, A., Varikoti, R. A., ... Sangamwar, A. T. (2015). Structure based virtual screening to identify selective phosphodiesterase 4B inhibitors. *Journal of Molecular Graphics & Modelling*, *57*, 89–98. doi:10.1016/j.jmgm.2015.01.007 PMID:25687765

Garber, M., Grabherr, M. G., Guttman, M., & Trapnell, C. (2011). Computational methods for transcriptome annotation and quantification using RNA-seq. *Nature Methods*, *8*(6), 469–477. doi:10.1038/nmeth.1613 PMID:21623353

Garg, A. X., Adhikari, N. K., McDonald, H., Rosas-Arellano, M. P., Devereaux, P. J., Beyene, J., ... Haynes, R. B. (2005). Effects of Computerized Clinical Decision Support Systems on Practitioner Performance and Patient Outcomes: A systematic Review. *Journal of the American Medical Association*, *293*(10), 1223–1238. doi:10.1001/jama.293.10.1223 PMID:15755945

Garg, P., & Verma, J. (2006). *In silico* prediction of blood brain barrier permeability: An artificial neural network model. *Journal of Chemical Information and Modeling*, *46*(1), 289–297. doi:10.1021/ci050303i PMID:16426064

Garg, R., Kurup, A., Mekapati, S. B., & Hansch, C. (2003). Searching for allosteric effects via QSAR. Part II. *Bioorganic & Medicinal Chemistry*, *11*(4), 621–628. doi:10.1016/S0968-0896(02)00382-6 PMID:12538028

Gasteiger & Marsili. (1980). Iterative Partial Equalization of Orbital Electronegativity—a Rapid Access to Atomic Charges. *Tetrahedron*, *36*(2), 3219–3228.

Gehlaar, D. K. (1995). *De novo* design of enzyme inhibitors by Monte Carlo ligand generation. *Journal of Medicinal Chemistry*, *38*(3), 466–472. doi:10.1021/jm00003a010 PMID:7853340

Gentles, A. J., & Gallahan, D. (2011). Systems biology: Confronting the complexity of cancer. *Cancer Research*, *71*(18), 5961–5964. doi:10.1158/0008-5472.CAN-11-1569 PMID:21896642

Ghanemi, A., He, L., & Yan, M. (2013). New factors influencing G protein coupled receptors' system functions. *Alexandria Journal of Medicine*, *49*(1), 1–5. doi:10.1016/j.ajme.2012.10.002

Gharaghani, S., Khayamian, T., & Ebrahimi, M. (2013). Molecular dynamics simulation study and molecular docking descriptors in structure-based QSAR on acetylcholinesterase (AChE) inhibitors. *SAR and QSAR in Environmental Research*, *24*(9), 773–794. doi:10.1080/1062936X.2013.792877 PMID:23863115

Ghosh, S., & Chan, C.-K. K. (2016). Analysis of RNA-Seq data using TopHat and Cufflinks. In Plant Bioinformatics (pp. 339-361). Academic Press.

Ghuloum, A. M., Sage, C. R., & Jain, A. N. (1999). Molecular hash keys: A novel method for molecular characterization and its application for predicting important pharmaceutical properties of molecules. *Journal of Medicinal Chemistry*, *42*(10), 1739–1748. doi:10.1021/jm980527a PMID:10346926

Gillet, V. J., Myatt, G., Zsoldos, Z., & Johnson, A. P. (1995). SPROUT, HIPPO AND CAESA: Tools for *de novo* structure generation and estimation of synthetic accessibility. *Perspectives in Drug Discovery and Design*, *3*(1), 34–50. doi:10.1007/BF02174466

Gleeson, M. P. (2008). Generation of a set of simple, interpretable ADMET rules of thumb. *Journal of Medicinal Chemistry*, *51*(4), 817–834. doi:10.1021/jm701122q PMID:18232648

Gleeson, M. P., Hersey, A., Montanari, D., & Overington, J. (2011). Probing the links between in vitro potency, ADMET and physicochemical parameters. *Nature Reviews. Drug Discovery*, *10*(3), 197–208. doi:10.1038/nrd3367 PMID:21358739

Glenn, M. P., Kahnberg, P., Boyle, G. M., Hansford, K. A., Hans, D., Martyn, A. C., ... Fairlie, D. P. (2004). Antiproliferative and phenotype-transforming antitumor agents derived from cysteine. *Journal of Medicinal Chemistry*, *47*(12), 2984–2994. doi:10.1021/jm030222i PMID:15163181

Glide. (n.d.). Retrieved from www.schrodinger.com

Glodek, M., Liebowitz, S., & McCarthy, R. (2006). Process robustness: A PQRI white paper. *Pharmaceutical Engineering*, 1-11.

Goel, R., Harsha, H. C., Pandey, A., & Prasad, T. S. K. (2012). Human Protein Reference Database and Human Proteinpedia as resources for phosphoproteome analysis. *Molecular BioSystems*, *8*(2), 453–463. doi:10.1039/C1MB05340J PMID:22159132

Gohlke, H., Hendlich, M., & Klebe, G. (2000). Knowledge-based scoring function to predict protein-ligand interactions. *Journal of Molecular Biology*, *295*(2), 337–356. doi:10.1006/jmbi.1999.3371 PMID:10623530

Gohlke, H., & Klebe, G. (2002). Approaches to the description and prediction of the binding affinity of small-molecule ligands to macromolecular receptors. *Angewandte Chemie International Edition*, *41*(15), 2644–2676. doi:10.1002/1521-3773(20020802)41:15<2644::AID-ANIE2644>3.0.CO;2-O PMID:12203463

Golebiowski, A., Klopfenstein, S. R., & Portlock, D. E. (2003). Lead compounds discovered from libraries: Part 2. *Current Opinion in Chemical Biology*, *7*(3), 308–325. doi:10.1016/S1367-5931(03)00059-0 PMID:12826118

Goodford, P. J. (1985). A computational procedure for determining energetically favorable binding sites on biologically important macromolecules. *Journal of Medicinal Chemistry*, *28*(7), 849–857. doi:10.1021/jm00145a002 PMID:3892003

Goodsell, D. S., Morris, G. M., & Olson, A. J. (1996). Automated docking of flexible ligands: Applications of AutoDock. *Journal of Molecular Recognition*, *9*(1), 1–5. doi:10.1002/(SICI)1099-1352(199601)9:1<1::AID-JMR241>3.0.CO;2-6 PMID:8723313

Goodwin, S., McPherson, J. D., & McCombie, W. R. (2016). Coming of age: Ten years of next-generation sequencing technologies. *Nature Reviews. Genetics*, *17*(6), 333–351. doi:10.1038/nrg.2016.49 PMID:27184599

Gorelik, B., & Goldblum, A. (2008). High quality binding modes in docking ligands to proteins. *Proteins*, *71*(3), 1373–1386. doi:10.1002/prot.21847 PMID:18058908

Gozalbes, R., & Pineda-Lucena, A. (2010). QSAR-based solubility model for drug-like compounds. *Bioorganic & Medicinal Chemistry*, *18*(19), 7078–7084. doi:10.1016/j.bmc.2010.08.003 PMID:20810286

Green, D. V. (2003). Virtual screening of virtual libraries. *Progress in Medicinal Chemistry*, *41*, 61–97. doi:10.1016/S0079-6468(02)41002-8 PMID:12774691

Greene, N. (2002). Computer systems for the prediction of toxicity: An update. *Advanced Drug Delivery Reviews*, *54*(3), 417–431. doi:10.1016/S0169-409X(02)00012-1 PMID:11922956

Gregory, S., Sandeep Kumar, K., Jens, M., Edward, W., & Lowe Eric, L. B. (2014). Computational methods in drug discovery. *Pharmacological Reviews*, *66*(1), 334–395. PMID:24381236

Gryder, B. E., Sodji, Q. H., & Oyelere, A. K. (2012). Targeted cancer therapy: Giving histone deacetylase inhibitors all they need to succeed. *Future Medicinal Chemistry*, *4*(4), 505–524. doi:10.4155/fmc.12.3 PMID:22416777

Grzybowski, B. A., Ishchenko, A. V., Shimada, J., Whitesides, G. M., & Shakhnovich, E. I. (2002). From knowledge-based potentials to combinatorial lead design *in silico. Accounts of Chemical Research*, *5*(5), 261–269. doi:10.1021/ar970146b PMID:12020163

Gund, P. (1977). Three-dimensional Pharmacophore Pattern Searching. *Progress in Molecular and Subcellular Biology*, *5*, 117–143. doi:10.1007/978-3-642-66626-1_4

Guner, O., Clement, O., & Kurogi, Y. (2004). Pharmacophore modelling and three-dimensional database searching for drug design using catalyst: Recent advances. *Current Medicinal Chemistry, 11*(22), 2991–3005. doi:10.2174/0929867043364036 PMID:15544485

Gupta, S. P., & Kumaran, S. (2005). A quantitative structure–activity relationship study on some aromatic/heterocyclic sulfonamides and their charged derivatives acting as carbonic anhydrase inhibitors. *Journal of Enzyme Inhibition and Medicinal Chemistry, 20*(3), 251–259. doi:10.1080/14756360500067439 PMID:16119196

Haider, S., Joseph, C. G., Neidle, S., Fierke, C. A., & Fuchter, M. J. (2011). On the function of the internal cavity of histone deacetylase protein 8: R37 is a crucial residue for catalysis. *Bioorganic & Medicinal Chemistry Letters, 21*(7), 2129–2132. doi:10.1016/j.bmcl.2011.01.128 PMID:21320778

Hajduk, P. (2005). *NMR-based screening in drug discovery and design. 230th ACS National Meeting*, Washington, DC.

Hajduk, P. J., & Greer, J. (2007). A decade of fragment-based drug design: Strategic advances and lessons learned. *Nature Reviews. Drug Discovery, 6*(3), 211–219. doi:10.1038/nrd2220 PMID:17290284

Hajduk, P. J., Huth, J. R., & Fesik, S. W. (2005). Druggability indices for protein targets derived from NMR-based screening data. *Journal of Medicinal Chemistry, 48*(7), 2518–2525. doi:10.1021/jm049131r PMID:15801841

Halakou, F., Kilic, E. S., Cukuroglu, E., Keskin, O., & Gursoy, A. (2017). Enriching Traditional Protein-protein Interaction Networks with Alternative Conformations of Proteins. *Scientific Reports*, 7. PMID:28775330

Halperin, I., Ma, B., Wolfson, H., & Nussinov, R. (2002). Principles of docking: An overview of search algorithms and a guide to scoring functions. *Proteins, 47,* 409–443.

Hann, M. M., & Oprea, T. I. (2004). Pursuing the leadlikeness concept in pharmaceutical research. *Current Opinion in Chemical Biology, 8*(3), 255–263. doi:10.1016/j.cbpa.2004.04.003 PMID:15183323

Hannu, R. (2011). *Insilico*toxicology–non-testingmethods. *Frontiers in Pharmacology, 2,* 1–8. PMID:21779246

Hansch, C., Leo, A., Mekapati, S. B., & Kurup, A. (2004). QSAR and ADME. *Bioorganic & Medicinal Chemistry, 12*(12), 3391–3400. doi:10.1016/j.bmc.2003.11.037 PMID:15158808

Hanyuan, D. (2011). On the Balaban Index of Trees. *Match (Mülheim an der Ruhr, Germany), 66*, 253–260.

Haq, I. (2002). Thermodynamics of drug-DNA interactions. *Archives of Biochemistry and Biophysics, 403*(1), 1–15. doi:10.1016/S0003-9861(02)00202-3 PMID:12061796

Haque, M., Sarmah, R., & Bhattacharyya, D. K. (2018). A common neighbor based technique to detect protein complexes in PPI networks. *Journal of Genetic Engineering and Biotechnology, 16*(1), 227–238. doi:10.1016/j.jgeb.2017.10.010

Hardy, L. W., & Malikayil, A. (2003). The impact of structure-guided drug design on clinical agents. *Feature*, 15-20. Retrieved from https://pdfs.semanticscholar.org/8685/8146bca4c33c19fc7b31ed0bd5b4ff1835fb.pdf

Hardy, L. W., & Malikayil, A. (2003). The impact of structure-guided drug design on clinical agents. *Current Drug Discovery, 3*, 15–20.

Hardy, L. W., & Peet, N. P. (2004). The multiple orthogonal tools approach to define molecular causation in the validation of druggable targets. *Drug Discovery Today, 9*(3), 117–126. doi:10.1016/S1359-6446(03)02969-6 PMID:14960389

Hartshorn, M. J., Murray, C. W., Cleasby, A., Frederickson, M., Tickle, I. J., & Jhoti, H. (2005). Fragment-based lead discovery using X-ray crystallography. *Journal of Medicinal Chemistry, 48*(2), 403–413. doi:10.1021/jm0495778 PMID:15658854

Harvey, M. J., & de Fabritiis, G. (2012). High-throughput molecular dynamics: The powerful new tool for drug discovery. *Drug Discovery Today*, *17*(19-20), 1059–1062. doi:10.1016/j.drudis.2012.03.017 PMID:22504137

Hasegawa, H., Yamada, Y., Tsukasaki, K., Mori, N., Tsuruda, K., Sasaki, D., ... Kamihira, S. (2011). LBH589, a deacetylase inhibitor, induces apoptosis in adult T-cell leukemia/ lymphoma cells via activation of a novel RAIDD-caspase-2 pathway. *Leukemia*, *25*(4), 575–587. doi:10.1038/leu.2010.315 PMID:21242994

Hastings, J., de Matos, P., Dekker, A., Ennis, M., Harsha, B., Kale, N., ... Steinbeck, C. (2013). The ChEBI reference database and ontology for biologically relevant chemistry: Enhancements for 2013. *Nucleic Acids Research*, *41*(Database issue), D456–D463. doi:10.1093/nar/gks1146 PMID:23180789

Havelka, A. M., Berndtsson, M., Olofsson, M. H., Shoshan, M. C., & Linder, S. (2007). Mechanisms of action of DNA-damaging anticancer drugs in treatment of carcinomas: Is acute apoptosis an "off-target" effect? *Mini-Reviews in Medicinal Chemistry*, *7*(10), 1035–1039. doi:10.2174/138955707782110196 PMID:17979806

He, W. (2013). Small molecular drug innovation & development. *Abstract: 2013 International bioeconomy conference, session 2: R&D in drug innovation*, 67–69.

Helen, W. (2015). Biological membranes. *Essays in Biochemistry, 59,* 43-69. doi:10.1042/bse0590043 PMID:26504250

Hendlich, M. (1998). Databases for protein-ligand complexes. *Acta Crystallographica. Section D, Biological Crystallography*, *54*(6), 1178–1182. doi:10.1107/S0907444998007124 PMID:10089494

Hermjakob, H. (2004). IntAct: An open source molecular interaction database. *Nucleic Acids Research*, *32*(90001), 452D–455. doi:10.1093/nar/gkh052 PMID:14681455

Hersey, A., Chambers, J., Bellis, L., Patrícia Bento, A., Gaulton, A., & Overington, J. P. (2015). Chemical databases: Curation or integration by user-defined equivalence? *Drug Discovery Today. Technologies*, *14*, 17–24. doi:10.1016/j.ddtec.2015.01.005 PMID:26194583

Hertzberg, R. P., & Pope, A. J. (2000). High-throughput screening: New technology for the 21st century. *Current Opinion in Chemical Biology*, *4*(4), 445–451. doi:10.1016/S1367-5931(00)00110-1 PMID:10959774

He, X., & Zhang, J. (2006). Why Do Hubs Tend to Be Essential in Protein Networks? *PLOS Genetics*, *2*(6), e88. doi:10.1371/journal.pgen.0020088 PMID:16751849

Hindle, S. A., Rarey, M., Buning, C., & Lengauer, T. (2002). Flexible docking under pharmacophore type constraints. *Journal of Computer-Aided Molecular Design*, *16*(2), 129–149. doi:10.1023/A:1016399411208 PMID:12188022

Hirashima, A., Eiraku, T., Kuwano, E., & Eto, M. (2004). Comparative receptor surface analysis of agonists for tyramine receptor which inhibit sex-pheromone production in Plodiainterpunctella. *Combinatorial Chemistry & High Throughput Screening*, *7*(2), 83–91. doi:10.2174/138620704773120775 PMID:15032656

Hit-to-lead (H2L) and Lead Optimization in Medicinal Chemistry. (n.d.). Retrieved from https://sk.ru/cfs.../Lead-Optimization-_2D00_-Ivan-Efre_7E00_.pdf

Hitzler, P., Krötzsch, M., & Rudolph, S. (2009). *Foundations of Semantic Web Technologies*. CRC Press.

Hlinak, A. J., Kuriyan, K., Morris, K. R., Reklaitis, G. W., & Basu, P. K. (2006). Understanding critical material properties for solid dosage form design. Journal of Pharmaceutical Innovation, 1, 12-17. doi:10.1007/BF02784876

Ho, C. M. W., & Marshall, G. R. (1990). Cavity search: An algorithm for the isolation and display of cavity-like binding regions. *Journal of Computer-Aided Molecular Design*, *4*(4), 337–354. doi:10.1007/BF00117400 PMID:2092080

Ho, C. M., & Marshall, G. R. (1993). FOUNDATION: A program to retrieve all possible structures containing a user-defined minimum number of matching query elements from three-dimensional databases. *Journal of Computer-Aided Molecular Design*, *7*, 623–647. doi:10.1007/BF00125322 PMID:8473917

Ho, C. M., & Marshall, G. R. (1995). DBMAKER: A set of programs designed to generate three-dimensional databases based upon user-specific criteria. *Journal of Computer-Aided Molecular Design*, *9*(1), 65–86. doi:10.1007/BF00117279 PMID:7751871

Hochstrasser, R. M. (2007). Two-dimensional spectroscopy at infrared and optical frequencies. *Proceedings of the National Academy of Sciences of the United States*, *104*(36), 14190–14196. doi:10.1073/pnas.0704079104 PMID:17664429

Hohman, M., Gregory, K., Chibale, K., Smith, P. J., Ekins, S., & Bunin, B. (2009). Novel web-based tools combining chemistry informatics, biology and social networks for drug discovery. *Drug Discovery Today*, *14*(5-6), 261–270. doi:10.1016/j.drudis.2008.11.015 PMID:19231313

Holmes, M. A., & Matthews, B. W. (1981). Binding of hydroxamic acid inhibitors to crystalline thermolysin suggests a pentacoordinate zinc intermediate in catalysis. *Biochemistry*, *20*(24), 6912–6920. doi:10.1021/bi00527a026 PMID:7317361

HomeD. I. P. (n.d.). Retrieved from http://dip.mbi.ucla.edu/dip

Honma, T., Hayashi, K., Aoyama, T., Hashimoto, N., Machida, T., Fukasawa, K., ... Morishima, H. (2001). Structure-based generation of a new class of potent Cdk4 inhibitors: New *de novo* design strategy and library design. *Journal of Medicinal Chemistry*, *44*(26), 4615–4627. doi:10.1021/jm0103256 PMID:11741479

Hou, T. J., Wang, J. M., Chen, L. R., & Xu, X. J. (1999). Automatic docking of peptides and proteins using a hybrid method combined with genetic algorithm and tabu search. *Protein Engineering*, *12*, 639–647. doi:10.1093/protein/12.8.639 PMID:10469824

Hou, T. J., & Xu, X. J. (2002). ADME Evaluation in Drug Discovery: Applications of genetic algorithms on the prediction of blood-brain partitioning of a large set drug. *Journal of Molecular Modeling*, *8*(12), 337–349. doi:10.100700894-002-0101-1 PMID:12541001

Hou, T. J., Zhu, L. L., Chen, L. R., & Xu, X. J. (2003). Mapping the binding site of a large set of quinazoline type EGF-R inhibitors using molecular field analyses and molecular docking studies. *Journal of Chemical Information and Computer Sciences*, *43*(1), 273–287. doi:10.1021/ci025552a PMID:12546563

Huang, S. Y., Grinter, S. Z., & Zou, X. (2010). Scoring functions and their evaluation methods for protein-ligand docking: Recent advances and future directions. *Physical Chemistry Chemical Physics*, *12*(40), 12899–12908. doi:10.1039/c0cp00151a PMID:20730182

Huang, S. Y., & Zou, X. (2006). An iterative knowledge-based scoring function to predict protein-ligand interactions: I. Derivation of interaction potentials. *Journal of Computational Chemistry*, *27*(15), 1866–1875. doi:10.1002/jcc.20504 PMID:16983673

Huang, W. J., Wang, Y. C., Chao, S. W., Yang, C. Y., Chen, L. C., Lin, M. H., ... Chang, C.-I. (2012). Synthesis and biological evaluation of orthoaryl N-hydroxycinnamides as potent histone deacetylase (HDAC) 8 isoform-selective inhibitors. *ChemMedChem*, *7*(10), 1815–1824. doi:10.1002/cmdc.201200300 PMID:22907916

Hu, E., Dul, E., Sung, C. M., Chen, Z., Kirkpatrick, R., & Zhang, G. F. (2003). Identification of novel isoform-selective inhibitors within class I histone deacetylases. *The Journal of Pharmacology and Experimental Therapeutics*, *307*(2), 720–728. doi:10.1124/jpet.103.055541 PMID:12975486

Hughes, J. P., Rees, S., Kalindjian, S. B., & Philpott, K. L. (2011). Principles of early drug Discovery. *British Journal of Pharmacology*, *162*(6), 1239–1249. doi:10.1111/j.1476-5381.2010.01127.x PMID:21091654

Huynen, M. A., Diaz-Lazcoz, Y., & Bork, P. (1997). Differential genome display. *Trends in Genetics*, *13*(10), 389–390. doi:10.1016/S0168-9525(97)01255-9 PMID:9351339

ICH endorsed guide for ICH Q8/Q9/Q10 implementation. Dec 2011.

Implementation of Quality by Design (QbD): status, challenges and next steps. (n.d.). FDA advisory committee for pharmaceutical sciences. Retrieved from http://slideplayer.com/slide/4127998/

Ingles-Prieto, A., Ibarra-Molero, B., Delgado-Delgado, A., Perez-Jimenez, R., Fernandez, J. M., & Gaucher, E. A. (2013). 2YOI: Crystal Structure of Ancestral Thioredoxin Relative to Last Eukaryotes Common Ancestor (Leca) From the Precambrian Period. *Structure (London, England)*, *21*, 1690–1697. doi:10.1016/j.str.2013.06.020

Ingolia, N. T., Ghaemmaghami, S., Newman, J. R., & Weissman, J. S. (2009). Genome-wide analysis in vivo of translation with nucleotide resolution using ribosome profiling. *Science*, *324*(5924), 218-223.

Insinga, A., Monestiroli, S., Ronzoni, S., Gelmetti, V., Marchesi, F., Viale, A., ... Pelicci, P. G. (2005). Inhibitors of histone deacetylases induce tumor-selective apoptosis through activation of the death receptor pathway. *Nature Medicine*, *11*(1), 71–76. doi:10.1038/nm1160 PMID:15619634

Irwin, J. J., & Shoichet, B. K. (2005). ZINC--a free database of commercially available compounds for virtual screening. *Journal of Chemical Information and Modeling*, *45*(1), 177–182. doi:10.1021/ci049714+ PMID:15667143

Irwin, J. J., Sterling, T., Mysinger, M. M., Bolstad, E. S., & Coleman, R. G. (2012). ZINC: A free tool to discover chemistry for biology. *Journal of Chemical Information and Modeling*, *52*(7), 1757–1768. doi:10.1021/ci3001277 PMID:22587354

Ischchenko, A. V., & Shakhnovich, E. I. (2002). Small molecular growth 2001 (SMoG2001): An improved knowledge-based scoring function for protein-ligand interactions. *Journal of Medicinal Chemistry*, *45*(13), 2770–2780. doi:10.1021/jm0105833 PMID:12061879

Ishikawa, T., Hirano, H., Saito, H., Sano, K., Ikegami, Y., Yamaotsu, N., & Hirono, S. (2012). QSAR analysis to predict drug-drug interactions of ABC transporter ABCG2. *Mini-Reviews in Medicinal Chemistry*, *12*(6), 505–514. doi:10.2174/138955712800493825 PMID:22587765

Ish, K. (2012). Drug discovery in pharmaceutical Industry: Productivity challenges and trends. *Drug Discovery Today*, *17*(19/20), 1088–1102. PMID:22627006

Ivanov, A. S., Veselovsky, A. V., Dubanov, A. V., & Skvortsov, V. S. (2006). Bioinformatics platform development: From gene to lead compound. *Methods in Molecular Biology (Clifton, N.J.)*, *316*, 389–431. PMID:16671411

Jahnke, W., Florsheimer, A., Blommers, M. J., Paris, C. G., Heim, J., Nalin, C. M., & Perez, L. (2003). Second-site NMR screening and linker design. *Current Tropical Medicinal Chemistry*, *3*(1), 69–80. doi:10.2174/1568026033392778

Jain, A. N. (2004). Ligand-based structural hypotheses for virtual screening. *Journal of Medicinal Chemistry*, *47*(4), 947–961. doi:10.1021/jm030520f PMID:14761196

Jain, A. N. (2006). Scoring functions for protein-ligand docking. *Current Protein & Peptide Science*, *7*(5), 407–420. doi:10.2174/138920306778559395 PMID:17073693

Jain, N., & Yalkowsky, S. H. (2001). Estimation of the aqueous solubility I: Application to organic nonelectrolytes. *Journal of Pharmaceutical Sciences*, *90*(2), 234–252. doi:10.1002/1520-6017(200102)90:2<234::AID-JPS14>3.0.CO;2-V PMID:11169540

Jajaga, E., & Ahmedi, L. (2017). C-SWRL: SWRL for Reasoning Over Stream Data. *11th International Conference on Semantic Computing (ICSC)*. 10.1109/ICSC.2017.64

Jaspers, M. W., Smeulers, M., Vermeulen, H., & Peute, L. W. (2011). Effects of Clinical Decision-Support Systems on Practitioner Performance and Patient Outcomes: A Synthesis of High-Quality Systematic Review Finding. *Journal of the American Medical Informatics Association*, *18*(3), 327–334. doi:10.1136/amiajnl-2011-000094 PMID:21422100

Jensen, L. J., Kuhn, M., Stark, M., Chaffron, S., Creevey, C., Muller, J., ... von Mering, C. (2009). STRING 8--a global view on proteins and their functional interactions in 630 organisms. *Nucleic Acids Research*, *37*(Database), D412–D416. doi:10.1093/nar/gkn760 PMID:18940858

Jia, P., Wang, L., Meltzer, H. Y., & Zhao, Z. (2010). Common variants conferring risk of schizophrenia: A pathway analysis of GWAS data. *Schizophrenia Research*, *122*(1), 38–42. doi:10.1016/j.schres.2010.07.001 PMID:20659789

Ji, T. T., Zhang, W. N., Zhang, M., Kudo, M., Aoyama, Y., Yoshida, Y., ... Zhu, J. (2003). Structure-based *de novo* design, synthesis, and biological evaluation of non-azole inhibitors specific for lanosterol 14α-demethylase of fungi. *Journal of Medicinal Chemistry*, *46*(4), 474–485. doi:10.1021/jm020362c PMID:12570370

Jo-Lene, L., Rudi, B., Patrick, C. C., & Mei-Lin, G. (2007). Quantitative structure-activity relationship (QSAR) of indoloacetamides as inhibitors of human isoprenylcysteine carboxyl methyltransferase. *Bioorganic & Medicinal Chemistry Letters*, *17*(4), 1025–1032. doi:10.1016/j.bmcl.2006.11.030 PMID:17157012

Jones, D. T. (1999). GenTHREADER: An efficient and reliable protein fold recognition method for genomic sequences. *Journal of Molecular Biology*, *287*(4), 797–815. doi:10.1006/jmbi.1999.2583 PMID:10191147

Jones, D. T., Taylort, W. R., & Thornton, J. M. (1992). A new approach to protein fold recognition. *Nature*, *358*(6381), 86–89. doi:10.1038/358086a0 PMID:1614539

Jones, G., Willett, P., Glen, R., Leach, A. R., & Taylor, R. (1997). Development and validation of a genetic algorithm for flexible docking. *Journal of Molecular Biology*, *267*(3), 727–748. doi:10.1006/jmbi.1996.0897 PMID:9126849

Jorgensen, W. L. (2004). The many roles of computation in drug discovery. *Science*, *303*(5665), 1813–1818. doi:10.1126cience.1096361 PMID:15031495

Jorgensen, W. L. (2009). Efficient Drug Lead Discovery and Optimization. *Accounts of Chemical Research*, *42*(6), 724–733. doi:10.1021/ar800236t PMID:19317443

Kahnberg, P., Lucke, A. J., Glenn, M. P., Boyle, G. M., Tyndall, J. D. A., Parsons, P. G., & Fairlie, D. P. (2006). Design, synthesis, potency and cytoselectivity of anticancer agents derived by parallel synthesis from α- amino suberic acid. *Journal of Medicinal Chemistry*, *49*(26), 7611–7622. doi:10.1021/jm050214x PMID:17181145

Kanehisa, M. (2004). The KEGG resource for deciphering the genome. *Nucleic Acids Research*, *32*(90001), 277D–280. doi:10.1093/nar/gkh063 PMID:14681412

Kanehisa, M., Goto, S., Sato, Y., Furumichi, M., & Tanabe, M. (2012). KEGG for integration and interpretation of large-scale molecular data sets. *Nucleic Acids Research*, *40*(Database issue), D109–D114. doi:10.1093/nar/gkr988 PMID:22080510

Kapetanovic, I. M. (2008). Computer-aided drug discovery and development (CADDD): *In silico*-chemico-biological approach. *Chemico-Biological Interactions*, *171*(2), 165–176. doi:10.1016/j.cbi.2006.12.006 PMID:17229415

Kawai, S., Kojima, F., & Kusunoki, N. (2005). Recent advances in nonsteroidal anti-inflammatory drugs. *Allergology International*, *54*(2), 209–215. doi:10.2332/allergolint.54.209

Keating, B. J., Tischfield, S., Murray, S. S., Bhangale, T., Price, T. S., Glessner, J. T., ... FitzGerald, G. A. (2008). Concept, design and implementation of a cardiovascular gene-centric 50 k SNP array for large-scale genomic association studies. *PLoS One*, *3*(10), e3583. doi:10.1371/journal.pone.0003583 PMID:18974833

Keet, C. M. (2011). The Use of Foundational Ontologies in Ontology Development: An Empirical Assessment. *8th Extended Semantic Web Conference.*

Kelder, J., Grootenhuis, P. D. J., Bayada, D. M., Delbressine, L. P. C., & Ploemen, J. P. (1999). Polarmolecular surface as a dominating determinant for oral absorption and brainpenetration of drugs. *Pharmaceutical Research*, *6*(10), 1514–1519. doi:10.1023/A:1015040217741 PMID:10554091

Kellogg, G. E., & Chen, D. L. (2004). The importance of being exhaustive. Optimization of bridging structural water molecules and water networks in models of biological systems. *Chemistry & Biodiversity*, *1*(1), 98–105. doi:10.1002/cbdv.200490016 PMID:17191777

Kerrien, S., Aranda, B., Breuza, L., Bridge, A., Broackes-Carter, F., Chen, C., ... Hermjakob, H. (2012). The IntAct molecular interaction database in 2012. *Nucleic Acids Research*, *40*(D1), D841–D846. doi:10.1093/nar/gkr1088 PMID:22121220

Keseru, G. M., & Makara, G. M. (2003). The influence of lead discovery strategies on the properties of drug candidates. *Nature Reviews. Drug Discovery*, *8*(3), 203–212. doi:10.1038/nrd2796 PMID:19247303

Keseru, G. M., & Makara, G. M. (2006). Hit discovery and hit-to-lead approaches. *Drug Discovery Today*, *11*(15/16), 741–748. doi:10.1016/j.drudis.2006.06.016 PMID:16846802

Keskin, O., Tuncbag, N., & Gursoy, A. (2016). Predicting Protein–Protein Interactions from the Molecular to the Proteome Level. *Chemical Reviews*, *116*(8), 4884–4909. doi:10.1021/acs.chemrev.5b00683 PMID:27074302

Khatri, Saini, Gangawat, & Gurubalaji. (2014). Pharmaceutical QbD: Concepts for Drug Product Development. *Int. J. Pharm. Sci., 13*, 84-91.

Khedkar, S. A., Malde, A. K., Coutinho, E. C., & Srivastava, S. (2007). Pharmacophore modeling in drug discovery and development: An overview. *Medicinal Chemistry (Shariqah, United Arab Emirates)*, *3*(2), 187–197. doi:10.2174/157340607780059521 PMID:17348856

Kier, L. B., & Hall, L. H. (1993). The generation of molecular-structures from a graph-based Qsar equation. *Molecular Informatics*, *12*, 383–388.

Kim, S., Thiessen, P. A., Bolton, E. E., Chen, J., Fu, G., Gindulyte, A., ... Bryant, S. H. (2016). PubChem Substance and Compound databases. *Nucleic Acids Research*, *44*(D1), D1202–D1213. doi:10.1093/nar/gkv951 PMID:26400175

King, R. D., Muggleton, S., Lewis, R. A., & Sternberg, M. J. E. (1992). Drug design by machine learning – the use of inductive logic programming to model the structure-activity relationships of trimethoprim analogues binding to dihydrofolate-reductase. *Proceedings of the National Academy of Sciences of the United States of America*, *89*(23), 11322–11326. doi:10.1073/pnas.89.23.11322 PMID:1454814

Kitano, H. (2002). Systems Biology: A Brief Overview. *Science*, *295*(5560), 1662–1664. doi:10.1126cience.1069492 PMID:11872829

Kitchen, D. B., Decornez, H., Furr, J. R., & Bajorath, J. (2004). Docking and scoring in virtual screening for drug discovery: Methods and applications. *Nature Reviews. Drug Discovery*, *3*(11), 935–949. doi:10.1038/nrd1549 PMID:15520816

Klebe, G. (2006). Virtual ligand screening: Strategies, perspectives and limitations. *Drug Discovery Today*, *11*(13-14), 580–594. doi:10.1016/j.drudis.2006.05.012 PMID:16793526

Klingstrom, T., & Plewczynski, D. (2011). Protein-protein interaction and pathway databases, a graphical review. *Briefings in Bioinformatics, 12*(6), 702–713. doi:10.1093/bib/bbq064 PMID:20851835

Klopman, G. (1992). MULTI-CASE. 1. A hierarchical computer automated structure evaluation program. *Molecular Informatics, 11*, 176–184.

Klopman, G., Chakravarti, S. K., Harris, N., Ivanov, J., & Saiakhov, R. D. (2003). *In silico* screening of high production volume chemicals for mutagenicity using the MCASE QSAR expert system. *SAR and QSAR in Environmental Research, 14*(2), 165–180. doi:10.1080/1062936031000073171 PMID:12747573

Knox, C., Law, V., Jewison, T., Liu, P., Ly, S., Frolkis, A., ... Wishart, D. S. (2011). DrugBank 3.0: A comprehensive resource for "omics" research on drugs. *Nucleic Acids Research, 39*(Database issue), D1035–D1041. doi:10.1093/nar/gkq1126 PMID:21059682

Koga, H., Itoh, A., Murayama, S., Suzue, S., & Irikura, T. (1980). Structure activity relationship of antibacterial 6,7 & 7,8 disubstituted 1-alkyl 1,4- dihydro 4-oxoquinolone, 3-carboxylic acid. *Journal of Medicinal Chemistry, 23*(12), 1358–1363. doi:10.1021/jm00186a014 PMID:7452690

Koh, G. C. K. W., Porras, P., Aranda, B., Hermjakob, H., & Orchard, S. E. (2012). Analyzing Protein–Protein Interaction Networks. *Journal of Proteome Research, 11*(4), 2014–2031. doi:10.1021/pr201211w PMID:22385417

Koh, J. (2003). Making virtual screening a reality. *Proceedings of the National Academy of Science*, 6902–6903.

Koide, Y., Tatsui, A., Hasegawa, T., Nurakami, A., Satoh, S., & Yamada, H. (2003). Identification of a stable chymase inhibitor using a pharmacophore-based database search. *Bioorganic & Medicinal Chemistry Letters, 13*(1), 25–29. doi:10.1016/S0960-894X(02)00853-3 PMID:12467610

Koki, A. T., Khan, N. K., Woerner, B. M., Seibert, K., Harmon, J. L., Dannenberg, A. J., ... Masferrer, J. L. (2002). Characterization of cyclooxygenase-2 (COX-2) during tumorigenesis in human epithelial cancers: Evidence for potential clinical utility of COX-2 inhibitors in epithelial cancers. *Prostaglandins, Leukotrienes, and Essential Fatty Acids, 66*(1), 13–18. doi:10.1054/plef.2001.0335 PMID:12051953

Kollman, P. A., Massova, I., Reyes, C., Kuhn, B., Huo, S. H., Chong, L., ... Cheatham, T. E. (2000). Calculating structures and free energies of complex molecules: Combining molecular mechanics and continuum models. *Accounts of Chemical Research, 33*(12), 889–897. doi:10.1021/ar000033j PMID:11123888

Kontogiorgis, C. A., & Hadjipavlou-Litina, D. (2003). Quantitative Structure - Activity Relationships (QSARs) of Thrombin Inhibitors: Review, Evaluation and Comparative Analysis. *Current Medicinal Chemistry, 10*(7), 525–577. doi:10.2174/0929867033457935 PMID:12678789

Koppen, H. (2009). Virtual screening - what does it give us? *Current Opinion in Drug Discovery & Development, 12*, 397–407. PMID:19396741

Kortagere, S., Krasowski, M. D., & Ekins, S. (2009, March). The importance of discerning shape in molecular pharmacology. *Trends in Pharmacological Sciences, 30*(3), 138–147. doi:10.1016/j.tips.2008.12.001 PMID:19187977

Kramer, B., Metz, G., Rarey, M., & Lengauer, T. (1999). Ligand docking and screening with FlexX. *Medicinal Chemistry Research, 9*, 463–478.

Kratochwil, N. A., Huber, W., Muller, F., Kansy, M., & Gerber, P. R. (2002). Predicting plasma protein binding of drugs: A new approach. *Biochemical Pharmacology, 64*(9), 1355–1374. doi:10.1016/S0006-2952(02)01074-2 PMID:12392818

Krennhrubec, K., Marshall, B. L., Hedglin, M., Verdin, E., & Ulrich, S. M. (2007). Design and evaluation of 'Linker-less' hydroxamic acids as selective HDAC8 inhibitors. *Bioorganic & Medicinal Chemistry Letters*, *17*(10), 2874–2878. doi:10.1016/j.bmcl.2007.02.064 PMID:17346959

Kubinyi, H. (2006). Success stories of computer-aided design. In Computer Applications in Pharmaceutical Research and Development. Wiley-Interscience. doi:10.1002/0470037237.ch16

Kujawski, J., Bernard, M. K., Janusz, A., & Kuzma, W. (2012). Prediction of log P – ALOGPS Application in Medicinal Chemistry Education. *Journal of Chemical Education*, *89*(1), 64–67. doi:10.1021/ed100444h

Kujawski, J., Popielarska, H., Myka, A., Drabinska, B., & Bernard, M. K. (2012). The log *P* parameter as a molecular descriptor in the Computer-aided Drug Design – an overview. *Computational Methods in Science and Technology*, *18*(2), 81–88. doi:10.12921/cmst.2012.18.02.81-88

Kujubu, D. A., Fletcher, B. S., Varnum, B. C., Lim, R. W., & Herschman, H. R. (1991). TIS10, a phorbol ester tumour-promoter-inducible mRNA from Swiss 3T3 cells, encodes a novel prostaglandin synthase. Cyclooxygenase homologue. *The Journal of Biological Chemistry*, *266*, 12866–12872.

Kukurba, K. R., & Montgomery, S. B. (2015). RNA sequencing and analysis. *Cold Spring Harbor Protocols*, *2015*(11).

Kulkarni, A., & Wilson, D. M. III. (2008). The involvement of DNA-damage and -repair defects in neurological dysfunction. *American Journal of Human Genetics*, *82*(3), 539–566. doi:10.1016/j.ajhg.2008.01.009 PMID:18319069

Kumalo, H. M., Bhakat, S., & Soliman, M. E. (2015). Theory and applications of covalent docking in drug discovery: Merits and pitfalls. *Molecules (Basel, Switzerland)*, *20*(2), 1984–2000. doi:10.3390/molecules20021984 PMID:25633330

Kumar & Gupta. (2015). A review of quality by design approach (QbD) for Pharmaceuticals. International of Drug Development and Research, 7(1), 52-60.

Kumar, N., Hendriks, B. S., Janes, K. A., de Graaf, D., & Lauffenburger, D. A. (2006). Applying computational modeling to drug discovery and development. *Drug Discovery Today*, *11*(17–18), 806–811. doi:10.1016/j.drudis.2006.07.010 PMID:16935748

Kumar, P. (2015). Survivin:Amolecular biomarker in cancer. *The Indian Journal of Medical Research*, *141*(4), 389–397. doi:10.4103/0971-5916.159250 PMID:26112839

Kunal, R. (2017). *Advances in QSAR modeling: applications in pharmaceutical, chemical, food agricultural and environmental sciences*. Springer.

Kuntz, I. D., Blaney, J. M., Oatley, S. J., Langridge, R., & Ferrin, T. E. (1982). A geometric approach to macromolecule-ligand interactions. *Journal of Molecular Biology*, *161*(2), 269–288. doi:10.1016/0022-2836(82)90153-X PMID:7154081

Kuntz, I. D., Meng, E. C., & Shoichet, B. K. (1994). Structure-based molecular design. *Accounts of Chemical Research*, *27*(5), 117–123. doi:10.1021/ar00041a001

Kunze, M. B. A., Wright, D. W., Werbeck, N. D., Kirkpatrick, J., Coveney, P. V., & Hansen, D. F. (2013). Loop interactions and dynamics tune the enzymatic activity of the human histone deacetylase 8. *Journal of the American Chemical Society*, *135*(47), 17862–17868. doi:10.1021/ja408184x PMID:24171457

Kurogi, Y., & Guner, O. F. (2001). Pharmacophore modeling and three-dimensional database searching for Drug Design using catalyst. *Current Medicinal Chemistry*, *8*(9), 1035–1055. doi:10.2174/0929867013372481 PMID:11472240

Kurup, A. (2003). C-QSAR: a database of 18,000 QSARs and associated biological and physical data. *Journal of Computer Aided Drug Design*, *17*, 187–196.

Lagerstrom, M. C., & Schioth, H. B. (2008). Structural diversity of G protein-coupled receptors and significance for drug discovery. *Nature Reviews. Drug Discovery*, *7*(4), 339–357. doi:10.1038/nrd2518 PMID:18382464

Lahlou, M. (2013). The Success of Natural Products in Drug Discovery. *Pharmacology & Pharmacy*, *4*(03), 17–31. doi:10.4236/pp.2013.43A003

Lakings, D. B. (2009). Drug development teams. In R. Guarino (Ed.), *New drug approval process* (Vol. 139, pp. 1–15). Marcel Dekker.

Lakshmana Prabu, S., Thirumurugan, R., Mahesh Vijay, P. & Shanmugarathinam, A. (2016, October). Applications of computer in Health Profession: From Drug Discovery to Market. *International Journal of Research in Pharmacology & Pharmacotherapeutics,* 46-54.

Lakshmana Prabu, S., Thirumurugan, R., & Suriya Prakash, T. N. K. (2014). The role of the drug discovery, clinical and regulatory affairs teams in turning a potent agent into a registered product. In J. Reedijk (Ed.), *Elsevier Reference Module in Chemistry, Molecular Sciences and Chemical Engineering*. Waltham, MA: Elsevier; doi:10.1016/B978-0-12-409547-2.11400-3

Lanevskij, K., Dapkunas, J., Juska, L., Japertas, P., & Didziapetris, R. (2011). QSAR analysis of blood-brain distribution: The influence of plasma and brain tissue binding. *Journal of Pharmaceutical Sciences*, *100*(6), 2147–2160. doi:10.1002/jps.22442 PMID:21271563

Langer, T., & Hoffmann, R. D. (2001). Virtual screening: An effective tool for lead structure discovery? *Current Pharmaceutical Design*, *7*(7), 509–527. doi:10.2174/1381612013397861 PMID:11375766

Langer, T., & Krovat, E. M. (2003). Chemical features based pharmacophore and virtual library screening for discovery of new leads. *Current Opinion in Drug Discovery & Development*, *6*, 370–376. PMID:12833670

Langer, T., & Wolber, G. (2004). Virtual combinatorial chemistry and in silico screening: Efficient tools for lead structure discovery? *Pure and Applied Chemistry*, *76*(5), 991–996. doi:10.1351/pac200476050991

Langmead, B. (2010). Aligning short sequencing reads with Bowtie. *Current Protocols in Bioinformatics.*

Langmead, B., & Salzberg, S. L. (2012). Fast gapped-read alignment with Bowtie 2. *Nature Methods*, *9*(4), 357–359. doi:10.1038/nmeth.1923 PMID:22388286

Langowski, J., & Long, A. (2002). Computer systems for the prediction of xenobiotic metabolism. *Advanced Drug Delivery Reviews*, *54*(3), 407–415. doi:10.1016/S0169-409X(02)00011-X PMID:11922955

Lappalainen, T., Sammeth, M., Friedländer, M. R., & C't Hoen, A. (2013). Transcriptome and genome sequencing uncovers functional variation in humans. *Nature*, *501*(7468), 506–511. doi:10.1038/nature12531 PMID:24037378

Larmuth, K. M., Masuyer, G., Douglas, R. G., Schwager, S. L., Acharya, K. R., & Sturrock, E. D. (2016). Kinetic and structural characterization of amyloid-β peptide hydrolysis by human angiotensin-1-converting enzyme. *The FEBS Journal*, *283*(6), 1060–1076. doi:10.1111/febs.13647 PMID:26748546

Larry, W.H. & Antony, M. (2003). The impact of structure-guided drug design on clinical agents. *Current Drug Discovery*, 15-20.

Launay-Vacher, V., Izzedine, H., Karie, S., Hulot, J. S., Baumelou, A., & Deray, G. (2006). Renal tubular drug transporters. *Nephron. Physiology*, *103*(3), 97–106. doi:10.1159/000092212 PMID:16554667

Laurie, A. T., & Jackson, R. M. (2005). Q-SiteFinder: An energy-based method for the prediction of protein-ligand binding sites. *Bioinformatics (Oxford, England)*, *21*(9), 1908–1916. doi:10.1093/bioinformatics/bti315 PMID:15701681

Lauri, G., & Barlett, P. A. (1994). CAVEAT: A program to facilitate the design of organic molecules. *Journal of Computer-Aided Molecular Design*, *8*(1), 51–66. doi:10.1007/BF00124349 PMID:8035213

Lawrence, X. Y. (2008). Pharmaceutical Quality by Design: Product and Process Development, Understanding, and Control. Pharmaceutical Research, 25(4).

Lawrence, X. Yu., Amidon, G., Khan, M. A., Hoag, S. W., Polli, J., Raju, G. K., & Woodcock, J. (2014). Understanding Pharmaceutical Quality by Design. The AAPS Journal, 16(4).

Lawrence, M. C., & Davis, P. C. (1992). CLIX: A search algorithm for finding novel ligands capable of binding proteins of known three-dimensional structure. *Proteins*, *12*(1), 31–41. doi:10.1002/prot.340120105 PMID:1313175

Law, V., Knox, C., Djoumbou, Y., Jewison, T., Guo, A. C., Liu, Y., ... Wishart, D. S. (2014). DrugBank 4.0: Shedding new light on drug metabolism. *Nucleic Acids Research*, *42*(D1), D1091–D1097. doi:10.1093/nar/gkt1068 PMID:24203711

Le, A. V., Phan, T. C. Q., & Nguyen, T. H. (2015). *In silico* Drug Design: Prospective for Drug Lead Discovery. *International Journal of Engineering Science Invention*, *4*(10), 60–70.

Leach, A. R., Shoichet, B. K., & Peishoff, C. E. (2006). Prediction of protein–ligand interactions. Docking and scoring: Successes and gaps. *Journal of Medicinal Chemistry*, *49*(20), 5851–5855. doi:10.1021/jm060999m PMID:17004700

Lea, K., Qu, L., Whitley, P., Schageman, J., Gu, J., & Bramlett, K. (2011). Transcriptome Analysis Using Next-Generation Sequencing Technology. *Journal of Biomolecular Techniques: JBT*, *22*(Suppl), S44.

Lee, G., Ramirez, C. N., Kim, H., Liu, N. Z. B., & Radu, C. (2012). Large-scale screening using familial dysautonomia induced pluripotent stem cells identifies compounds that rescue IKBKAP expression. *Nature Biotechnology*, *30*(12), 1244–1248. doi:10.1038/nbt.2435 PMID:23159879

Leeson, P. D., & Springthorpe, B. (2007). The influence of drug-like concepts on decision-making in medicinal chemistry. *Nature Reviews. Drug Discovery*, *6*(11), 881–890. doi:10.1038/nrd2445 PMID:17971784

Lee, W., & Kim, R. B. (2004). Transporters and renal drug elimination. *Annual Review of Pharmacology and Toxicology*, *44*(1), 137–166. doi:10.1146/annurev.pharmtox.44.101802.121856 PMID:14744242

Lehmann, J. (2009). DL-Learner: Learning Concepts in Description Logics. *Journal of Machine Learning Research*, *10*, 2639–2642.

Lehne, B., & Schlitt, T. (2009). Protein-protein interaction databases: Keeping up with growing interactomes. *Human Genomics*, *3*, 291–297. PMID:19403463

Lengauer, T. (2004). *Bioinformatics from genome to drugs*. Weinheim, Germany: Wiley- VCH.

Leo, A. J., & Hansch, C. (1999). Role of hydrophobic effects in mechanistic QSAR. *Perspectives in Drug Discovery and Design*, *17*, 1–25.

Leonardo, G. F., Ricardo, N. S., Glaucius, O., & Adriano, D. A. (2015). Molecular Docking and Structure-Based Drug Design Strategies. *Molecules (Basel, Switzerland)*, *20*(7), 13384–13421. doi:10.3390/molecules200713384 PMID:26205061

Leuenberger, H., Puchkov, M., Krausbauer, E., & Betz, G. (2009). Manufacturing pharmaceutical granules, Is the granulation end-point a myth. Powder Technology, 189, 141–148.

Lewis, C. V. F., Ioannides, C., & Parke, D. V. (1998). An improved and updated version of the compact procedure for the evaluation of P450-mediated activation. *Drug Metabolism Reviews*, *30*(4), 709–737. doi:10.3109/03602539808996328 PMID:9844807

Lewis, D. F., Ioannides, C., & Parke, D. V. (1998). A combined COMPACT and HazardExpert study of 40 chemicals for which information on mutagenicity and carcinogenicity is known, including the results of human epidemiological studies. *Human & Experimental Pharmacology*, *17*, 577–586. PMID:9821022

Lewis, D. V. F. (2001). COMPACT: A structural approach to the modelling of cytochromes P450 and their interactions with xenobiotics. *Journal of Chemical Technology and Biotechnology (Oxford, Oxfordshire)*, *76*(3), 237–244. doi:10.1002/jctb.363

Li, A. P. (2005). Preclinical in Vitro Screening Assays for Drug- Like Properties. *Drug Discovery Today*, *2*(2), 179–185. doi:10.1016/j.ddtec.2005.05.024 PMID:24981846

Liang, J., Edelsbrunner, H., & Woodward, C. (1998). Anatomy of protein pockets and cavities: Measurement of binding site geometry and implications for ligand design. *Protein Science*, *7*(9), 1884–1887. doi:10.1002/pro.5560070905 PMID:9761470

Liebeschuetz, J. W., Jones, S. D., Morgan, P. J., Murray, C. W., Rimmer, A. D., Roscoe, J. M. E., ... Wilkinson, K. (2002). PRO_SELECT: Combining structure-based Drug Design and array-based chemistry for rapid lead discovery 2 the development of a series of highly potent and selective factor Xa inhibitors. *Journal of Medicinal Chemistry*, *45*(6), 1221–1232. doi:10.1021/jm010944e PMID:11881991

Li, H., Handsaker, B., Wysoker, A., Fennell, T., Ruan, J., Homer, N., ... Durbin, R. (2009). The sequence alignment/map format and SAMtools. *Bioinformatics (Oxford, England)*, *25*(16), 2078–2079. doi:10.1093/bioinformatics/btp352 PMID:19505943

Lindert, S., Zhu, W., Liu, Y. L., Pang, R., Oldfield, E., & McCammon, J. A. (2013). Non-Bisphosphonate Inhibitors of Isoprenoid Biosynthesis Identified via Computer-Aided Drug Design. *Chemical Biology & Drug Design*, *81*, 742–748. doi:10.1111/cbdd.12121 PMID:23421555

Lin, S. K. (2005). Pharmacophore Perception, Development and Use in Drug Design. *Molecules (Basel, Switzerland)*, *5*(12), 987–989. doi:10.3390/50700987

Lionberger, Lee, Lee, Raw, & Yu. (2008). Quality by design: concepts for ANDAs. The AAPS Journal, 10, 268-276.

Lionta, E., Spyrou, G., Vassilatis, D. K., & Cournia, Z. (2014). Structure-based virtual screening for drug discovery: Principles, applications and recent advances. *Current Topics in Medicinal Chemistry*, *14*(16), 1923–1938. doi:10.2174/1568026614666140929124445 PMID:25262799

Lipinski, C. A. (2000). Druglike properties and the causes of poor solubility and poor permeability. *Journal of Pharmacological and Toxicological Methods*, *44*(1), 235–249. doi:10.1016/S1056-8719(00)00107-6 PMID:11274893

Lipinski, C. A., Lombardo, F. M., Dominy, B. W., & Feeney, P. J. (2001). Experimental and computational approaches to estimate solubility and permeability in drug discovery and development settings. *Advanced Drug Delivery Reviews*, *46*(1-3), 3–26. doi:10.1016/S0169-409X(00)00129-0 PMID:11259830

Lipinski, C. A., Lombardo, F., Dominy, B. W., & Feeney, P. J. (1997). Experimental and Computational Approaches to Estimate Solubility and Permeability in Drug Discovery and Development Settings. *Advanced Drug Delivery Reviews*, *23*(1-3), 3–25. doi:10.1016/S0169-409X(96)00423-1 PMID:11259830

Li, R., Fan, W., Tian, G., Zhu, H., He, L., Cai, J., ... Wang, J. (2010). The sequence and de novo assembly of the giant panda genome. *Nature*, *463*(7279), 311–317. doi:10.1038/nature08696 PMID:20010809

Liu, B., Luo, W., Zhang, Y., Li, H., Zhu, N., Huang, D., & Zhou, Y. (2012). Role of cyclooxygenase-1-mediated prostacyclin synthesis in endothelium-dependent vasoconstrictor activity of porcine interlobular renal arteries. *American Journal of Physiology. Renal Physiology*, *302*(9), F1133–F1140. doi:10.1152/ajprenal.00604.2011 PMID:22301626

Liu, C. X. (2013). Rethinking on research and development in innovation of biomedicines. *Drugs Clinic*, *28*, 469–475.

Liu, L. L., Lu, J., Lu, Y., Zheng, M. Y., Luo, X. M., Zhu, W. L., ... Chen, K. (2014). Novel Bayesian classification models for predicting compounds blocking hERG potassium channels. *Acta Pharmacologica Sinica*, *35*(8), 1093–1102. doi:10.1038/aps.2014.35 PMID:24976154

Liu, L., Li, Y., Li, S., Hu, N., He, Y., & Pong, R. (2012a). Comparison of Next-Generation Sequencing Systems. *Journal of Biomedicine & Biotechnology*, *11*. doi:10.1155/2012/251364 PMID:22829749

Liu, L., Li, Y., Li, S., Hu, N., He, Y., & Pong, R. (2012b). Comparison of next-generation sequencing systems. *BioMed Research International*. PMID:22829749

Loew, G. H., Villar, H. O., & Alkorta, I. (1993). Strategies for Indirect Computer-Aided Drug Design. *Pharmaceutical Research*, *10*(4), 475–486. doi:10.1023/A:1018977414572 PMID:8483829

Lombardino, J. G., & Lowe, J. A. (2004). The role of the medicinal chemist in drug discovery--then and now. *Nature Reviews. Drug Discovery*, *3*(10), 853–862. doi:10.1038/nrd1523 PMID:15459676

López, Y., Nakai, K., & Patil, A. (2015). HitPredict version 4: Comprehensive reliability scoring of physical protein–protein interactions from more than 100 species. *Database*, *2015*, bav117. doi:10.1093/database/bav117 PMID:26708988

Lyne, P. D. (2002). Structure-based virtual screening: An overview. *Drug Discovery Today*, *7*(20), 1602178. doi:10.1016/S1359-6446(02)02483-2 PMID:12546894

Mahadevan, D., Powis, G., Mash, E. A., George, B., Gokhale, V. M., Zhang, S., ... Jana, U. (2008). Discovery of a novel class of AKT pleckstrin homology domain inhibitors. *Molecular Cancer Therapeutics*, *7*(9), 2621–2632. doi:10.1158/1535-7163.MCT-07-2276 PMID:18790745

Majeed & Prakash. (2000). The medicinal uses of pepper. *The International Pepper News*, *1*, 23-31.

Makino, S., & Kuntz, I. D. (1997). Automated flexible ligand docking method and its application for database search. *Journal of Computational Chemistry*, *18*(14), 1812–1825. doi:10.1002/(SICI)1096-987X(19971115)18:14<1812::AID-JCC10>3.0.CO;2-H

Małgorzata, J., Katarzyna, S., & Anna, P. (2012). Quantification of Lipophilicity of 1, 2, 4-Triazoles Using Micellar Chromatography. *Chromatographia*, *75*(9), 449–456. PMID:22593604

Mandagere, A. K., Thompson, T. N., & Hwang, K. K. (2002). A graphical model for estimating oral bioavailability of drugs in humans and other species from their Caco-2 permeability and *in vitro* liver enzyme metabolic stability rates. *Journal of Medicinal Chemistry*, *45*(2), 304–311. doi:10.1021/jm010152k PMID:11784135

Mannhold, R., & van de Waterbeemd, H. (2001). Substructure and whole molecule approaches for calculating log P. *Journal of Computer-Aided Molecular Design*, *15*(4), 337–354. doi:10.1023/A:1011107422318 PMID:11349816

Ma, P., & Zemmel, R. (2002). Value of Novelty? *Nature Reviews. Drug Discovery*, *1*(8), 571–572. doi:10.1038/nrd884 PMID:12402497

Mardis, E. R. (2008). The impact of next-generation sequencing technology on genetics. *Trends in Genetics*, *24*(3), 133–141. doi:10.1016/j.tig.2007.12.007 PMID:18262675

Mardis, E. R. (2013). Next-generation sequencing platforms. *Annual Review of Analytical Chemistry (Palo Alto, Calif.)*, *6*(1), 287–303. doi:10.1146/annurev-anchem-062012-092628 PMID:23560931

Margulies, M., Egholm, M., Altman, W. E., Attiya, S., Bader, J. S., Bemben, L. A., ... Rothberg, J. M. (2005). Genome sequencing in microfabricated high-density picolitre reactors. *Nature*, *437*(7057), 376–380. doi:10.1038/nature03959 PMID:16056220

Martinez-Mancilla, M., Rosa, Z. G., & Gomez, R. E. (2006). Molecular haemoto-oncology and new specific treatment strategies for leukemia. *Gaceta Medica de Mexico*, *142*, 145–150. PMID:16711549

Martin, M., Srinivasaraghavan, K., Alexander-Thomas, H., Marina, M. M., Stephanie, C., & Vincent, C. (2013). Structural basis for the inhibition of histone deacetylases 8 (HDAC8), a key epigenetic player in the blood fluke Schistosomamansoni. *PLoS Pathogens*, *9*(9), e1003645. doi:10.1371/journal.ppat.1003645 PMID:24086136

Marvin, C. (1978). Composition of the steric parameter as a function of alkyl branching. *The Journal of Organic Chemistry*, *43*(21), 3995–4001. doi:10.1021/jo00415a002

Maryanoff, B. E. (2004). Inhibitors of serine proteases as potential therapeutic agents: The road from thrombin totryptase to cathepsin G. *Journal of Medicinal Chemistry*, *47*(4), 769–787. doi:10.1021/jm030493t PMID:14761180

Masferrer, J. L., & Leahy, K. M. (2000). Antiangiogenic and Antitumor Activities of Cyclooxygenase-2 Inhibitors. *Cancer Research*, *60*(5), 1306–1311. PMID:10728691

Mason, J. S., Good, A. C., & Martin, E. J. (2001). 3-D pharmacophores in drug discovery. *Current Pharmaceutical Design*, *7*(7), 567–597. doi:10.2174/1381612013397843 PMID:11375769

Mata, P., Gillet, V. J., Johnson, A. P., Lampreia, J., Myatt, G. J., Sike, S., & Stebbings, A. L. (1995). SPROUT-3D structure generation using templates. *Journal of Chemical Information and Computer Sciences*, *35*(3), 479–493. doi:10.1021/ci00025a016

Mathieu, M. (Ed.). (2002). *New drug development: A regulatory overview* (6th ed.). Waltham: Parexel International Corporation.

Mc Guire, J. J. (2003). Anticancer antifolates: Current status and future directions. *Current Pharmaceutical Design*, *9*(31), 2593–2613. doi:10.2174/1381612033453712 PMID:14529544

McGann, M. (2012). FRED and HYBRID docking performance on standardized datasets. *Journal of Computer-Aided Molecular Design*, *26*(8), 897–906. doi:10.100710822-012-9584-8 PMID:22669221

McGleenon, B. M., Dynan, K. B., & Passmore, A. P. (1999). Acetylcholinesterase inhibitors in Alzheimer's disease. *British Journal of Clinical Pharmacology*, *48*(4), 471–480. doi:10.1046/j.1365-2125.1999.00026.x PMID:10583015

McGuffin, L. J. (2008). Protein Fold Recognition and Threading. *Computational Structural Biology*, 37–60. doi:10.1142/9789812778789_0002

McLaren, D., Gorba, T., Rotrou, A. M., Pillai, G., Chappell, C., Stacey, A., & ... . (2013). Automated large-scale culture and medium-throughput chemical screen for modulators of proliferation and viability of human induced pluripotent stem cell-derived neuroepithelial-like stem cells. *Journal of Biomolecular Screening*, *18*(3), 258–268. doi:10.1177/1087057112461446 PMID:23042076

McMartin, C., & Bohacek, R. S. (1997). QXP: Powerful, rapid computer algorithms for structure-based Drug Design. *Journal of Computer-Aided Molecular Design*, *11*(4), 333–344. doi:10.1023/A:1007907728892 PMID:9334900

Meanwell, N. A. (2012). Synopsis of some recent tactical application of bioisosteres. *Journal of Medicinal Chemistry*, *54*(8), 2529–2591. doi:10.1021/jm1013693 PMID:21413808

Meireles, L. M., Domling, A. S., & Camacho, C. J. (2010). ANCHOR: A web server and database for analysis of protein-protein interaction binding pockets for drug discovery. *Nucleic Acids Research*, *38*(Web Server), W407–W411. doi:10.1093/nar/gkq502 PMID:20525787

Melesina, J., Robaa, D., Pierce, R. J., Romier, C., & Sippl, W. (2015). Homology modeling of parasite histone deacetylases to guide the structure-based design of selective inhibitors. *Journal of Molecular Graphics & Modelling*, *62*, 342–361. doi:10.1016/j.jmgm.2015.10.006 PMID:26595183

Mendenhall, J. & Meiler, J. (2016). Improving quantitative structure-activity relationship models using Artificial Neural Networks trained with dropout. *Journal of Computer Aided Drug Design, 30*, 177–189.

Meng, X. Y., Zhang, H. X., Mezei, M., & Cui, M. (2011). Molecular docking: A powerful approach for structure-based drug discovery. *Current Computer-aided Drug Design*, *7*(2), 146–157. doi:10.2174/157340911795677602 PMID:21534921

Mestres, J., & Veeneman, G. H. (2003). Identification of "latent hits" in compound screening collections. *Journal of Medicinal Chemistry. Medicinal Chemistry (New York)*, *46*, 3441–3444. PMID:12877579

Mhadhb, L., Akaichi, J., Karray, M. H., & Archimde, B. (2015, April). Ontologies for Location Based Services Quality Enhancement: The Case of Emergency Services. *Second International Conference on Edemocracy & Egovernment (Icedeg)*. 10.1109/ICEDEG.2015.7114469

Michael, H., David, W. T., Craighead, J. L., Economides, C., & Rosenthal, J. (2014). Clinical development success rates for investigational drugs. *Nature Biotechnology*, *32*(1), 40–51. doi:10.1038/nbt.2786 PMID:24406927

Michelini, E., Cevenini, L., Mezzanotte, L., Coppa, A., & Roda, A. (2010). Cell Based Assays: Fuelling drug discovery. *Analytical Biochemistry*, *397*, 1–10. PMID:19761747

Michel, J., Tirado-Rives, J., & Jorgensen, W. L. (2009). Energetics of displacing water molecules from protein binding sites: Consequences for ligand optimization. *Journal of the American Chemical Society*, *131*(42), 15403–15411. doi:10.1021/ja906058w PMID:19778066

Mihaylova, M. M., & Shaw, R. J. (2013). Metabolic reprogramming by class I and II histone deacetylases. *Trends in Endocrinology and Metabolism*, *24*(1), 48–57. doi:10.1016/j.tem.2012.09.003 PMID:23062770

Miller, M. A. (2002). Chemical database techniques in drug discovery. *Nature Reviews. Drug Discovery*, *1*(3), 220–227. doi:10.1038/nrd745 PMID:12120506

Milne, J. R., Hellestrand, K. J., Bexton, R. S., Burnett, P. J., Debbas, N. M., & Camm, A. J. (1984). Class 1 antiarrhythmic drugs characteristic electrocardiographic differences when assessed by atrial and ventricular pacing. *European Heart Journal*, *5*(2), 99–107. doi:10.1093/oxfordjournals.eurheartj.a061633 PMID:6723689

Miranker, A., & Karplus, M. (1991). Functionality maps of binding sites: A multiple copy simultaneous search method. *Proteins*, *11*(1), 29–34. doi:10.1002/prot.340110104 PMID:1961699

Miranker, A., & Karplus, M. (1995). An automated-method for dynamic ligand design. *Proteins*, *23*(4), 472–490. doi:10.1002/prot.340230403 PMID:8749844

Mitchell, J. B. O., Laskowski, R. A., Alex, A., & Thornton, J. M. (1999). BLEEP-potential of mean force describing protein-ligand interactions: I generating potential. *Journal of Computational Chemistry*, *20*(11), 1165–1176. doi:10.1002/(SICI)1096-987X(199908)20:11<1165::AID-JCC7>3.0.CO;2-A

Moazed, D., & Noller, H. F. (1987). Interaction of antibiotics with functional sites in 16S ribosomal RNA. *Nature*, *327*(6121), 389–394. doi:10.1038/327389a0 PMID:2953976

Moitessier, N., Englebienne, P., Lee, D., Lawandi, J., & Corbeil, C. (2008). Towards the development of universal, fast and highly accurate docking/scoring methods: A long way to go. *British Journal of Pharmacology*, *153*(S1), S7–S26. doi:10.1038j.bjp.0707515 PMID:18037925

Moon, J., & Howe, W. (1991). Computer design of bioactive molecules: A method for receptor-based *de novo* ligand design. *Proteins*, *11*(4), 314–328. doi:10.1002/prot.340110409 PMID:1758885

Moreton. (2009). Functionality and Performance of Excipients in Quality-by-Design World Part V: Changes in the Sourcing and Supply of Pharmaceutical Excipients. *American Pharmaceutical Review*. Retrieved from https://www.americanpharmaceuticalreview.com/Featured-Articles/118926-Functionality-and-Performance-of-Excipients-in-Quality-by-Design-World-Part-V-Changes-in-the-Sourcing-and-Supply-of-Pharmaceutical-Excipients/

Morgan, S., Grootendorst, P., Lexchin, J., Cunningham, C., & Greyson, D. (2011). The cost of drug development: A systematic review. *Health Policy (Amsterdam)*, *100*(1), 4–17. doi:10.1016/j.healthpol.2010.12.002 PMID:21256615

Morris, G. M., Goodsell, D. S., Halliday, R. S., Huey, R., Hart, W. E., Belew, R. K., & Olson, A. J. (1999). Automated docking using a Lamarckian genetic algorithm and an empirical binding free energy function. *Journal of Computational Chemistry*, *19*(14), 1639–1662. doi:10.1002/(SICI)1096-987X(19981115)19:14<1639::AID-JCC10>3.0.CO;2-B

Morris, G. M., Goodsell, D. S., Huey, R., & Olson, A. J. (1996). Distributed automated docking of flexible ligands to proteins: Parallel applications of AutoDock 2.4. *Journal of Computer-Aided Molecular Design*, *10*(4), 293–304. doi:10.1007/BF00124499 PMID:8877701

Mortazavi, A., Williams, B. A., McCue, K., Schaeffer, L., & Wold, B. (2008). Mapping and quantifying mammalian transcriptomes by RNA-Seq. *Nature Methods*, *5*(7), 621–628. doi:10.1038/nmeth.1226 PMID:18516045

Moses, S. A., Ali, M. A., Zuohe, S., Du-Cuny, L., Zhou, L. L., Lemos, R., ... Meuille, E. J. (2009). In vitro and in vivo activity of novel small-molecule inhibitors targeting the pleckstrin homology domain of protein kinase B/AKT. *Cancer Research*, *69*(12), 5073–5081. doi:10.1158/0008-5472.CAN-08-3839 PMID:19491272

Muegge, I., & Martin, Y. C. (1999). A general and fast scoring function for protein-ligand interactions: A simplified potential approach. *Journal of Medicinal Chemistry*, *42*(5), 791–804. doi:10.1021/jm980536j PMID:10072678

Muhuo, L., & Bolian, L. (2010). Some properties of the first general Zagreb index. *Australasian Journal of Combinatorics*, *47*, 285–294.

Munos, B. (2009). Lessons from 60 years of pharmaceutical innovation. *Nature Reviews. Drug Discovery*, *8*(12), 959–968. doi:10.1038/nrd2961 PMID:19949401

Murcko, M. (1997). Recent advances in ligand design methods. *Reviews in Computational Chemistry*, *11*, 1–66.

Murray, C., Auton, T. R., & Eldridge, M. D. (1998). Empirical scoring functions. II. The testing of an empirical scoring function for the prediction of ligand-receptor binding affinities and the use of Bayesian regression to improve the quality of the model. *Journal of Computer-Aided Molecular Design*, *12*(5), 503–519. doi:10.1023/A:1008040323669 PMID:9834910

Myers, M., Richmond, R. C., & Oakeshott, J. G. (1988). On the origins of esterases. *Molecular Biology and Evolution*, *5*(2), 113–119. PMID:3163407

Narke, R. M., & Singh, R. P. (2014). Qverview of QbD: A challenge to the Pharmaceuticval industry. Asian Journal of Pharmaceutical Research and Development, 2, 42-53.

Naseem, A. C. (2012). A Case Study of Dispersible Tablets. *Quality by Design Approach for Formulation Development, 423*, 167–178.

Nassar, A. E. F., Kamel, A. M., & Clarimont, C. (2004). Improving the decision-making process in structural modification of drug candidates: Reducing toxicity. *Drug Discovery Today, 9*(24), 1055–1064. doi:10.1016/S1359-6446(04)03297-0 PMID:15582794

NCBI Resource Coordinators. (2013). Database resources of the National Center for Biotechnology Information. *Nucleic Acids Research, 41*(Database issue), D8–D20. doi:10.1093/nar/gks1189 PMID:23193264

Neuberger, T., Burton, B., Clark, H., & Van Goor, F. (2011). Use of primary cultures of human bronchial epithelial cells isolated from cystic fibrosis patients for the pre-clinical testing of CFTR modulators. *Methods in Molecular Biology (Clifton, N.J.), 741*, 39–54. doi:10.1007/978-1-61779-117-8_4 PMID:21594777

Neumann, S., Huang, W., Titus, S., Krause, G., Kleinau, G., Alberobello, A. T., ... Gershengorn, M. C. (2009). Small-molecule agonists for the thyrotropin receptor stimulate thyroid function in human thyrocytes and mice. *Proceedings of the National Academy of Sciences of the United States of America, 106*(30), 12471–12476. doi:10.1073/pnas.0904506106 PMID:19592511

Nichols, S. E., Baron, R., Ivetac, A., & McCammon, J. A. (2011). Predictive power of molecular dynamics receptor structures in virtual screening. *Journal of Chemical Information and Modeling, 51*(6), 1439–1446. doi:10.1021/ci200117n PMID:21534609

Nienaber, V. L., Richardson, P. L., Klighofer, V., Bouska, J. J., Giranda, V. L., & Greer, J. (2000). Discovering novel ligands for macromolecules using Xray crystallographic screening. *Nature Biotechnology, 18*(10), 1105–1108. doi:10.1038/80319 PMID:11017052

Nishibata, Y., & Itai, A. (1991). Automatic creation of drug candidate structures based on receptor structure-starting point for artificial lead generation. *Tetrahedron, 47*(43), 8985–8990. doi:10.1016/S0040-4020(01)86503-0

Nolte-'t Hoen, E. N., Buermans, H. P., Waasdorp, M., Stoorvogel, W., Wauben, M. H., & 't Hoen, P. A. (2012). Deep sequencing of RNA from immune cell-derived vesicles uncovers the selective incorporation of small non-coding RNA biotypes with potential regulatory functions. *Nucleic Acids Research, 40*(18), 9272–9285. doi:10.1093/nar/gks658 PMID:22821563

Nosal, R. (2006). Industry perspective of risk based CMC assessment under QbD. *AAPS Annual Meeting*.

Nuez, A., & Rodriguez, R. (2008). Current methodology for the assessment of ADME-Tox properties on drug candidate molecules. *Biotecnología Aplicada, 25*, 97–110.

Oehme, I., Oehme, I., Deubzer, H. E., Wegener, D., Pickert, D., Linke, J. P., & ... . (2009). Histone deacetylase 8 in neuro blasto matumorigenesis. *Clinical Cancer Research, 15*(1), 91–99. doi:10.1158/1078-0432.CCR-08-0684 PMID:19118036

Oh, W. S., Kim, D. N., Jung, J., Cho, K. H., & No, K. T. (2008). New combined model for the prediction of regioselectivity in cytochrome P450/3A4 mediated metabolism. *Journal of Chemical Information and Modeling, 48*(3), 591–601. doi:10.1021/ci7003576 PMID:18290640

Olivier, R., Daniel, I., & Elizabeth, D. (2003). Constitutive nuclear localization and initial cytoplasmic apoptotic activation of endogenous caspase-3 evidenced by confocal microscopy. *International Journal of Experimental Pathology, 84*(2), 75–81. doi:10.1046/j.1365-2613.2003.00339.x PMID:12801281

Olson, D. E., Wagner, F. F., Kaya, T., Gale, J. P., Aidoud, N., Davoine, E. L., ... Holson, E. B. (2013). Discovery of the first histone deacetylase 6/8 dual inhibitors. *Journal of Medicinal Chemistry*, *56*(11), 4816–4820. doi:10.1021/jm400390r PMID:23672185

Ononye, S. N., Heyst, M. V., Falcone, E. M., Anderson, A. C., & Wright, D. L. (2012). Toward isozyme-selective inhibitors of histone deacetylase as therapeutic agents for the treatment of cancer. *Pharmaceutical Patent Analyst*, *1*(2), 207–221. doi:10.4155/ppa.12.21 PMID:24163736

OpenHelix. (n.d.). *IntAct protein interaction database*. Retrieved from http://www.openhelix.com/tutorialInfo.cgi?id=55

Oprea, T. I., Allu, T. K., Fara, D. C., Rad, R. F., Ostopovici, L., & Bologa, C. G. (2007). Lead-like, drug-like or "pub-like": How different are they? *Journal of Computer-Aided Molecular Design*, *21*(1-3), 113–119. doi:10.100710822-007-9105-3 PMID:17333482

Oprea, T. I., & Matter, H. (2004). Integrating virtual screening in lead discovery. *Current Opinion in Chemical Biology*, *8*(4), 349–358. doi:10.1016/j.cbpa.2004.06.008 PMID:15288243

Ortore, G., Colo, F. D., & Martinelli, A. (2009). Docking of hydroxamic acids into HDAC1 and HDAC8: A rationalization of activity trends and selectivities. *Journal of Chemical Information and Modeling*, *49*(12), 2774–2785. doi:10.1021/ci900288e PMID:19947584

Osterberg, F., Morris, G. M., Sanner, M. F., Olson, A. J., & Goodsell, D. S. (2002). Automated docking to multiple target structures: Incorporation of protein mobility and structural water heterogeneity in Auto Dock. *Proteins*, *46*(1), 34–40. doi:10.1002/prot.10028 PMID:11746701

Ouyang, X., Zhou, S., Su, C. T. T., Ge, Z., Li, R., & Kwoh, C. K. (2013). Covalent Dock: Automated covalent docking with parameterized covalent linkage energy estimation and molecular geometry constraints. *Journal of Computational Chemistry*, *34*(4), 326–336. doi:10.1002/jcc.23136 PMID:23034731

Ouzounis, C. A. (2012). Rise and Demise of Bioinformatics? Promise and Progress. *PLoS Computational Biology*, *8*(4), e1002487. doi:10.1371/journal.pcbi.1002487 PMID:22570600

Overington, J. P., Al-Lazikani, B., & Hopkins, A. L. (2006). How many drug targets are there? *Nature Reviews. Drug Discovery*, *5*(12), 993–996. doi:10.1038/nrd2199 PMID:17139284

Pacák, P. (1989). Molar refractivity and interactions in solutions I. Molar refractivity of some monovalent ions in aqueous and dimethyl sulfoxide solutions. *Chemical Papers*, *43*(4), 489–500.

Pairet, M., Churchill, L., Trummlitz, G., & Engelhardt, G. (1996). Differential inhibition of cyclooxygenase-1(COX-1) and −2 (COX2) by NSAIDS: Consequences on anti-inflammatory activity versus gastric and renal safety. In Side Effects of Anti-Inflammatory Drugs IV (pp. 223-232). Kluwer Academic Publishers.

Pajeva, I. K., & Wiese, M. (2002). Pharmacophore model of drugs involved in P-glycoprotein multidrug resistance: Explanation of structural variety (hypothesis). *Journal of Medicinal Chemistry*, *45*(26), 5671–5686. doi:10.1021/jm020941h PMID:12477351

Palm, K., Stenberg, P., Luthman, K., & Artursson, P. I. (1997). Polar molecular surface properties predict the intestinal absorption of drugs in human. *Pharmaceutical Research*, *14*(5), 568–571. doi:10.1023/A:1012188625088 PMID:9165525

Pammolli, F., Magazzini, L. & Riccaboni, M. (2011). The productivity crisis in pharmaceutical R&D. *Nature Reviews Drug Discovery*, *10*, 428–38.

Pang, Y. P., Perola, E., Xu, K., & Prendergast, F. G. (2001). Predergast FG. EDUDOC: A computer program for identification of drug interaction sites in macromolecules and drug leads from chemical databases. *Journal of Computational Chemistry*, *22*(15), 1750–1771. doi:10.1002/jcc.1129 PMID:12116409

Pang, Y. P., Xu, K., Kollmeyer, T. M., Perola, E., McGrath, W. J., Green, D. T., & Mangel, W. F. (2001). Discovery of a new inhibitor lead of adenovirus proteinase: Steps towards selective, irreversible inhibitors of cysteine proteinases. *FEBS Letters*, *502*(3), 93–97. doi:10.1016/S0014-5793(01)02672-2 PMID:11583118

Papadatos, G., Davies, M., Dedman, N., Chambers, J., Gaulton, A., Siddle, J., ... Overington, J. P. (2016). SureChEMBL: A large-scale, chemically annotated patent document database. *Nucleic Acids Research*, *44*(D1), D1220–D1228. doi:10.1093/nar/gkv1253 PMID:26582922

Parvu, L. (2003). QSAR – a piece of drug design. *Journal of Cellular and Molecular Medicine*, *7*(3), 333–335. doi:10.1111/j.1582-4934.2003.tb00235.x PMID:14594559

Passin, T. B. (2004). *Explorer's Guide to the Semantic Web.* Manning Publication.

PAT - A Framework for Innovative Pharmaceutical Development, Manufacturing, and Quality Assurance. (2004). U.S. Department of Health and Human Services Food and Drug Administration Guidance.

Patel, C. K., &Sen, D. J. (2009). COX-1 and COX-2 inhibitors: Current status and prospects over COX-3 inhibitors. *International Journal of Drug Development and Research*, 136-145.

Patel, Y., Gillet, V. J., Bravi, G. & Leach, A. R. (2002). A comparison of the pharmacophore identification programme CATALYST, DISCO and GASP. *Journal of Computer Aided Drug Design, 16*, 653–681.

Patel, R. K., & Jain, M. (2012). NGS QC Toolkit: A toolkit for quality control of next generation sequencing data. *PLoS One*, *7*(2), e30619. doi:10.1371/journal.pone.0030619 PMID:22312429

Patel-Schneider, P. F., Hayes, P., & Horrocks, I. (2004). *OWL Web Ontology Language Semantics and Abstract Syntax.* W3c Recommendation.

Patodar, A.A., Selvam, G., Jayakandan, M., Mobiya, A.K., Bagherwal, A. & Sanadya, G. *et al.*, (2011). Lead discovery and lead optimization: A useful strategy in molecular modification of lead compound in analog design. *International Journal of Drug Design and Discovery, 2*(2), 458-463.

Paul, N., & Rognan, D. (2002). ConsDock: A new program for the consensus analysis of protein-ligand interactions. *Proteins*, *47*(4), 521–533. doi:10.1002/prot.10119 PMID:12001231

Pearlman, D. A., & Murcko, M. A. (1993). CONCEPTS: New dynamics algorithm for *de novo* drug suggestions. *Journal of Computer-Aided Molecular Design, 14*, 1184.

Pearlman, D. A., & Murcko, M. A. (1996). CONCERTS: Dynamics connection of fragments as an approach to *De novo* ligand design. *Journal of Computer-Aided Molecular Design*, *39*, 1651–1663. PMID:8648605

Peng, J., Li, J., & Hamann, M. (2005). The Marine Bromotyrosine Derivatives. *The Alkaloids. Chemistry and Biology*, *6*, 59–262. doi:10.1016/S1099-4831(05)61002-4 PMID:16173400

Pengyu, R., Jaehun, C., Dennis, G. T., Michael, J. S., Marcelo, M., Jiajing, Z., & Nathan, A. B. (2012). Biomolecular electrostatics and solvation: A computational perspective. *Quarterly Reviews of Biophysics*, *45*(4), 427–491. doi:10.1017/S003358351200011X PMID:23217364

Penning, T. D., Talley, J. J., Bertenshaw, S. R., Carter, J. S., Collins, P. W., Docter, S., ... Isakson, P. C. (1997). Synthesis and Biological Evaluation of the 1,5-Diarylpyrazole Class of Cyclooxygenase-2 Inhibitors: Identification of 4-[5-(4-Methylphenyl)-3- (trifluoromethyl)-1 *H* -pyrazol-1-yl]benzenesulfonamide (SC-58635, Celecoxib). *Journal of Medicinal Chemistry*, *40*(9), 1347–1365. doi:10.1021/jm960803q PMID:9135032

Perkins, J. R., Diboun, I., Dessailly, B. H., Lees, J. G., & Orengo, C. (2010). Transient Protein-Protein Interactions: Structural, Functional, and Network Properties. *Structure (London, England)*, *18*(10), 1233–1243. doi:10.1016/j.str.2010.08.007 PMID:20947012

Perkins, R., Fang, H., Tong, W. D., & Welsh, W. J. (2003). Quantitative structure-activity relationship methods: Perspectives on drug discovery and toxicology. *Environmental Toxicology and Chemistry*, *2*(8), 1666–1679. doi:10.1897/01-171 PMID:12924569

Peter, I., Christian, S., & Achim, M. (2006). Drugs, their targets and the nature and number of drug targets. *Nature Reviews. Drug Discovery*, *5*(10), 821–834. doi:10.1038/nrd2132 PMID:17016423

Polamarasetty, A., Kakularam, K. R., & Pallu, R. (2012). Structure and ligand based drug design strategies in the development of novel 5-LOX inhibitors. *Current Medicinal Chemistry*, *19*(22), 3763–3778. doi:10.2174/092986712801661112 PMID:22680930

Pollock, J. T. (2009). *Semantic Web for Dummies*. Wiley.

Popa-Burke, I. G., Issakova, O., Arroway, J. D., Bernasconi, P., Chen, M., Coudurier, L., ... Hodge, C. N. (2004). Streamlined system for purifying and quantifying a diverse library of compounds and the effect of compound concentration measurements on the accurate interpretation of biological assay results. *Analytical Chemistry*, *76*(24), 7278–7287. doi:10.1021/ac0491859 PMID:15595870

Prasit, P., & Riendeau, D. (1997). Selective cyclooxygenase-2 inhibitors. In Annual Reports in Medicinal Chemistry (pp. 211-220). Elsevier Publishing.

Prieto, P., Kinsner-Ovaskainen, A., Stanzel, S., Albella, B., Artursson, P., Campillo, N., ... Kopp-Schneider, A. (2013). The value of selected in vitro and in silico methods to predict acute oral toxicity in a regulatory context: Results from the European project ACuteTox. *Toxicology In Vitro*, *27*(4), 1357–1376. doi:10.1016/j.tiv.2012.07.013 PMID:22922246

Prija, P., Shikhar, G., Madhu, C., Rashmi, T., Anil, S. B., Garima, G., ... Hanumantharao, G. R. (2012). 2D-QSAR, docking studies, and in silico ADMET Prediction of polyphenolic acetates as substrates for protein acetyltransferasefunction of glutamine synthetase of Mycobacterium tuberculosis. *ISRN Structural Biology*.

Pritchard, J. F., Romet, M. J., Reimer, M. L. J., Mortimer, E., Rolfe, B., & Cayen, M. N. (2003). Making better drugs: Decision gates in non-clinical drug development. *Nature Reviews. Drug Discovery*, *2*(7), 542–553. doi:10.1038/nrd1131 PMID:12815380

Prival, M. J. (2001). Evaluation of the TOPKAT system for predicting the carcinogenicity of chemicals. *Environmental and Molecular Mutagenesis*, *37*(1), 55–69. doi:10.1002/1098-2280(2001)37:1<55::AID-EM1006>3.0.CO;2-5 PMID:11170242

Profile Biopharmaceutical Industry. (2016). Retrieved from http://phrma-docs.phrma.org/sites/default/files/pdf/biopharmaceutical-industry-profile.pdf

Proudfoot, J. R. (2002). Drugs, leads, and drug-likeness: An analysis of some recently launched drugs. *Bioorganic & Medicinal Chemistry Letters*, *12*(12), 1647–1650. doi:10.1016/S0960-894X(02)00244-5 PMID:12039582

PubChem Docs. (n.d.). Retrieved March 10, 2018, from https://pubchemdocs.ncbi.nlm.nih.gov/data-organization

PubChem. (n.d.). Retrieved from https://pubchem.ncbi.nlm.nih.gov/#

Pueyo, M. E., Arnal, J. F., Rami, J., & Michel, J. B. (1998). Angiotensin II stimulates the production of NO and peroxynitrite in endothelial cells. *The American Journal of Physiology*, *274*(1), C214–C220. doi:10.1152/ajpcell.1998.274.1.C214 PMID:9458730

QikProp. (n.d.). Retrieved from http://www.schrodinger.com

R&D Organizational Structure. (n.d.). Retrieved from https://www.slideshare.net/teresatreasures/drug-development-biotechnology

Rabbani, B., Nakaoka, H., Akhondzadeh, S., Tekin, M., & Mahdieh, N. (2016). Next generation sequencing: Implications in personalized medicine and pharmacogenomics. *Molecular BioSystems*, *12*(6), 1818–1830. doi:10.1039/C6MB00115G PMID:27066891

Raies, A. B., & Bajic, V. B. (2016). *In silico* toxicology: Computational methods for the prediction of chemical toxicity. *WIREs Computational Molecular Science.*, *6*(2), 147–172. doi:10.1002/wcms.1240 PMID:27066112

Ranganatha, N., & Kuppast, I. J. (2012). A review on alternatives to animal testing methods in drug development. *International Journal of Pharmacy and Pharmaceutical Sciences*, *4*(5), 28–32.

Rao, V. S., Srinivas, K., Sujini, G. N., & Kumar, G. N. S. (2014). Protein-Protein Interaction Detection: Methods and Analysis. *International Journal of Proteomics*, *2014*, 1–12. doi:10.1155/2014/147648 PMID:24693427

Rarey, M., Kramer, B., Lengauer, T., & Klebe, G. A. (1996). Fast Flexible Docking Method using an Incremental Construction Algorithm. *Journal of Molecular Biology*, *261*(3), 470–489. doi:10.1006/jmbi.1996.0477 PMID:8780787

Rastelli, G., Ferrari, A. M., Costantino, L., & Gamberini, M. C. (2002). Discovery of new inhibitors of aldose reductase from molecular modeling and database searching. *Bioorganic & Medicinal Chemistry*, *10*(5), 1437–1450. doi:10.1016/S0968-0896(01)00410-2 PMID:11886806

Ravichandran, V., Harish, R., Abhishek, J., Shalini, S., Christapher, P. V., & Ram, K. A. (2011).. . *International Journal of Drug Design and Discovery*, *2*(3), 511–519.

Reddy, M. R., & Erion, M. D. (1998). Structure-based drug design approaches for predicting binding affinities of HIV1 protease inhibitors. *Journal of Enzyme Inhibition*, *14*(1), 1–14. doi:10.3109/14756369809036542 PMID:10520756

Regulatory control of active pharmaceutical ingredients. Version 1, Appendix 14. (n.d.). Retrieved from https://npra.moh.gov.my/images/Announcement/2011/Regulatory-Control-of-Active-Pharmaceutical-Ingredients/API_Guideline_VERSION_1_-_PBKD.pdf

Reich, D., Green, R. E., Kircher, M., Krause, J., Patterson, N., Durand, E. Y., ... Pääbo, S. (2010). Genetic history of an archaic hominin group from Denisova Cave in Siberia. *Nature*, *468*(7327), 1053–1060. doi:10.1038/nature09710 PMID:21179161

Rester, U. (2008). From virtuality to reality - virtual screening in lead discovery and lead optimization: A medicinal chemistry perspective. *Current Opinion in Drug Discovery & Development*, *11*, 559–568. PMID:18600572

Rhodes, D. R., Yu, J., Shanker, K., Deshpande, N., Varambally, R., Ghosh, D., ... Chinnaiyan, A. M. (2004). Large-scale meta-analysis of cancer microarray data identifies common transcriptional profiles of neoplastic transformation and progression. *Proceedings of the National Academy of Sciences of the United States of America*, *101*(25), 9309–9314. doi:10.1073/pnas.0401994101 PMID:15184677

Riañoa, D., Reala, F., López-Vallverdúa, J. A., Campanab, F., Ercolanic, S., Mecoccic, P., ... Caltagironed, C. (2012). An Ontology-Based Personalization of Health-Care Knowledge to Support Clinical Decisions for Chronically Ill Patients. *Journal of Biomedical Informatics*, *45*(3), 429–446. doi:10.1016/j.jbi.2011.12.008 PMID:22269224

Ristoski, P., & Paulheim, H. (2016). Semantic Web in Data Mining and Knowledge Discovery: A Comprehensive Survey. *Journal of Web Semantics*, *36*, 1–22. doi:10.1016/j.websem.2016.01.001

Roche, O., & Guba, W. (2005). Computational chemistry as an integral component of lead generation. *Mini-Reviews in Medicinal Chemistry*, *7*(7), 677–683. doi:10.2174/1389557054368826 PMID:16026314

Rockville, M. D. (2011). Good manufacturing practice for bulk pharmaceutical excipients. *USP*, *2011*, 1415–1420.

Rockville, M. D. (2011). USP and NF Excipients, Listed by Category. *USP*, *2011*, 583–595.

Rohland, N., Reich, D., Mallick, S., Meyer, M., Green, R. E., Georgiadis, N. J., ... Hofreiter, M. (2010). Genomic DNA sequences from mastodon and woolly mammoth reveal deep speciation of forest and savanna elephants. *PLoS Biology*, *8*(12), e1000564. doi:10.1371/journal.pbio.1000564 PMID:21203580

Roncaglioni, A., Toropov, A. A., Toropova, A. P., & Benfenati, E. (2013). *In silico* methods to predict drug toxicity. *Current Opinion in Pharmacology*, *13*(5), 802–806. doi:10.1016/j.coph.2013.06.001 PMID:23797035

Rose, P. W., Bi, C., Bluhm, W. F., Christie, C. H., Dimitropoulos, D., Dutta, S., ... Bourne, P. E. (2013). The RCSB Protein Data Bank: New resources for research and education. *Nucleic Acids Research*, *41*(Database issue), D475–D482. doi:10.1093/nar/gks1200 PMID:23193259

Rotstein, S. H., & Murcko, M. A. (1993). GenStar: A method for *de novo* Drug Design. *Journal of Computer-Aided Molecular Design*, *7*(1), 23–43. doi:10.1007/BF00141573 PMID:8473916

Rotstein, S. H., & Murcko, M. A. (1993). Group Build: A fragment-based method for *de novo* Drug Design. *Journal of Medicinal Chemistry*, *36*(12), 1700–1710. doi:10.1021/jm00064a003 PMID:8510098

Roy, K., & Mitra, I. (2012). Electrotopological state atom (E-state) index in drug design, QSAR, property prediction and toxicity assessment. *Current Computer-aided Drug Design*, *8*(2), 135–158. doi:10.2174/157340912800492366 PMID:22497469

Ruth, Morris, Olson, & Goodsell. (2007). A Semiempirical Free Energy Force Field with Charge-Based Desolvation. *Journal of Computational Chemistry, 28*(6), 1145–52.

Rydberg, P., Gloriam, D. E., Zaretzki, J., Breneman, C., & Olsen, L. (2010). SMARTCyp: A 2D method for prediction of Cytochrome P450-mediated drug metabolism. *ACS Medicinal Chemistry Letters*, *1*(3), 96–100. doi:10.1021/ml100016x PMID:24936230

Safari-Alighiarloo, N., Taghizadeh, M., Rezaei-Tavirani, M., Goliaei, B., & Peyvandi, A. A. (2014). Protein-protein interaction networks (PPI) and complex diseases. *Gastroenterology and Hepatology from Bed To Bench*, *7*, 17–31. PMID:25436094

Saito, R., Smoot, M. E., Ono, K., Ruscheinski, J., Wang, P. L., Lotia, S., ... Ideker, T. (2012). A travel guide to Cytoscape plugins. *Nature Methods*, *9*(11), 1069–1076. doi:10.1038/nmeth.2212 PMID:23132118

Salisbury, C. M., & Cravatt, B. F. (2007). Activity-based probes for proteomic profiling of histone deacetylase complexes. *Proceedings of the National Academy of Sciences of the United States of America*, *104*(4), 1171–1176. doi:10.1073/pnas.0608659104 PMID:17227860

Sallam, A. A., Ramasahayam, S., Meyer, S. A., & El Sayed, K. A. (2010). Design, synthesis, and biological evaluation of dibromotyrosine analogues inspired by marine natural products as inhibitors of human prostate cancer proliferation, invasion, and migration. *Bioorganic & Medicinal Chemistry*, *18*(21), 7446–7457. doi:10.1016/j.bmc.2010.08.057 PMID:20884214

Salsbury, F. R. Jr. (2010). Molecular dynamics simulations of protein dynamics and their relevance to drug discovery. *Current Opinion in Pharmacology*, *10*(6), 738–744. doi:10.1016/j.coph.2010.09.016 PMID:20971684

Sanderson, D. M., & Earnshaw, C. G. (1991). Computer prediction of possible toxic action from chemical structure; the DEREK system. *Human and Experimental Toxicology*, *10*(4), 261–273. doi:10.1177/096032719101000405 PMID:1679649

Sarmiento, M., Wu, L., Keng, Y. F., Song, L., Luo, Z. W., Huang, Z. W., ... Zhang, Z.-Y. (2000). Structure-based discovery of small inhibitors targeted to protein tyrosine phosphatase 1B. *Journal of Medicinal Chemistry*, *3*(2), 146–155. doi:10.1021/jm990329z PMID:10649970

Satya, P. G. (2003). Quantitative structure activity relationships of renin inhibitors. *Mini-Reviews in Medicinal Chemistry*, *3*(4), 315–321. doi:10.2174/1389557033488051 PMID:12678825

Scannell, J. W., Alex, B., Helen, B., & Brian, W. (2012). Diagnosing the decline in pharmaceutical R&D efficiency. *Nature Reviews. Drug Discovery*, *11*(3), 191–200. doi:10.1038/nrd3681 PMID:22378269

Schapira, M., Raaka, B. M., Samuels, H. H., & Abagyan, R. (2000). Rational discovery of novel nuclear hormone receptor antagonists. *Proceedings of the National Academy of Sciences of the United States of America*, *97*(3), 1008–1013. doi:10.1073/pnas.97.3.1008 PMID:10655475

Schnecke, V., & Kuln, L. A. (2000). Virtual screening with solvation and ligand-induced complementarity. *Perspect Drug Des Discov*, *20*(1), 171–190. doi:10.1023/A:1008737207775

Schneider, G., & Böhm, H. J. (2002). Virtual screening and fast automated docking methods. *Drug Discovery Today*, *7*, 63–70. doi:10.1016/S1359-6446(02)00004-1 PMID:11790605

Schneider, G., Lee, M. L., Stahl, M., & Schneider, P. (2000). *De novo* design of molecular architectures by evolutionary assembly of drug-derived building blocks. *Journal of Computer-Aided Molecular Design*, *14*(5), 487–494. doi:10.1023/A:1008184403558 PMID:10896320

Schwede, T., Kopp, J., Guex, N., & Peitsch, M. C. (2003). SWISS-MODEL: An automated protein homology-modeling server. *Nucleic Acids Research*, *31*(13), 3381–3385. doi:10.1093/nar/gkg520 PMID:12824332

Scior, T., Bender, A., Tresadern, G., Medina-Franco, J. L., Martínez-Mayorga, K., Langer, T., ... Agrafiotis, D. K. (2012). Recognizing pitfalls in virtual screening: A critical review. *Journal of Chemical Information and Modeling*, *52*(4), 867–881. doi:10.1021/ci200528d PMID:22435959

Scott, A. W., & Gordon, M. C. (2002). Three-dimensional molecular descriptors and a novel QSAR method. *Journal of Molecular Graphics & Modelling*, *21*(3), 161–170. doi:10.1016/S1093-3263(02)00147-X PMID:12463634

Seierstad, M., & Agrafiotis, D. K. (2006). A QSAR model of hERG binding using a large, diverse, and internally consistent training set. *Chemical Biology & Drug Design*, *67*(4), 284–296. doi:10.1111/j.1747-0285.2006.00379.x PMID:16629826

Shah. (2009). Quality by Design in Pharmaceutical Manufacturing. American Association of Pharmaceutical Scientist.

Shaikh, S. A., Jain, T., Sandhu, G., Latha, N., & Jayaram, B. (2007). From drug target to leads--sketching a physicochemical pathway for lead molecule design in silico. *Current Pharmaceutical Design*, *13*(34), 3454–3470. doi:10.2174/138161207782794220 PMID:18220783

Sharma, P. C., Sharma, S. V., Archana, S., & Suresh, B. (2008). 3D-QSAR CoMFA study of some heteroarylpyrroles as possible anticandida agents. *Indian Journal of Pharmaceutical Sciences*, *70*(2), 154–158. doi:10.4103/0250-474X.41447 PMID:20046704

Shoichet, B. K., & Kuntz, I. D. (1991). Protein docking and complementarity. *Journal of Molecular Biology*, *221*(1), 327–346. doi:10.1016/0022-2836(91)80222-G PMID:1920412

Siddiqua, Kumar, & Kumar. (2013). QBD – A challenge to the Pharma industry. *International Journal of Innovative Pharmaceutical Sciences and Research*, *1*, 1-21.

Sikos, L. F. (2015). *Mastering Structured Data On The Semantic Web.* A Press.

Sim, G., Gorman, P., Greenes, R. A., Haynes, R. B., Kaplan, B., Lehmann, H., & Tang, P. C. (2001). Clinical Decision Support Systems for the Practice of Evidence-Based Medicine. *Journal of the American Medical Informatics Association*, *8*(6), 527–534. doi:10.1136/jamia.2001.0080527 PMID:11687560

Singh, Singh, Mishra, Patel, Kamalesh, & Yadav. (2014). Piperine: Delightful surprise to the biological world, made by plant pepper and a great bioavailability enhancer for our drugs and supplements. *World Journal of Pharmaceutical Research*, *3*(6), 2084-2098.

Singh, S. B., Shen, L. Q., Walker, M. J., & Sheridan, R. P. (2003). A model for predicting likely sites of CYP3A4-mediated metabolism on drug like molecules. *Journal of Medicinal Chemistry*, *46*(8), 1330–1336. doi:10.1021/jm020400s PMID:12672233

Singh, S. K., Saibaba, V., Ravikumar, V., Rudrawar, S. V., Daga, P., Rao, C. S., ... Rao, Y. K. (2004). Synthesis and biological evaluation of 2,3-diarylpyrazines and quinoxalines as selective COX-2 inhibitors. *Bioorganic & Medicinal Chemistry*, *12*(8), 1881–1893. doi:10.1016/j.bmc.2004.01.033 PMID:15051057

Singh, S., Malik, B. K., & Sharma, D. K. (2006). Molecular drug targets and structure based drug design: A holistic approach. *Bioinformation*, *1*(8), 314–320. doi:10.6026/97320630001314 PMID:17597912

Singletary, K. (2010). Black Pepper and health. *Nutrition Today*, *45*(1), 43–47. doi:10.1097/NT.0b013e3181cb4539

Sippl, W. (2002). Development of biologically active compounds by combining 3D QSAR and structure-based design methods. *Journal of Computer Aided Drug Design*, *16*, 825–830.

Slovakova, A., & Hutt, A. J. (1999). Chiral compounds and their pharmacologic effects [in Slovak]. *Ceska a Slovenska Farmacie*, *48*, 107–112. PMID:10422348

Smil, D. V., Manku, S., Chantigny, Y. A., Leit, S., Wahhab, A., Yan, T. P., ... Déziel, R. (2009). Novel HDAC6 isoform selective chiral small molecule histone deacetylase inhibitors. *Bioorganic & Medicinal Chemistry Letters*, *19*(3), 688–692. doi:10.1016/j.bmcl.2008.12.045 PMID:19111466

Smith, J. B., & Willis, A. L. (1971). Aspirin selectively inhibits prostaglandin production in human platelets. *Nature: New Biology*, *231*(25), 235–237. doi:10.1038/newbio231235a0 PMID:5284361

Smith, P. A., Sorich, M. J., McKinnon, R. A., & Miners, J. O. (2002). Pharmacophore and quantitative structure activity relationship (QSAR) modelling: Complemetary approaches to the rationalization and prediction of UDP glucuronosyltransferase 1A4 (UGT1A4) substrate selectivity. *Journal of Medicinal Chemistry*, *46*(9), 1617–1626. doi:10.1021/jm020397c PMID:12699380

Soding, J., Biegert, A., & Lupas, A. N. (2005). The HHpred interactive server for protein homology detection and structure prediction. *Nucleic Acids Research*, *33*(Web Server), W244–W248. doi:10.1093/nar/gki408 PMID:15980461

Sohn, H. Y., Raff, U., Hoffmann, A., Gloe, T., Heermeier, K., Galle, J., & Pohl, U. (2000). Differential role of angiotensin II receptor subtypes on endothelial superoxide formation. *British Journal of Pharmacology*, *131*(4), 667–672. doi:10.1038j.bjp.0703566 PMID:11030714

Somoza, J. R., Skene, R. J., Katz, B. A., Mol, C., Ho, J. D., Jennings, A. J., ... Tari, L. W. (2004). Structural snapshots of human HDAC8 provides insights into the class I histone deacetylases. *Structure (London, England)*, *12*(7), 1325–1334. doi:10.1016/j.str.2004.04.012 PMID:15242608

Song, J., Noh, J. H., Lee, J. H., Eun, J. W., Ahn, Y. M., Kim, S. Y., ... Nam, S. W. (2005). Increased expression of histone deacetylase 2 is found in human gastric cancer. *APMIS*, *113*(4), 264–268. doi:10.1111/j.1600-0463.2005.apm_04.x PMID:15865607

Sorich, M. J., Smith, P. A., McKinnon, R. A., & Miners, J. O. (2002). Pharmacophore and quantitative structure activity relationship modelling of UDP-glucuronosyl transferase 1A1 (UGT1A1) substrates. *Pharmacogenetics*, *12*(8), 635–645. doi:10.1097/00008571-200211000-00008 PMID:12439224

Sotriffer, C. A., Gohlke, H., & Klebe, G. (2002). Docking into knowledge-based potential fields: A comparative evaluation of DrugScore. *Journal of Medicinal Chemistry*, *45*(10), 1967–1970. doi:10.1021/jm025507u PMID:11985464

Sousa, S. F., Fernandes, P. A., & Ramos, M. J. (2006). Protein-ligand docking: Current status and future challenges. *Proteins*, *65*(1), 15–26. doi:10.1002/prot.21082 PMID:16862531

Sreenivasa Reddy, P. E., Sreenivasulu Reddy, T., & Krushna, G. S. (2011). Advantages of Bio and Cheminformatics tools in drug design. *Current Research in Drug Targeting*, *1*(2), 6–17.

Stahura, F. L., & Bajorath, J. (2004). Virtual screening methods that complement HTS. *Combinatorial Chemistry & High Throughput Screening*, *7*(4), 259–269. doi:10.2174/1386207043328706 PMID:15200375

Stark, C. (2006). BioGRID: A general repository for interaction datasets. *Nucleic Acids Research*, *34*(90001), D535–D539. doi:10.1093/nar/gkj109 PMID:16381927

Steinauer, K. K., Gibbs, I., Ning, S., French, J. N., Armstrong, J., & Knox, S. J. (2000). Radiation induces upregulation of cyclooxygenase-2 (COX-2) protein in PC-3 cells. *International Journal of Radiation Oncology, Biology, Physics*, *48*(2), 325–328. doi:10.1016/S0360-3016(00)00671-4 PMID:10974444

Stelzer, G., Dalah, I., Stein, T. I., Satanower, Y., Rosen, N., & Nativ, N. … Lancet, D. (2011). In-silico human genomics with GeneCards. *Human Genomics, 5*(6), 709–17. Retrieved from http://www.ncbi.nlm.nih.gov/pubmed/22155609

Stenberg, P., Norinder, U., Luthman, K., & Artursson, P. (2001). Experimental and computational screening models for the prediction of intestinal drug absorption. *Journal of Medicinal Chemistry*, *44*(12), 1927–1937. doi:10.1021/jm001101a PMID:11384238

Sterling, T., & Irwin, J. J. (2015). ZINC 15--Ligand Discovery for Everyone. *Journal of Chemical Information and Modeling*, *55*(11), 2324–2337. doi:10.1021/acs.jcim.5b00559 PMID:26479676

Steven, M. P., Daniel, S. M., Christopher, T. D., Charles, C. P., Bernard, H. M., Stacy, R. L., & … . (2010). How to improve R&D productivity: The pharmaceutical industry's grand challenge. *Nature Reviews. Drug Discovery*, *9*(3), 203–214. doi:10.1038/nrd3078 PMID:20168317

Stewart, B., & Wild, C. P. (2014). *World Cancer Report*. Lyon, France: International Agency for Research on Cancer.

Stolfa, D. A., Marek, M., Lancelot, J., Hauser, A. T., Walter, A., Leproult, E., ... Jung, M. (2014). Molecular basis for the antiparasitic activity of a mercaptoacetamide derivative that inhibits histone deacetylase 8 (HDAC8) from the human pathogen Schistosomamansoni. *Journal of Molecular Biology*, *426*(20), 3442–3453. doi:10.1016/j.jmb.2014.03.007 PMID:24657767

Subbaramaiah, K., & Dannenberg, A. J. (2003). Cyclooxygenase 2: A molecular target for cancer prevention and treatment. *Trends in Pharmacological Sciences*, *24*(2), 96–102. doi:10.1016/S0165-6147(02)00043-3 PMID:12559775

Subramaniam, S., Mehrotra, M., & Gupta, D. (2008). Virtual high throughput screening (vhts) - a perspective. *Bioinformation*, *3*(1), 14–17. doi:10.6026/97320630003014 PMID:19052660

Sumithira, G., & Sujatha, M. (2013). Drug chirality & its clinical significance evident, future for the development/separation of single enantiomer drug from racemates - The chiral switch. *International Journal of Advanced Pharmaceutical Genuine Research*, *1*(1), 1–19.

Sumudu, P. L., & Steffen, L. (2016). Computational methods in drug discovery. *Beilstein Journal of Organic Chemistry*, *12*, 2694–2718. doi:10.3762/bjoc.12.267 PMID:28144341

Sun, H. (2006). An accurate and interpretable Bayesian classification model for prediction of hERG liability. *ChemMedChem*, *1*(3), 315–322. doi:10.1002/cmdc.200500047 PMID:16892366

Sushko, I., Salmina, E., Potemkin, V. A., Poda, G., & Tetko, I. V. (2012). ToxAlerts: A web server of structural alerts for toxfic chemicals and compounds with potential adverse reactions. *Journal of Chemical Information and Modeling*, *52*(8), 2310–2316. doi:10.1021/ci300245q PMID:22876798

Sussman, J. L., Cygler, M., Harel, M., Silman, I., Schrag, J. D., Doctor, B. P., & Gentry, M. K. (1993). Relationship between sequence conservation and three-dimensional structure in a large family of esterases, lipases, and related proteins. *Protein Science*, *2*(3), 366–382. PMID:8453375

Suzuki, T., Muto, N., Bando, M., Itoh, Y., Masaki, A., Ri, M., ... Miyata, N. (2014). Design, synthesis, and biological activity of NCC149 derivatives as histone deacetylase 8-selective inhibitors. *ChemMedChem*, *9*(3), 657–664. doi:10.1002/cmdc.201300414 PMID:24403121

Swaan, P. W., Szoka, F. C. Jr, & Oie, S. (1997). Molecular modeling of the intestinal bile acid carrier: A comparative molecular field analysis study. *Journal of Computer Aided Drug Design*, *11*(6), 581–588. doi:10.1023/A:1007919704457 PMID:9491350

Szklarczyk, D., Franceschini, A., Wyder, S., Forslund, K., Heller, D., Huerta-Cepas, J., ... von Mering, C. (2015). STRING v10: Protein–protein interaction networks, integrated over the tree of life. *Nucleic Acids Research*, *43*(D1), D447–D452. doi:10.1093/nar/gku1003 PMID:25352553

Talley, J. J. (1999). 5 Selective inhibitors of cyclooxygenase-2 (COT-2). *Progress in Medicinal Chemistry*, *36*, 201–234. doi:10.1016/S0079-6468(08)70048-1 PMID:10818674

Talley, J. J., Bertenshaw, S. R., Brown, D. L., Carter, J. S., Graneto, M. J., Koboldt, C. M., ... Seibert, K. (1999). 4,5-Diaryloxazole inhibitors of cyclooxygenase-2 (COX-2). *Medicinal Research Reviews*, *19*(3), 199–208. doi:10.1002/(SICI)1098-1128(199905)19:3<199::AID-MED1>3.0.CO;2-7 PMID:10232649

Tang, L. D. (2013). Drug discovery & development: strategies and management. *Abstract: 2013 International Bioeconomy Conference, session 2: R&D in drug innovation*, 59–60.

Tang, W. P., Luo, T. P., Greenberg, E. F., Bradner, J. E., & Schreiber, S. L. (2011). Discovery of histone deacetylase 8 selective inhibitors. *Bioorganic & Medicinal Chemistry Letters*, *21*(9), 2601–2605. doi:10.1016/j.bmcl.2011.01.134 PMID:21334896

Taylor, R. D., Jewsbury, P. J., & Essex, J. W. (2002). A review of protein-small molecule docking methods. *Journal of Computer-Aided Molecular Design*, *16*(3), 151–166. doi:10.1023/A:1020155510718 PMID:12363215

Terstappen, G. C., Schlüpen, C., Raggiaschi, R., & Gaviraghi, G. (2007). Target deconvolution strategies in drug discovery. *Nature Reviews. Drug Discovery*, *6*(11), 891–903. doi:10.1038/nrd2410 PMID:17917669

Tessier, P., Smil, D. V., Wahhab, A., Leit, S., Rahil, J., Li, Z., ... Besterman, J. M. (2009). Diphenylmethylenehydroxamic acids as selective class IIa histone deacetylase inhibitors. *Bioorganic & Medicinal Chemistry Letters*, *19*(19), 5684–5688. doi:10.1016/j.bmcl.2009.08.010 PMID:19699639

Tetko, I. V. (n.d.). *Associative Neural Network, CogPrints archive code: cog00001441*. Retrieved from http://www.vc-clab.org/lab/alogps/library.html

Tetko, I. V., Gasteiger, J., Todeschini, R., Mauri, A., Livingstone, D., Ertl, P., ... Prokopenko, V. V. (2005). Virtual Computational Chemistry Laboratory – Design and Description. *Journal of Computer-Aided Molecular Design*, *19*(6), 453–463. doi:10.100710822-005-8694-y PMID:16231203

Tetko, I. V., Tanchuk, V. Y., Chentsova, N. P., Antonenko, S. V., Poda, G. I., Kukhar, V. P., & Luik, A. I. (1994). Hiv-1 reverse-transcriptase inhibitor design using artificial neural networks. *Journal of Medicinal Chemistry*, *37*(16), 2520–2526. doi:10.1021/jm00042a005 PMID:7520081

Thayer, A. M. (2011). Emerging strategies. *Chemical and Engineering News*, *89*(42), 15–20. doi:10.1021/cen-v089n042.p015

The Molecular INTeraction Database. (n.d.). *An ELIXIR Core Resource*. Retrieved from https://mint.bio.uniroma2.it/

The Pharmaceutical Innovation Platform. (2004). International Federation of Pharmaceutical Manufacturers Associations.

Thomas, M. T., Roger, M., Larry, S., & David, K. (2006). *R&D structure in a changing world*. Industrial Research Institute, Inc.

Thomas, S., Brightman, F., Gill, H., Lee, S., & Pufong, B. (2008). Simulation modelling of human intestinal absorption using Caco-2 permeability and kinetic solubility data for early drug discovery. *Journal of Pharmaceutical Sciences*, *97*(10), 4557–4574. doi:10.1002/jps.21305 PMID:18300298

Thorn, C. F., Klein, T. E., & Altman, R. B. (2013). PharmGKB: The Pharmacogenomics Knowledge Base. *Methods in Molecular Biology (Clifton, N.J.)*, *1015*, 311–320. doi:10.1007/978-1-62703-435-7_20 PMID:23824865

Tintori, C., Manetti, F., & Botta, M. (2010). Pharmacophoric models and 3D QSAR studies of the adenosine receptor ligands. *Current Topics in Medicinal Chemistry*, *10*(10), 1019–1035. doi:10.2174/156802610791293118 PMID:20370655

Titus, S. A., Southall, N., Marugan, J., Austin, C. P., & Zheng, W. (2012). High-throughput multiplexed quantitation of protein aggregation and cytotoxicity in a Huntington's disease model. *Current Chemical Genomics*, *6*, 79–86. doi:10.2174/1875397301206010079 PMID:23346268

Tollman, P. (2001). *A Revolution in R&D: How Genomics and Genetics are Transforming the Biopharmaceutical Industry*. Academic Press.

Trainor, G. L. (2007). The importance of plasma protein binding in drug discovery. *Expert Opinion on Drug Discovery*, *2*(1), 51–64. doi:10.1517/17460441.2.1.51 PMID:23496037

Trapnell, C., Pachter, L., & Salzberg, S. L. (2009). TopHat: Discovering splice junctions with RNA-Seq. *Bioinformatics (Oxford, England)*, *25*(9), 1105–1111. doi:10.1093/bioinformatics/btp120 PMID:19289445

Trapnell, C., Roberts, A., Goff, L., Pertea, G., Kim, D., Kelley, D. R., ... Pachter, L. (2012). Differential gene and transcript expression analysis of RNA-seq experiments with TopHat and Cufflinks. *Nature Protocols*, *7*(3), 562–578. doi:10.1038/nprot.2012.016 PMID:22383036

Trapnell, C., Williams, B. A., Pertea, G., Mortazavi, A., Kwan, G., van Baren, M. J., ... Pachter, L. (2010). Transcript assembly and quantification by RNA-Seq reveals unannotated transcripts and isoform switching during cell differentiation. *Nature Biotechnology*, *28*(5), 511–515. doi:10.1038/nbt.1621 PMID:20436464

Tropsha, A., & Zhang, W. F. (2001). Identification of the descriptor pharmacophoresusing Variable selection QSAR: Applications to database mining. *Current Pharmaceutical Design*, *7*, 599–612.

Tsai, C. J., Ma, B., & Nussinov, R. (2009). Protein–protein interaction networks: How can a hub protein bind so many different partners? *Trends in Biochemical Sciences*, *34*(12), 594–600. doi:10.1016/j.tibs.2009.07.007 PMID:19837592

Tschinke, V., & Cohen, N. C. (1993). The NEWLEAD program: A new method for the design for the design of candidate structures from pharmacophoric hypotheses. *Journal of Medicinal Chemistry*, *36*(24), 3863–3870. doi:10.1021/jm00076a016 PMID:8254618

Tsuji, S., Tsuji, M., Kawano, S., & Hori, M. (2001). Cyclooxygenase-2 Upregulation as a Perigenetic Change in Carcinogenesis. *Journal of Experimental and Clinical Cancer Research*, *20*(1),117-130.

Tushman, M., & O'Reilly, C. III. (1996). Ambidextrous Organizations: Managing Evolutionary and Revolutionary Change. *California Management Review*, *38*(4), 8–30. doi:10.2307/41165852

U. S. Food and Drug Administration. (1995). *Guidance for industry: immediate release solid oral dosage forms scale-up and post approval changes: chemistry, manufacturing, and controls, in vitro dissolution testing, and in vivo bioequivalence documentation*. Author.

U. S. Food and Drug Administration. (1997). *Guidance for industry: modified release solid oral dosage forms scale-up and post approval changes: chemistry, manufacturing, and controls, in vitro dissolution testing, and in vivo bioequivalence documentation*. Author.

U. S. Food and Drug Administration. (2011). *Quality by design for ANDs: an example for modified-release dosage forms*. Author.

U. S. Food and Drug Administration. (2012). *Quality by design for ANDs: an example for immediate-release dosage forms*. Author.

U. S. Food and Drug Administration. Guidance for industry. (2014). *CMC post approval manufacturing changes to be documented in annual reports*. Author.

U.S. Food and Drug Administration CDER. (2004). *Guidance for industry: PAT—a framework for innovative pharmaceutical development, manufacturing, and quality assurance*. Author.

Umamaheswari, A., Irfan, N., & Puratchikody, A. (2015). *In silico* molecular interaction studies of chiral heterocyclic analogs of SAHA as selective histone deacetylase 8 inhibitors. *Letters in Drug Design & Discovery*, *12*(9), 711–727. doi:10.2174/1570180812666150326004848

Ungerstedt, J. S., Sowa, Y., Xu, W. S., Shao, Y., Dokmanovic, M., Perez, G., ... Marks, P. A. (2005). Role of thioredoxin in the response of normal and transformed cells to histone deacetylase inhibitors. *Proceedings of the National Academy of Sciences of the United States of America*, *102*(3), 673–678. doi:10.1073/pnas.0408732102 PMID:15637150

UniProt Consortium. (2013). Update on activities at the Universal Protein Resource (UniProt) in 2013. *Nucleic Acids Research*, *41*(Database issue), D43–D47. doi:10.1093/nar/gks1068 PMID:23161681

Valen, E., Pascarella, G., Chalk, A., Maeda, N., Kojima, M., Kawazu, C., ... Carninci, P. (2009). Genome-wide detection and analysis of hippocampus core promoters using DeepCAGE. *Genome Research*, *19*(2), 255–265. doi:10.1101/gr.084541.108 PMID:19074369

Valerio, L. G. Jr. (2009). *In silico* toxicology for the pharmaceutical sciences. *Toxicology and Applied Pharmacology*, *241*(3), 356–370. doi:10.1016/j.taap.2009.08.022 PMID:19716836

Van Arnum. (2007). A FDA Perspective on Quality by Design. Advancing Development & Manufacturing Pharmaceutical Technology, 3(12).

van de Waterbeemd, H., & Gifford, E. (2003). ADMET *in silico* modeling: Towards prediction paradise? *Nature Reviews. Drug Discovery*, *2*, 192–204. PMID:12612645

Van der Greef, J., & McBurney, R. N. (2005). Innovation: Rescuing drug discovery: *in vivo* systems pathology and systems pharmacology. *Nature Reviews. Drug Discovery*, *4*(12), 961–967. doi:10.1038/nrd1904 PMID:16341061

Vane, J. R. (1971). Inhibition of prostaglandin synthesis as a mechanism of action for aspirin-like drugs. Nature (London). *Nature: New Biology*, *231*(25), 232–235. doi:10.1038/newbio231232a0 PMID:5284360

Vannini, A., Volpari, C., Gallinari, P., Jones, P., Mattu, M., Carfí, A., ... Di Marco, S. (2007). Substrate bindingto histone deacetylases as shown by the crystal structure of the HDAC8-substrate complex. *The EMBO Journal*, *8*(9), 879–884. doi:10.1038j.embor.7401047 PMID:17721440

Vastrik, I., D'Eustachio, P., Schmidt, E., Joshi-Tope, G., Gopinath, G., Croft, D., ... de. (2007). Reactome: A knowledge base of biologic pathways and processes. *Genome Biology*, *8*(3), R39. doi:10.1186/gb-2007-8-3-r39 PMID:17367534

Vaughan Williams, E. M. (1984). Subgroups of class 1 antiarrhythmic drugs. *European Heart Journal*, *5*(2), 96–98. doi:10.1093/oxfordjournals.eurheartj.a061632 PMID:6373262

Venkatachalam, C. M., Jiang, X., Oldfield, T., & Waldman, M. (2003). LigandFit: A novel method for the shape-directed rapid docking of ligands to protein active sites. *J Mol Graphics Mol Mod*, *21*(4), 289–307. doi:10.1016/S1093-3263(02)00164-X PMID:12479928

Venkatapathy, R., & Wang, N. C. Y. (2013). Developmental toxicity prediction. In B. Reisfeld & A. N. Mayeno (Eds.), *Computational Toxicology* (pp. 305–340). New York: Humana Press.

Venter, J. C., Remington, K., Heidelberg, J. F., Halpern, A. L., Rusch, D., Eisen, J. A. *et al.*, (2004). Environmental genome shotgun sequencing of the Sargasso Sea. *Science*, *304*(5667), 66-74.

Verdica, M. A., Huang, H., Dutil, E., Kaiser, D. A., Hunter, T., & Noel, J. P. (2000). Structure of the human anti-apoptotic protein surviving reveals a dimeric arrangement. *Nature Structural & Molecular Biology*, *7*(7), 602–608. doi:10.1038/76838

Verkhiver, G., Appelt, K., Freer, S. T., & Villafrancda, J. E. (1995). Empirical free energy calculations of protein-ligand crystallographic complexes I knowledge-based ligand-protein interaction potentials applied to the prediction of human immunodeficiency virus 1 protease binding affinity. *Protein Engineering*, *8*(7), 677–691. doi:10.1093/protein/8.7.677 PMID:8577696

Verma, J., Khedkar, V. M., & Coutinho, E. C. (2010). 3D-QSAR in drug design – A review. *Current Topics in Medicinal Chemistry*, *10*(1), 95–115. doi:10.2174/156802610790232260 PMID:19929826

Verma, R. P., & Hansch, C. (2009). Camptothecins: A SAR/QSAR Study. *Chemical Reviews*, *109*(1), 213–235. doi:10.1021/cr0780210 PMID:19099450

Vernon, J. A., Golec, J. H., & Dimasi, J. A. (2010). Drug development costs when financial risk is measured using the Fama-French three-factor model. *Health Economics*, *19*(8), 1002–1005. doi:10.1002/hec.1538 PMID:19655335

Vijayakumar, B., Umamaheswari, A., Puratchikody, A., & Velmurugan, D. (2011). Selection of an improved HDAC8 inhibitor through structure-based drug design. *Bioinformation*, *7*(3), 134–141. doi:10.6026/97320630007134 PMID:22125384

Vikramjeet, J., Rakesh, N., Deepika, S., Balasubramanian, N., & Pradeep, K. (2011). Hansch analysis for the prediction of antimycobacterial activity of ofloxacin derivatives. *Medicinal Chemistry Research*, *20*(7), 826–837. doi:10.100700044-010-9400-8

Villar, H. O., Yan, J., & Hansen, M. R. (2004). Using NMR for ligand discovery and optimization. *Current Opinion in Chemical Biology*, *8*(4), 387–391. doi:10.1016/j.cbpa.2004.05.002 PMID:15288248

Vogt, M., & Bajorath, J. (2011). Predicting the performance of fingerprint similarity searching. In J. Bajorath (Ed.), *Chemoinformatics and Computational Chemical Biology* (pp. 159–173). Totowa, NJ: Humana Press.

Voronkov, A., Holsworth, D. D., Waaler, J., Wilson, S. R., Ekblad, B., Perdreau-dahl, H., ... Krauss, S. (2013). Structural basis and SAR for G007-LK, a lead stage 1,2,4-triazole based specific tankyrase 1/2 inhibitor. *Journal of Medicinal Chemistry*, *56*(7), 3012–3023. doi:10.1021/jm4000566 PMID:23473363

Votano, J. R., Parham, M., Hall, L. M., Hall, L. H., Kier, L. B., Oloff, S., & Tropsha, A. (2006). QSAR Modelling of Human Serum Protein Binding with Several Modelling Techniques Utilizing Structure? Information Representation. *Journal of Medicinal Chemistry*, *49*(24), 7169–7181. doi:10.1021/jm051245v PMID:17125269

Vukić, V., Vukić, D., Milanović, S., Iličić, M., Kanurić, K. (2016). Molecular docking and stimulation through the angiotensin converting enzyme by inhibition by milk peptides. *Food Technology Quality and Safety*, *10*, 42-45.

Walters, W. P., Stahl, M. T., & Murcko, M. A. (1998). Virtual screening-an overview. *Drug Discovery Today*, *3*(4), 160–178. doi:10.1016/S1359-6446(97)01163-X

Waltregny, D., Glenisson, W., Tran, S. L., North, B. J., Verdin, E., Colige, A., & Castronovo, V. (2005). Histone deacetylase HDAC8 associates with smooth muscle alpha-actin and is essential for smooth muscle cell contractility. *Federation of American Societies for Experimental Biology Journal*, *19*(8), 966–968. doi:10.1096/fj.04-2303fje PMID:15772115

Wang, H., Zhou, T., Tian, L., Qian, Y., & Li, J. (2014). Creating Hospital-Specific Customized Clinical Pathways By Applying Semantic Reasoning To Clinical Data. *Journal of Biomedical Informatics*, *52*, 354–363. doi:10.1016/j.jbi.2014.07.017 PMID:25109270

Wang, S. C., Li, Y. Y., Wang, J. M., Chen, L., Zhang, L. L., Yu, H. D., & Hou, T. (2012). ADMET evaluation in drug discovery. 12. Development of binary classification models for prediction of hERG potassium channel blockage. *Molecular Pharmaceutics*, *9*(4), 996–1010. doi:10.1021/mp300023x PMID:22380484

Wang, S. C., Li, Y. Y., Xu, L., Li, D., & Hou, T. J. (2013). Recent developments in computational prediction of hERG blockage. *Current Topics in Medicinal Chemistry*, *13*(11), 1317–1326. doi:10.2174/15680266113139990036 PMID:23675938

Wang, X., Wei, X., Thijssen, B., Das, J., Lipkin, S. M., & Yu, H. (2012). Three-dimensional reconstruction of protein networks provides insight into human genetic disease. *Nature Biotechnology*, *30*(2), 159–164. doi:10.1038/nbt.2106 PMID:22252508

Wang, Y., Shaikh, S. A., & Tajkhorshid, E. (2010). Exploring transmembrane diffusion pathways with molecular dynamics. *Physiology (Bethesda, MD)*, *25*(3), 142–154. doi:10.1152/physiol.00046.2009 PMID:20551228

Wang, Y., Xing, J., Xu, Y., Zhou, N., Peng, J., Xiong, Z., ... Jiang, H. (2015). *In silico* ADME/T modelling for rational drug design. *Quarterly Reviews of Biophysics*, *48*(4), 488–515. doi:10.1017/S0033583515000190 PMID:26328949

Waring, M. J. (2010). Lipophilicity in drug discovery. *Expert Opinion on Drug Discovery*, *5*(3), 235–248. doi:10.1517/17460441003605098 PMID:22823020

Watson, J. D., & Crick, F. H. (1953). *The structure of DNA*. Paper presented at the Cold Spring Harbor symposia on quantitative biology. 10.1101/SQB.1953.018.01.020

Welch. (2008). Angiotensin II dependent superoxide effects on hypertension and vascular dysfunction. *Hypertension*, *52*, 51-56.

Wells, J. A., & McClendon, C. L. (2007). Reaching for high-hanging fruit in drug discovery at protein-protein interfaces. *Nature*, *450*(7172), 1001–1009. doi:10.1038/nature06526 PMID:18075579

Welter, D., MacArthur, J., Morales, J., Burdett, T., Hall, P., Junkins, H., ... Parkinson, H. (2013). The NHGRI GWAS Catalog, a curated resource of SNP-trait associations. *Nucleic Acids Research*, *42*(D1), D1001–D1006. doi:10.1093/nar/gkt1229 PMID:24316577

Wenbo, Y., & Alexander, D. M. (2017). Computer-aided drug design methods. *Methods in Molecular Biology (Clifton, N.J.)*, *1520*, 85–106. doi:10.1007/978-1-4939-6634-9_5 PMID:27873247

Whalen, E. J., Rajagopal, S., & Lefkowitz, R. J. (2011). Therapeutic potential of beta-arrestin and G protein-biased agonists. *Trends in Molecular Medicine*, *17*(3), 126–139. doi:10.1016/j.molmed.2010.11.004 PMID:21183406

What is Reactome? (n.d.). *Reactome Pathway Database*. Retrieved from https://reactome.org/what-is-reactome

Whitehead, L., Dobler, M. R., Radetich, B., Zhu, Y., Atadja, P. W., Claiborne, T., ... Stams, T. (2011). Human HDAC isoform selectivity achieved via exploitation of the acetate release channel with structurally unique small molecule inhibitors. *Bioorganic & Medicinal Chemistry*, *19*(15), 4626–4634. doi:10.1016/j.bmc.2011.06.030 PMID:21723733

Wichmann, K., Diedenhofen, M., & Klamt, A. (2007). Prediction of blood-brain partitioning and human serum albumin binding based on COSMO-RS sigma-moments. *Journal of Chemical Information and Modeling*, *47*(1), 228–233. doi:10.1021/ci600385w PMID:17238268

Wiese, M., & Pajeva, I. K. (2001). Structure-activity relationships of multidrug resistance reversers. *Current Medicinal Chemistry*, *8*(6), 685–713. doi:10.2174/0929867013373138 PMID:11281849

Wiggins, S. N. (1987). *The Cost of Developing a New Drug*. Washington, DC: Pharmaceutical Manufacturers Association.

Williams, J. A., Hyland, R., Jones, B. C., Smith, D. A., Hurst, S., & Goosen, T. C. (2004). Drug-drug interactions for UDP-glucuronosyl transferase substrates: A pharmacokinetic explanation for typically observed low exposure (AUCi/AUC) ratios. *Drug Metabolism and Disposition: the Biological Fate of Chemicals*, *32*(11), 1201–1208. doi:10.1124/dmd.104.000794 PMID:15304429

Wishart, D. S., Knox, C., Guo, A. C., Cheng, D., Shrivastava, S., Tzur, D., ... Hassanali, M. (2008). DrugBank: A knowledgebase for drugs, drug actions and drug targets. *Nucleic Acids Research*, *36*(Database issuesuppl_1), D901–D906. doi:10.1093/nar/gkm958 PMID:18048412

Wishart, D. S., Knox, C., Guo, A. C., Shrivastava, S., Hassanali, M., Stothard, P., ... Woolsey, J. (2006). DrugBank: A comprehensive resource for in silico drug discovery and exploration. *Nucleic Acids Research*, *34*(Database issue), D668–D672. doi:10.1093/nar/gkj067 PMID:16381955

Witt, O., Deubzer, H. E., Milde, T., & Oehme, I. (2009). HDAC family: What are the cancer relevant targets? *Cancer Letters*, *277*(1), 8–21. doi:10.1016/j.canlet.2008.08.016 PMID:18824292

Woodcock, J. (2004). The concept of pharmaceutical quality. *American Pharmaceutical Review*, 1–3.

Wu, Tawakkul, White, & Khan. (2009). Quality-by-design (QbD): and integrated multivariate approach for the component quantification of powder blends. *International Journal of Pharmaceutics, 372*(1-2).

Wu, G., Robertson, D. H., Brooks, C. L., & Vieth, M. (2003). Detailed Analysis of Grid-Based Molecular Docking: A Case Study of CDOCKER - ACHARMm-Based MD Docking Algorithm. *Journal of Computational Chemistry*, *24*(13), 1549–1562. doi:10.1002/jcc.10306 PMID:12925999

Wu, H., & Khan, M. A. (2009). Quality-by-design (QbD): An integrated approach for evaluation of powder blending process kinetics and determination of powder blending end-point. *Journal of Pharmaceutical Sciences*, *98*(8), 2784–2798. doi:10.1002/jps.21646 PMID:19116952

Wunberg, T., Hendrix, M., Hillisch, A., Lobell, M., Meier, H., Schmeck, C., ... Hinzen, B. (2006). Improving the Hit-to-Lead Process: Data-Driven Assessment of Drug-Like and Lead-Like Screening Hits. *Drug Discovery Today*, *11*(3-4), 175–180. doi:10.1016/S1359-6446(05)03700-1 PMID:16533716

Xenarios, I. (2000). DIP: The Database of Interacting Proteins. *Nucleic Acids Research*, *28*(1), 289–291. doi:10.1093/nar/28.1.289 PMID:10592249

Xiang, Z. (2006). Advances in homology protein structure modeling. *Current Protein & Peptide Science*, *7*(3), 217–227. doi:10.2174/138920306777452312 PMID:16787261

Xiao, J., Marugan, J. J., Zheng, W., Titus, S., Southall, N., Cherry, J. J., ... Austin, C. P. (2011). Discovery, synthesis, and biological evaluation of novel SMN protein modulators. *Journal of Medicinal Chemistry*, *54*(18), 6215–6233. doi:10.1021/jm200497t PMID:21819082

Xia, X., Maliski, E. G., Gallant, P., & Rogers, D. (2004). Classification of kinase inhibitors using a Bayesian model. *Journal of Medicinal Chemistry*, *47*(18), 4463–4470. doi:10.1021/jm0303195 PMID:15317458

Xie, W. L., Chipman, J. G., Robertson, D. L., Erikson, R. L., & Simmons, D. L. (1991). Expression of a mitogen-responsive gene encoding prostaglandin synthase is regulated by mRNA splicing. *Proceedings of the National Academy of Sciences of the United States*, *88*(7), 2692–2696. doi:10.1073/pnas.88.7.2692 PMID:1849272

Xin, L., Yu-Ze, Z., Zhi, J., Wen-Qing, J., Shu-Qing, W., Wei-Ren, X., & Xian-Chao, C. (2017). Molecular docking, 3D-QSAR and structural optimization of indolebiphenylcarboxylic acids as PPARγ antagonists. *Letters in Drug Design & Discovery*, *14*(8).

Yamashita, F., & Hashida, M. (2004). *In silico* approaches for predicting ADME properties of drugs. *Drug Metabolism and Pharmacokinetics*, *19*(5), 327–338. doi:10.2133/dmpk.19.327 PMID:15548844

Yamauchi, Y., Boukari, H., Banerjee, I., Sbalzarini, I. F., Horvath, P., & Helenius, A. (2011). Histone deacetylase 8 is required for centrosome cohesion and influenza A virus entry. *PLoS Pathogens*, *7*(10), e1002316. doi:10.1371/journal.ppat.1002316 PMID:22046129

Yan-Fen, D., & Xing-Ming, Z. (2015). *A Survey on the Computational Approaches to Identify Drug Targets in the Post-genomic Era*. BioMed Research International.

Yang, S. S. O., Lu, J. Y., Kong, X. Q., Ling, Z. J., Luo, C., & Jiang, H. (2012). Computational drug discovery. *Acta Pharmacologica Sinica*, *33*(9), 1131–1140. doi:10.1038/aps.2012.109 PMID:22922346

Yang, Y., Adelstein, S. J., & Kassis, A. I. (2009). Target discovery from data mining approaches. *Drug Discovery Today*, *14*(3-4), 147–154. doi:10.1016/j.drudis.2008.12.005 PMID:19135549

Yan, W., Liu, S., Xu, E., Zhang, J., Zhang, Y., Chen, X., & Chen, X. (2012). Histone deacetylase inhibitors suppress mutant p53 transcription via histone deacetylase 8. *Oncogene*, *32*(5), 599–609. doi:10.1038/onc.2012.81 PMID:22391568

Yap, C. W. (2011). PaDEL-descriptor: An open source software to calculate molecular descriptors and fingerprints. *Journal of Computational Chemistry*, *32*(7), 1466–1474. doi:10.1002/jcc.21707 PMID:21425294

Yoh, D., Akiteru, G., Maiko, K., & Tomoyuki, N. (2012). Molecularly Targeted Therapy: Past, Present and Future. *Chemotherapy*, *1*, 105.

Yoshica, F., & Toplss, J. G. (2000). QSAR model for drug human oral bioavailability. *Journal of Medicinal Chemistry*, *43*(13), 2575–2585. doi:10.1021/jm0000564 PMID:10891117

Yoshida, K., & Niwa, T. (2006). Quantitative Structure–Activity Relationship Studies on Inhibition of HERG Potassium Channels. *Journal of Chemical Information and Modeling*, *46*(3), 1371–1378. doi:10.1021/ci050450g PMID:16711756

Young, D. (2009). *Computational drug design*. John Wiley & Sons. doi:10.1002/9780470451854

Yu, L. X. (2008). Pharmaceutical quality by design: product and process development, understanding, and control. Pharmaceutical Research, 25, 781-791.

Yuan, H. Z., Michael, H. A., & Andreas, M. Z. (2003). Fast calculation of van der waals volume as a sum of atomic and bond contributions and its application to drug compounds. *The Journal of Organic Chemistry*, *68*(19), 7368–7373. doi:10.1021/jo034808o PMID:12968888

Yuan, H., Myers, S., Wang, J., Zhou, D., Woo, J. A., Kallakury, B., ... Schlegel, R. (2012). Use of reprogrammed cells to identify therapy for respiratory papillomatosis. *The New England Journal of Medicine*, *367*(13), 1220–1227. doi:10.1056/NEJMoa1203055 PMID:23013073

Yuhong, X., Liang, Z., & Zhuoyong, Z. (2012). QSAR and Docking studies on different series of histone deacetylase inhibitors (HDACIs). *Letters in Drug Design & Discovery*, *9*(4), 367–378. doi:10.2174/157018012799860033

Yu, L. (2014). *A Developer's Guide to the Semantic Web* (2nd ed.). Springer.

Yuriev, E., Agostino, M., & Ramsland, P. A. (2011). Challenges and advances in computational docking: 2009 in review. *Journal of Molecular Recognition*, *24*(2), 149–164. doi:10.1002/jmr.1077 PMID:21360606

Zarghi, A., & Arfaei, S. (2011). Selective COX-2 Inhibitors: A Review of Their Structure-Activity Relationships. *Iranian Journal of Pharmaceutical Research*, *10*, 655–683. PMID:24250402

Zenuni, X., Raufi, B., Ismaili, F., & Ajdari, J. (2015). State Of The Art of Semantic Web For Healthcare. *Procedia: Social and Behavioral Sciences*, *195*, 1990–1998. doi:10.1016/j.sbspro.2015.06.213

Zhang, L., & Mao, S. (2017). Application of quality by design in the current drug development. Asian Journal of Pharmaceutical Sciences, 12, 1-8.

Zhang, S., Ying, W. S., Siahaan, T. J., & Jois, S. D. S. (2003). Solution structure of a peptide derived from the beta subunit of LFA-1. *Peptides*, *4*, 827–835. PMID:12948834

Zhang, X. F., Ou-Yang, L., Hu, X., & Dai, D. Q. (2015). Identifying binary protein-protein interactions from affinity purification mass spectrometry data. *BMC Genomics*, 16. PMID:26438428

Zhao, S., & Li, S. (2010). Network-based relating pharmacological and genomic spaces for drug target identification. *PLoS One*, *5*(7), e11764. doi:10.1371/journal.pone.0011764 PMID:20668676

Zheng, P. P., Li, J., & Kros, J. M. (2017). Breakthroughs in modern cancer therapy and elusive cardiotoxicity: Critical research-practice gaps, challenges, and insights. *Medicinal Research Reviews*, *00*, 1–49. PMID:28862319

Zheng, W., Thorne, N., & McKew, J. C. (2013). Phenotypic screens as a renewed approach for drug discovery. *Drug Discovery Today*, *18*(21-22), 1067–1073. doi:10.1016/j.drudis.2013.07.001 PMID:23850704

Zhu, H. (2013). From QSAR to QSIIR: searching for enhanced computational toxicology models. In B. Reisfeld & A. N. Mayeno (Eds.), *Computational Toxicology* (pp. 53–65). New York: Humana Press. doi:10.1007/978-1-62703-059-5_3

Zhu, P., Martin, E., Mengwasser, J., Schlag, P., Janssen, K. P., & Gottlicher, M. (2004). Induction of HDAC2 expression upon loss of APC in colorectal tumorigenesis. *Cancer Cell*, *5*(5), 455–463. doi:10.1016/S1535-6108(04)00114-X PMID:15144953

Zhu, W., Zhang, Y., Sinko, W., Hensler, M. E., Olson, J., Molohon, K. J., ... Oldfield, E. (2013). Antibacterial drug leads targeting isoprenoid biosynthesis. *Proceedings of the National Academy of Sciences of the United States of America*, *110*(1), 123–128. doi:10.1073/pnas.1219899110 PMID:23248302

Zhu, Y., Li, H. F., Lu, S., Zheng, Y. X., Wu, Z., Tang, W. F., ... Lu, T. (2010). Investigation on the isoform selectivity of histone deacetylase inhibitors using chemical feature based pharmacophore and docking approaches. *European Journal of Medicinal Chemistry*, *45*(5), 1777–1791. doi:10.1016/j.ejmech.2010.01.010 PMID:20153566

ZINC12. (n.d.). Retrieved from http://zinc.docking.org/

ZINC15. (n.d.). Retrieved from http://zinc15.docking.org/

Zou, X., Sun, Y., & Kuntz, I. D. (1999). Inclusion of solvation in ligand binding free energy calculations using the generalized-Born model. *Journal of the American Chemical Society*, *121*(35), 8033–8043. doi:10.1021/ja984102p

Zsila, F., Bikadi, Z., Malik, D., Hari, P., Pechan, I., Berces, A., & Hazai, E. (2011). Evaluation of drug-human serum albumin binding interactions with support vector machine aided online automated docking. *Bioinformatics (Oxford, England)*, *27*(13), 1806–1813. doi:10.1093/bioinformatics/btr284 PMID:21593135

Zsoldos, Z., Johnson, A. P., Simon, A., & Szabo, I. (2002). *eHiTS: Novel algorithm for fast, exhaustive flexible ligand docking and scoring*. Presentation at the *224th ACS National Meeting*, Boston, MA.

Zsoldos, Z., Reid, D., Simon, A., Sadjad, S. B., & Johnson, A. P. (2007). eHiTS: A new fast, exhaustive flexible ligand docking system. *Journal of Molecular Graphics & Modelling*, *26*(1), 198–212. doi:10.1016/j.jmgm.2006.06.002 PMID:16860582

Zuegge, J., Fechner, U., Roche, O., Parratt, N. J., Engkvist, O., & Schneider, G. (2002). A fastvirtual screening filter for cytochrom450 3A4 inhibition liability of compound libraries. *QSAR*, *21*, 249–256.

About the Contributors

Ayarivan Puratchikody has completed her M.Pharm., degree from the Tamilnadu Dr. MGR. Medical University, Chennai, Tamil Nadu, India in the year 1996. She has completed her Ph.D., in the area of Chemistry-Pharmaceutical Chemistry from Bharthidasan University, Tiruchirappalli, Tamil Nadu, India in the year 2006. Currently, she is working as an Associate Professor in the Department of Pharmaceutical Technology, Bharathidasan Institute of Technology, Tiruchirapplli Campus, Anna University, Chennai-600025, Tamil Nadu, India. She has a total experience of 22 years in teaching and research. She has qualified GATE, and was the best outgoing student in M.Pharmacy for which she was awarded Thiru. Gnana Sebastian-Theresa Educational Endowment award. She is very committed to her research career and had been offered the Tamil Nadu Young Women Scientist Award 2008, Prof. S.P.Thyagarajan - Prof.S.Rajarajan endowment award 2011, Innovation award 2015 by Anna University Chennai for her research credits. She has guided more than 52 two UG projects and 63 PG projects so far and few received financial assistance from Tamilnadu Government Science and Technology- Chennai, DBT New Delhi and TEQIP New Delhi. In her credits so far, nine scholars were awarded Ph.D and other two pursuing their research in interdisciplinary approach. She has presented several research findings in the national and international conferences. Being a continuous researcher, she was sanctioned a research project entitled "Isolation and characterization of bioactive molecules from marine organisms" by the Department of Science and Technology (DST), New Delhi during the year 2006-09. Again, for the year, 2013-16, she had received a DST project entitled "Design, synthesis and evaluation of novel COX-2 inhibitors of dibromotyrosine derivatives as anti-inflammatory drugs". She is also a co-investigator for a UGC sponsored project. She has been advisor of student forum called MANANM since 2011. Manam forum is a group of students organized for the purpose furthering their common interests in an activity through participation and competition. Manam forum is meant to be a learning experience for the members through their involvement in public reactions, organization, administration and scheduling, as well as, through the development of skills in their particular area of interest. Involvement in a group and team environment helps enhance a student's overall education while living in the collegiate setting. She has organized short term programme, conferences and workshops with the support of various research funding agencies in India. She has authored two books in her area of research, discovery and development of novel lead molecules. Apart from her role of academician, she has many feathers in her hat. She has held various administrative positions of Anna University, Tiruchirappalli.

Appavoo Umamaheswari received the Bachelor of Pharmacy degree in Pharmacy from The Tamil Nadu Dr. MGR Medical University Chennai. She is a recipient of Thiru Gnana Sebastian Endowment Award for securing highest in M. Pharmacy. She was offered Management Gold medal by Periyar College of Pharmaceutical Sciences for girls, Tiruchirappalli. She earned the Doctor of Philosophy in

Pharmaceutical Technology degree from Anna University Chennai. Dr. A. Umamaheswari has served as a full-time tenured faculty as an Assistant Professor at University College of Engineering (BIT Campus), Anna University, Tiruchirappalli. She has a good number of research publications to her credit on pharmacy and technology-related topics. Dr. A. Umamaheswari authored five book chapters from her research expertise. Her areas of interest include Drug Design and Development using organic synthetic strategies and Cancer Biology. She has been given multiple presentations at National and International conferences. She is an active member of many professional bodies. Dr. A. Umamaheswari is a co-investigator in government funded project sponsored by DST, New Delhi.

S. Lakshmana Prabu, associated with Anna University since 2009 is a GATE qualified personality and secured 110th rank at all India level. He pursued his Ph.D from Manipal University and Post Graduate Diploma in Intellectual Property Rights Law from National Law School of India University, Bangalore. Dr. S. Lakshmana Prabu, is one of the editors of Computer Applications in Drug Discovery and Development, Publisher: IGI Global, Hershey, USA; Intellectual Property Rights, InTech, Croatia and authored thirteen book chapters from his research expertise. He has filled 3 international patents, 97 peer reviewed publication. authored 13 book chapters. One of his major achievement is evidenced in a book chapter entitled "Extraction of Drug from the Biological Matrix: A Review", InTech Publication, Croatia that was downloaded more than 22,000 times worldwide. He is having great experience in reputed Pharmaceutical Industries and University. He has special expertise in the field of quality assurance, validation and formulation development. He has 97 research publications in his credit and has given many presentation in both International and National Conferences. He serves as reviewer for eight reputed journals and is an editorial board member for five journals. He has organized various national and international conferences, hands on training, workshops and symposium and added to his credit. Dr. S. Lakshmana Prabu is a Principal investigator in government funded project sponsored by DBT, New Delhi.

* * *

Muthuswamy Anusuyadevi's research is to gain insight knowledge in the prolongation of life expectancy and improving noble cognitive capability during aging and to understand the neuro-biological processes and biochemical changes between normal physiology to pathological forms in the brain regions during aging process. This prompted him to intrude on the molecular cascade leading to neurodegeneration, senescence, dementia and cognitive impairments.

Subramani Arunkumar is College first in B.Pharm. He has 21 years of teaching experience. He has guided17 M.Pharm Students. He is doctoral committee member for Ph.D students in various Universities. His field of research includes synthesis of various heterocyclic structures, screening their Pharmacological activity and performing QSAR analysis. He has 35 national and international publications in reputed journals.

Saleena B. is currently working as an Associate Professor in School of Computing Science and Engineering, VIT-Chennai, India. She has completed her Ph.D in Computer Science from VIT Vellore, India. She has published more than 25 papers in reputed journals and conferences. Her current research interests include Data Mining, Software Engineering, Machine Learning and Semantic web Technologies.

Sakthivel Balasubramaniyan is a Ph.D. candidate in the Drug Discovery and Development Research Group, Dept. of Pharmaceutical Technology, University College of Engineering, Anna University – BIT Campus, Tiruchirappalli. He did his M.Phil from Gandhigram Rural Institute (Deemed University)-Dindigul, Tamilnadu and M.Sc Chemistry from Periyar E.V.R College Trichy. His Research work is focused on drug development against raising antibiotic resistance. His expertise is in design and synthesis of novel drugs by using both structure and ligand-based drug designing method and applying various virtual screening method (molecular docking, dynamics, structure, ligand-based pharmacophore, 3D QSAR, ADMET and toxicity predictions).

Virupaksha Ajit Bastikar is a Pharmaceutical Sciences (B.Pharm) graduate and correspondingly pursued Post Graduate Diploma in Bioinformatics as well as Master of Science in Bioinformatics focusing on the concepts of Molecular Modelling and Computer aided Drug Design and conventional drug developmental aspects. He obtained is research degree PhD in Bioinformatics by receiving "Erasmus Mundus - Mobility for Life Fellowship" at University of Rome, Tor Vergata, Italy as his host University. Further he was awarded "Erasmus Mundus – EUPHRATES" Post-Doctoral fellowship at Proteomics Centre, Vilnius University, Lithuania. He is working as a Computational Medicinal Chemist with primary expertise in the areas of Molecular Modeling, proteomics, Ligand based and Structure based drug design. He is a Principal Researcher and Consultant with in-depth exposure in the field of Drug Discovery, Therapeutic Application, Molecular design and lead Discovery Proficient at developing novel ways to implement and integrate computational tools; applied acquaintance of lead optimization, development and discovery. He has competency to work with a wide variety of computational chemistry software's like – Vlife-MDS, TRIPOS- Sybyl, Schrodinger, MOE, Accelrys and techniques associated with spectrometry, chromatography. He has core competency in execution of research projects, designing and development of Drugs.

Santosh Chhajed is working at Mumbai Education Trust's Institute of Pharmacy, Adgaon, Nashik. Dr. Santosh Chhajed is having teaching experience of 12 years of various pharmaceutical chemistry subjects at undergraduate as well postgraduate level. He has completed two funded minor research projects funded by Savitribai Phule Pune University Pune. Professor Chhajed has to his credit 05 book on pharmacy and has published twenty papers in national and international journal of repute. He is nominated as "Focal Point" by European commission for Horizon 2020 projects. Also he is acted as reviewer for proposals submitted to the 2017 FONDECYT regular competition, by Chilean National Science and Technology Commission Santiago, Chile. He is recipient of best research guide award at state level conference "METRxplore."

Pramodkumar P. Gupta is working with School of Biotechnology and Bioinformatics, D Y Patil Deemed to be University, having 10 years of teaching experience of various bioinformatics and cheminformatics subjects at undergraduate and post graduate level. Professor Gupta has contributed numerous book chapters and research articles in national, international and has chaired organizing committee member, national advisory board member to national and international scientific events. Currently he is working in the field of "Protein kinase and drug discovery", "Metabolic pathway mapping and analysis". He is a recipient of Erasmus Mundus Doctoral Fellowship year (2016 – 2017) under Erasmus Mundus Euphrates Program, by European Union Commission, has completed his work at Proteomic Center, Vilnius University, Lithuania, Europe. He is a reviewer and editorial board member to numerous scientific journal and life member to various scientific society national and international.

Afzal Hussain completed his research work from NIT, Bhopal, He worked in the field of medicinal chemistry using a bioinformatics approach for searching out novel anticancer agents as well as using advanced next-generation sequencing for analysis cancer gene expression. He has more than nine years experience in this field, in which he has found novel compounds for the specific kinases for reducing harmful death-leading effects. Afzal is currently collaborating with many organizations to design anti-inflammatory molecules against cancer. He is working as Advisory board member & Commissioning Editor in Cambridge Scholar Publishing and selected for continuing further research from Harvard. He has received the prestigious Young Scientist Award and has twice been the recipient of the Young Scientist Fellowship from the Ministry of Science and Technology, India, for showing their best involvement in research work. He has also worked in the Ministry of Science and Technology in Junior Research Fellow projects. His scientific work has been published in high impact journals including the European Journal of Medicinal Chemistry, Biomedical Research and the SJBC. His areas of expertise include bioinformatics, drug designing, next-generation sequencing data analysis, and phylogenetic analysis.

Navabshan Irfan is a medicinal chemist. He is interested in sharing and updating his knowledge and likes to face challenges with full confidence. His prime object is to impart basic knowledge of the subject in theoretical, practical and research aspects. His discipline and sincerity with the students to make them successful in their academic career and produce them as industrial and research-oriented persons in the pharma profession.

Kesavan Swaminathan Jayachandran's research interest is to analyze molecular mechanism behind myocardial ischemia/reperfusion injury and find better drugs by identifying therapeutic targets. The main goal of his research is to transform bench to bedside medicine. The main focus of his research is about Molecular basis of Cardiovascular Diseases and Structure-Based Drug Designing.

Anju Kumari is working as Assistant Professor in St. Mary's College of Pharmacy, Secunderabad, Telangana. Currently she is doing her research work on Zebrafish as an animal model. She is also a life member of Indian Science Congress Association and Indian Pharmaceutical Association.

Gurusamy Mariappan is working as Associate Professor in St. Mary's College of Pharmacy, Secunderabad, Telangana. He obtained his degree Ph.D. from University of North Bengal and Post doctorate from Augusta University, USA. He published more than 35 Research papers in International Journal of repute. He is also a life member of Association of Chemistry Teachers, Indian Cancer Research Association and also a Fellow of Institution of Chemist (FIC), India.

Thenmozhi Marudhadurai is working as an Assistant Professor, Department of Biotechnology, Selvam College of Technology, Namakkal. She completed her Doctoral degree in the field of bioinformatics from Department of Bioinformatics, Bharathidasan University. She completed her Master of technology from SASTRA University and obtained her Bachelor of Technology from School of Engineering and Technology, Bharathidasan University. She has 5 journal publications and also received Best Faculty Award for academic performance and results in Selvam College of Technology and also received Best Scientist Award from Indian Academic Research Association.

N. Ramalakshmi is Gold medalist in M.Pharm at University level and College first in B.Pharm. She has 21 years of teaching experience. She has guided 35 M.Pharm Students. She is doctoral committee member for Ph.D students in various Universities. Her field of research includes synthesis of various heterocyclic structures, screening their Pharmacological activity and performing QSAR analysis. She has 35 national publications and 10 international publications in various reputed journals like *Chemical Biology and Drug Design, Medicinal Chemistry*, etc.

Thirumurugan Rathinasabapathy is a Postdoctoral Research Scholar in North Carolina State University since 2016. He pursued his Ph.D from Birla Institute of Technology and Science (BITS), Pilani. He has 14 years research experience in Pharmaceutical industry as well as in Academia and his expertise is in design and synthesis of small molecules for the treatment of MetS and also multistep synthesis of macrolides and ketolides. He has been awarded 1 international patent, 25 peer reviewed publications and authored 5 book chapters. He developed 3 preclinical candidates for the treatment of cancer (Histone Deacetylase 1 inhibitor) and also he developed a nutritional supplement like chilitenoids from red chili as well as zealutein from marigold flower.

Shridevi S. is currently working as Assistant Professor(SG) in VIT, Chennai. She has completed her Ph.D from MS University. She has published many papers in reputed Journals and in International Conferences. Her research areas of interest include Semantic Web Technology, Semantic Big Data and Semantic Web Services.

Viswanathan V. completed his doctoral degree from Anna University, Chennai, India, by contributing his ideas to the field of semantic web technologies and social media marketing. He has a teaching experience of over 20 years in the field of computer applications. His research interests include data mining, semantic web, and social network analysis. He has authored articles in semantic web technologies for renowned publications.

Sundaramurthy Vivekanandan is Postgraduate in Pharmacy from Annamalai university, having around 17 years of experience in Formulation Research and Development from various Pharmaceutical industries. Currently working as Head of Research and Development at Bluefish Pharmaceuticals Pvt. Ltd., heading team of scientists from the formulation, analytical, Clinical and Intellectual Property Rights, etc. Developed different type of dosage forms like immediate release, modified release, delayed release dosage forms etc., with successful completion of critical bio-equivalence studies. Strong technical skills to address technical challenges at different stages of product development like development scale, pilot scale, technology transfer and commercial scale, etc. Expertise in implementation of ICH Q8, Q9 and Q10 requirements and QbD, DoE concepts etc., in development of generics drug products of Niche molecules for various regulatory markets.

Index

T

U

V

www.ingramcontent.com/pod-product-compliance
Lightning Source LLC
LaVergne TN
LVHW060303011026
849161LV00011B/2767
* 9 7 8 1 5 2 2 5 7 3 2 6 5 *